Injury & Tr...

Learning Disabilities Sourcebook, 4th Edition

Leukemia Sourcebook

Liver Disorders Sourcebook

Medical Tests Sourcebook, 4th Edition

Men's Health Concerns Sourcebook, 4th Edition

Mental Health Disorders Sourcebook, 5th Edition

Mental Retardation Sourcebook

Movement Disorders Sourcebook, 2nd Edition

Multiple Sclerosis Sourcebook

Muscular Dystrophy Sourcebook

Obesity Sourcebook

Osteoporosis Sourcebook

Pain Sourcebook, 3rd Edition

Pediatric Cancer Sourcebook

Physical & Mental Issues in Aging Sourcebook

Podiatry Sourcebook, 2nd Edition

Pregnancy & Birth Sourcebook, 3rd Edition

Prostate & Urological Disorders Sourcebook

Prostate Cancer Sourcebook

Rehabilitation Sourcebook

Respiratory Disorders Sourcebook, 2nd Edition

Sexually Transmitted Diseases Sourcebook, 5th
  Edition

Sleep Disorders Sourcebook, 3rd Edition

Smoking Concerns Sourcebook

Sports Injuries Sourcebook, 4th Edition

Stress-Related Disorders Sourcebook, 3rd Edition

Stroke Sourcebook, 2nd Edition

Surgery Sourcebook, 2nd Edition

Thyroid Disorders Sourcebook

Transplantation Sourcebook

Traveler's Health Sourcebook

Urinary Tract & Kidney Diseases & Disorders Sourcebook, 2nd Edition

Vegetarian Sourcebook

Women's Health Concerns Sourcebook, 3rd Edition

Workplace Health & Safety Sourcebook

Worldwide Health Sourcebook

Teen Health Series

Abuse & Violence Information for Teens

Accident & Safety Information for Teens

D0712744

Body Information for Teens

Cancer Information for Teens,
  2nd Edition

Complementary & Alternative
  Medicine Information for Teens

Diabetes Information for Teens,
  2nd Edition

Diet Information for Teens, 3rd Edition

Drug Information for Teens, 3rd Edition

Eating Disorders Information for Teens,
  2nd Edition

Fitness Information for Teens,
  3rd Edition

Learning Disabilities Information for
  Teens

Mental Health Information for Teens,
  3rd Edition

Pregnancy Information for Teens,
  2nd Edition

Sexual Health Information for Teens,
  3rd Edition

Skin Health Information for Teens,
  2nd Edition

Sleep Information for Teens

Sports Injuries Information for Teens,
  3rd Edition

Stress Information for Teens

Suicide Information for Teens,
  2nd Edition

Tobacco Information for Teens,
  2nd Edition

Sexually Transmitted Diseases

SOURCEBOOK

Fifth Edition

Health Reference Series

Fifth Edition

Sexually Transmitted Diseases

SOURCEBOOK

Basic Consumer Health Information about Sexual Health and the Screening, Diagnosis, Treatment, and Prevention of Common Sexually Transmitted Diseases (STDs), Including Chancroid, Chlamydia, Gonorrhea, Herpes, Hepatitis, Human Immunodeficiency Virus/Acquired Immunodeficiency Syndrome (HIV/AIDS), Human Papillomavirus (HPV), Syphilis, and Trichomoniasis

Along with Facts about Risk Factors and Complications, Trends and Disparities in Infection Rates, Tips for Discussing STDs with Sexual Partners, a Glossary of Related Terms, and Resources for Additional Help and Information

Edited by
Amy L. Sutton

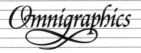

155 W. Congress, Suite 200, Detroit, MI 48226

Bibliographic Note
Because this page cannot legibly accommodate all the copyright notices, the Bibliographic
Note portion of the Preface constitutes an extension of the copyright notice.

Edited by Amy L. Sutton

Health Reference Series

Karen Bellenir, *Managing Editor*
David A. Cooke, MD, FACP, *Medical Consultant*
Elizabeth Collins, *Research and Permissions Coordinator*
Cherry Edwards, *Permissions Assistant*
EdIndex, Services for Publishers, *Indexers*

* * *

Omnigraphics, Inc.
Matthew P. Barbour, *Senior Vice President*
Kevin M. Hayes, *Operations Manager*

* * *

Peter E. Ruffner, *Publisher*

Copyright © 2013 Omnigraphics, Inc.

ISBN 978-0-7808-1281-9

E-ISBN 978-0-7808-1282-6

Library of Congress Cataloging-in-Publication Data

Sexually transmitted diseases sourcebook : basic consumer health information about
sexual health and the screening, diagnosis, treatment, and prevention of common
sexually transmitted diseases (STDs), including chancroid, chlamydia, gonorrhea,
herpes, hepatitis, human immunodeficiency virus/acquired immunodeficiency syndrome
(HIV/AIDS), human papillomavirus (HPV), syphilis, and trichomoniasis; along with
facts about risk factors and complications, trends and disparities in infection rates,
tips for discussing stds with sexual partners, a glossary of related terms, and
resources for additional help and information / edited by Amy L. Sutton. -- 5th ed.
     p. cm.
   Includes bibliographical references and index.
   Summary: "Provides basic consumer health information about risk factors, symptoms,
testing, and treatment of sexually transmitted diseases and related complications,
along with facts about prevention strategies. Includes index, glossary of related
terms, and other resources"-- Provided by publisher.
   ISBN 978-0-7808-1281-9 (hardcover : alk. paper) 1. Sexually transmitted
diseases--Popular works. I. Sutton, Amy L.
   RC200.2.S387 2012
   616.95'1--dc23
                                                              2012030809

Table of Contents

Visit www.healthreferenceseries.com to view *A Contents Guide to the Health Reference Series*, a listing of more than 16,000 topics and the volumes in which they are covered.

Preface xiii

Part I: Introduction to Sexually Transmitted Diseases (STDs)

Chapter 1—Overview of Sexual Health and
the Reproductive System 3

Section 1.1—Female Reproductive System 4

Section 1.2—Male Reproductive System 11

Chapter 2—What Is an STD? 17

Chapter 3—Trends in STD Infection in the United States 27

Chapter 4—Trends in STD Infection Worldwide 35

Section 4.1—Trends in STDs Other
Than HIV/AIDS 36

Section 4.2—The Global HIV/AIDS
Epidemic 41

Chapter 5—Women and STDs 43

Section 5.1—Ten Ways STDs Impact
Women Differently Than Men 44

Section 5.2—STDs in Women 46

Section 5.3—STDs in Women Who Have
Sex with Women 49

Chapter 6—Men and STDs 55

    Section 6.1—HPV in Men 56

    Section 6.2—HIV/AIDS in Men 62

    Section 6.3—STDs in Men Who Have
                Sex with Men 64

Chapter 7—STDs in Children 67

    Section 7.1—Child Sexual Abuse
                and STDs 68

    Section 7.2—Child Abuse Survivors
                Have Higher Risk for STDs
                in Adulthood 71

Chapter 8—STDs in Adolescents and Young Adults 73

Chapter 9—STDs in Older Adults 79

Chapter 10—Racial Disparities in STD Rates 83

    Section 10.1—Overview of STD
                 Racial Disparities 84

    Section 10.2—African Americans
                 Disproportionately
                 Affected by STDs 89

    Section 10.3—Latinos Bear a
                 Disproportionate Burden
                 of the HIV Epidemic 93

Chapter 11—STDs in People in Correctional Facilities 97

Chapter 12—Recent STD Research Findings 101

Part II: Types of STDs

Chapter 13—Common Symptoms of STDs 107

Chapter 14—Chancroid 115

Chapter 15—Chlamydia 119

    Section 15.1—What Is Chlamydia? 120

    Section 15.2—Chlamydia Is the Most
                 Common Cause of
                 Nongonococcal Urethritis 123

    Section 15.3—Chlamydia Treatment 127

Chapter 16—Donovanosis (Granuloma Inguinale).................. 133

Chapter 17—Gonorrhea 137

    Section 17.1—What Is Gonorrhea?................. 138

    Section 17.2—Gonorrhea Treatment 141

    Section 17.3—Antibiotic-Resistant
                    Gonorrhea Infections 144

Chapter 18—Herpes 147

    Section 18.1—Genital Herpes 148

    Section 18.2—Oral Herpes 151

    Section 18.3—Treating and Managing
                    Herpes...................................... 155

Chapter 19—Hepatitis... 161

    Section 19.1—What Is Hepatitis? 162

    Section 19.2—Hepatitis and HIV
                    Coinfection............................... 174

    Section 19.3—Treating Hepatitis.................... 178

Chapter 20—HIV/AIDS 183

    Section 20.1—How HIV Causes AIDS 184

    Section 20.2—How the Immune
                    System Reacts
                    to HIV 198

    Section 20.3—Questions and Answers
                    about HIV Transmission.......... 200

    Section 20.4—HIV Signs and
                    Symptoms 212

    Section 20.5—Testing for HIV........................ 214

    Section 20.6—HIV and Its Treatment 219

    Section 20.7—Living with HIV 232

    Section 20.8—How Can I Pay for
                    HIV Care? 241

    Section 20.9—The Affordable Care Act
                    and People Living with
                    HIV/AIDS................................. 245

Chapter 21—Human Papillomavirus (HPV) 247

    Section 21.1—What Is Genital HPV
                Infection and How Does
                It Affect Women? 248

    Section 21.2—HPV and Men 254

    Section 21.3—Recurrent Respiratory
                Papillomatosis 259

    Section 21.4—Pap Tests and Cervical
                Cancer Screening to
                Check for HPV 262

    Section 21.5—Making Sense of
                Your HPV Test
                Results 264

    Section 21.6—What You Should
                Know When You Are
                Diagnosed with
                Genital Warts 271

    Section 21.7—Treating HPV and
                Related Problems 273

    Section 21.8—HPV Infection and Cancer 276

Chapter 22—Lymphogranuloma Venereum 281

Chapter 23—Syphilis 285

    Section 23.1—What Is Syphilis? 286

    Section 23.2—Treating Syphilis 289

Chapter 24—Trichomoniasis 291

Part III: Complications That May Accompany STD Infection

Chapter 25—Infections and Syndromes That Develop
                after Sexual Contact 297

    Section 25.1—Bacterial Vaginosis 298

    Section 25.2—Cytomegalovirus 302

    Section 25.3—Fungal (Yeast) Infection 305

    Section 25.4—Intestinal Parasites 309

    Section 25.5—Molluscum Contagiosum 311

Section 25.6—Proctitis, Proctocolitis,
and Enteritis: Sexually
Transmitted Gastro-
intestinal Syndromes 314

Section 25.7—Pubic Lice 316

Section 25.8—Scabies 320

Chapter 26—Cervicitis 327

Chapter 27—Epididymitis.. 331

Chapter 28—Infertility Linked to STD Infection...................... 335

Chapter 29—Neurosyphilis 339

Chapter 30—Pelvic Inflammatory Disease.............................. 343

Chapter 31—Pregnancy Complications and STDs.................... 349

Chapter 32—Vaginitis 353

Part IV: STD Testing and Treatment Concerns

Chapter 33—Frequently Asked Questions about
STD and HIV Testing 359

Chapter 34—Talking to Your Health Care Professional
about STDs.. 365

Section 34.1—Talking about Your
Health 366

Section 34.2—Questions to Ask Your
Health Care Professional
about STDs 370

Section 34.3—For Teens: How Do I Discuss
Embarrassing Things with
My Doctor?................................ 372

Chapter 35—Confidentiality Issues Associated with
STD Testing.. 377

Section 35.1—Anonymous Testing for
STDs Like HIV 378

Section 35.2—Confidentiality for
Adolescents Who Seek
STD Testing and Care.............. 380

Section 35.3—At-Home/Mail Order STD
Tests Protect Patient
Confidentiality........................... 381

Chapter 36—Testing for STDs 385

Section 36.1—Where to Go and
How It Works.......................... 386

Section 36.2—Diagnostic Laparoscopy:
A Way to Test for STD
Complications........................... 390

Chapter 37—Understanding Antibiotic Resistance
and STD Treatment.. 393

Chapter 38—Unproven STD Treatment Products.................... 397

Part V: STD Risks and Prevention

Chapter 39—Sexual Behaviors That Increase the
Likelihood of STD Transmission........................... 403

Section 39.1—Overview of Risky
Sexual Behaviors...................... 404

Section 39.2—Choosing High-Risk
Partners Increases
STD Risk.................................. 405

Section 39.3—Oral Sex and HIV Risk 408

Chapter 40—Sexually Transmitted Diseases and
Substance Use... 411

Chapter 41—Other Behaviors That Increase STD Risk........... 415

Section 41.1—Douching May Increase
Risk of STDs 416

Section 41.2—Body Art Allows Exposure
to Bloodborne Pathogens
Such as HIV.............................. 419

Section 41.3—Injection Drug Use 421

Chapter 42—Talking to Sexual Partners Can Reduce
STD Risk 425

Section 42.1—Talking to Your Partner
about Condoms........................ 426

Section 42.2—Telling Your Partner
You Have an STD 429

Section 42.3—Sharing Your HIV Status 432

Chapter 43—Talking to Your Child or Teen about STDs 435

Chapter 44—Sex Education and STD Prevention 439

Section 44.1—Overview of Sex Education 440

Section 44.2—What Programs Effectively
Prevent STDs in Youth? 448

Section 44.3—Are Abstinence Only Sexual
Education Programs
Effective? 450

Section 44.4—Behavioral Intervention
May Reduce STD Rates 460

Chapter 45—Preventing STDs with Safer Sex 463

Section 45.1—What Is "Safer" Sex? 464

Section 45.2—Condoms: Do They Work
to Prevent STDs? 470

Section 45.3—Tips for Using Condoms
and Dental Dams to Prevent
STDs 475

Section 45.4—Spermicides Alone Do Not
Protect against STDs 479

Chapter 46—Preventing STDs after Possible or
Certain Exposure 483

Section 46.1—Expedited Partner Therapy 484

Section 46.2—Preventing STDs after
a Sexual Assault 488

Section 46.3—Post-Exposure Prophylaxis:
Taking HIV Drugs If You've
Been Exposed to the Virus
through Blood or Sexual
Contact 492

Chapter 47—Preventing Mother-to-Child HIV Transmission ... 495

Chapter 48—Needle Exchange Programs: Preventing
STDs in Injection Drug Users 507

Chapter 49—STD Vaccines and Microbicides 519

    Section 49.1—Anti-HIV Drug Acts to
                 Block Herpes Virus................... 520

    Section 49.2—Herpevac Trial.......................... 522

    Section 49.3—Shutting Down the
                 Genital Herpes Virus
                 with Microbicides 526

    Section 49.4—Preventive HIV Vaccines.......... 528

    Section 49.5—Therapeutic HIV Vaccines 531

    Section 49.6—Understanding the HPV
                 Vaccine 533

    Section 49.7—HPV Vaccine Information
                 for Preteens and Teens............. 538

    Section 49.8—HPV Vaccine Soon to Be
                 Recommended for Preteen
                 Boys as Well as Girls................ 541

Part VI: Additional Help and Information

Chapter 50—Glossary of Terms Related to Sexually
              Transmitted Diseases.. 547

Chapter 51—Directory of Organizations That Provide
              Information about Sexually Transmitted
              Diseases... 553

Index.. **563**

Preface

About This Book

Every year, more than 19 million people in the United States are diagnosed with sexually transmitted diseases (STDs), and the Centers for Disease Control and Prevention reports that diagnosing, treating, and preventing these potentially life-threatening STDs is one of the greatest public health challenges today. For some STDs, such as the easily treatable chlamydia, the rates of reported cases are on the rise, especially among adolescent girls and young women. The diagnosis rates of other STDs, such as HIV (human immunodeficiency virus), have decreased in recent years due to increased education and prevention efforts. Regardless of prevalence or severity, all STDs have significant health consequences if they are not diagnosed and treated.

Sexually Transmitted Diseases Sourcebook, Fifth Edition offers basic information about sexual health and the screening, diagnosis, treatment, and prevention of common sexually transmitted diseases, including chancroid, chlamydia, gonorrhea, herpes, hepatitis, human immunodeficiency virus (HIV/AIDS), human papillomavirus (HPV), syphilis, and trichomoniasis. It discusses trends in STD rates, developments in STD vaccine research, tips on talking to doctors and sexual partners, a glossary of related terms, and resources for additional help and information.

How to Use This Book

This book is divided into parts and chapters. Parts focus on broad areas of interest. Chapters are devoted to single topics within a part.

Part I: Introduction to Sexually Transmitted Diseases identifies the parts of the male and female reproductive system and discusses trends in STD rates in the United States and worldwide. It also examines the impact of these diseases on women, men, children and teens, and older adults. The part concludes with statistical information on minorities disproportionately affected by STDs and recent STD research findings.

Part II: Types of STDs identifies the symptoms, diagnoses, and treatments of common types of STDs, including chancroid, chlamydia, donovanosis, gonorrhea, herpes, hepatitis, HPV, lymphogranuloma venereum, syphilis, and trichomoniasis. The part also includes information on how HIV causes AIDS and the disease's transmission, testing, and treatment, as well as strategies for living with HIV and paying for medical care.

Part III: Complications That May Accompany STD Infection provides information about infections and syndromes that may develop after sexual contact, such as bacterial vaginosis, cytomegalovirus, yeast infection, intestinal parasites, molluscum contagiosum, sexually transmitted gastrointestinal syndromes, pubic lice, and scabies. The part also provides information about conditions related to STDs that can cause long-term health complications for men and women, including cervicitis, epididymitis, infertility and pregnancy complications, pelvic inflammatory disease, and vaginitis.

Part IV: STD Testing and Treatment Concerns offers information about how medical professionals test patients for STDs and addresses common issues associated with STD testing, such as maintaining confidentiality and discussing STDs with healthcare providers. Information about unproven STD treatment products is also included.

Part V: STD Risks and Prevention discusses sexual behaviors that increase the likelihood of STD transmission, such as choosing high-risk partners and using illegal substances. The part also offers tips on talking to sexual partners and adolescents about STDs and addresses the effectiveness of sexual and abstinence education as forms of STD prevention. The part concludes with information about preventing STDs by using safer sex and barrier methods such as condoms, by using medication after a known exposure to STDs, by preventing the transmission of these diseases from a pregnant woman to her child, and by using STD vaccines and microbicides.

Part VI: Additional Help and Information provides a glossary of important terms related to sexually transmitted diseases and a directory of organizations that offer information to people with STDs or their sexual partners.

Bibliographic Note

This volume contains documents and excerpts from publications issued by the following U.S. government agencies: Agency for Healthcare Research and Quality (AHRQ); Centers for Disease Control and Prevention (CDC); National Cancer Institute (NCI); National Institute of Allergy and Infectious Diseases (NIAID); National Institute of Mental Health (NIMH); National Institute of Neurological Disorders and Stroke (NINDS); National Institute on Aging (NIA); National Institute on Deafness and Other Communication Disorders (NIDCD); National Institutes of Health (NIH); National Library of Medicine (NLM); Office on Women's Health (OWH); Substance Abuse and Mental Health Services Administration (SAMHSA); U.S. Department of Health and Human Services (HHS); U.S. Department of Justice (DOJ); U.S. Department of Veterans Affairs (VA); and the U.S. Food and Drug Administration (FDA).

In addition, this volume contains copyrighted documents from the following organizations: A.D.A.M., Inc.; AVERT; Center for Young Women's Health–Boston Children's Hospital; Cleveland Clinic Foundation; Hepatitis B Foundation; Johns Hopkins Medicine; Henry J. Kaiser Family Foundation; Nemours Foundation; New Jersey Department of Health and Senior Services; Planned Parenthood Federation of America; State of Illinois; and the World Health Organization.

Full citation information is provided on the first page of each chapter or section. Every effort has been made to secure all necessary rights to reprint the copyrighted material. If any omissions have been made, please contact Omnigraphics to make corrections for future editions.

Acknowledgements

Thanks go to the many organizations, agencies, and individuals who have contributed materials for this *Sourcebook* and to medical consultant Dr. David Cooke and prepress service provider WhimsyInk.

Special thanks go to managing editor Karen Bellenir and research and permissions coordinator Liz Collins for their help and support.

About the Health Reference Series

The *Health Reference Series* is designed to provide basic medical information for patients, families, caregivers, and the general public. Each volume takes a particular topic and provides comprehensive coverage. This is especially important for people who may be dealing with a newly diagnosed disease or a chronic disorder in themselves or in a family member. People looking for preventive guidance, information about disease warning signs, medical statistics, and risk factors for health problems will also find answers to their questions in the *Health Reference Series.* The *Series*, however, is not intended to serve as a tool for diagnosing illness, in prescribing treatments, or as a substitute for the physician/patient relationship. All people concerned about medical symptoms or the possibility of disease are encouraged to seek professional care from an appropriate health care provider.

A Note about Spelling and Style

Health Reference Series editors use *Stedman's Medical Dictionary* as an authority for questions related to the spelling of medical terms and the *Chicago Manual of Style* for questions related to grammatical structures, punctuation, and other editorial concerns. Consistent adherence is not always possible, however, because the individual volumes within the *Series* include many documents from a wide variety of different producers and copyright holders, and the editor's primary goal is to present material from each source as accurately as is possible following the terms specified by each document's producer. This sometimes means that information in different chapters or sections may follow other guidelines and alternate spelling authorities. For example, occasionally a copyright holder may require that eponymous terms be shown in possessive forms (Crohn's disease *vs.* Crohn disease) or that British spelling norms be retained (leukaemia *vs.* leukemia).

Locating Information within the Health Reference Series

The *Health Reference Series* contains a wealth of information about a wide variety of medical topics. Ensuring easy access to all the fact sheets, research reports, in-depth discussions, and other material contained within the individual books of the *Series* remains one of our highest priorities. As the *Series* continues to grow in size and scope, however, locating the precise information needed by a reader may become more challenging.

A Contents Guide to the Health Reference Series was developed to direct readers to the specific volumes that address their concerns. It presents an extensive list of diseases, treatments, and other topics of general interest compiled from the Tables of Contents and major index headings. To access *A Contents Guide to the Health Reference Series*, visit www.healthreferenceseries.com.

Medical Consultant

Medical consultation services are provided to the *Health Reference Series* editors by David A. Cooke, MD, FACP. Dr. Cooke is a graduate of Brandeis University, and he received his M.D. degree from the University of Michigan. He completed residency training at the University of Wisconsin Hospital and Clinics. He is board-certified in Internal Medicine. Dr. Cooke currently works as part of the University of Michigan Health System and practices in Ann Arbor, MI. In his free time, he enjoys writing, science fiction, and spending time with his family.

Our Advisory Board

We would like to thank the following board members for providing guidance to the development of this *Series*:

- Dr. Lynda Baker, Associate Professor of Library and Information Science, Wayne State University, Detroit, MI

- Nancy Bulgarelli, William Beaumont Hospital Library, Royal Oak, MI

- Karen Imarisio, Bloomfield Township Public Library, Bloomfield Township, MI

- Karen Morgan, Mardigian Library, University of Michigan-Dearborn, Dearborn, MI

- Rosemary Orlando, St. Clair Shores Public Library, St. Clair Shores, MI

Health Reference Series *Update Policy*

The inaugural book in the *Health Reference Series* was the first edition of *Cancer Sourcebook* published in 1989. Since then, the

Series has been enthusiastically received by librarians and in the medical community. In order to maintain the standard of providing high-quality health information for the layperson the editorial staff at Omnigraphics felt it was necessary to implement a policy of updating volumes when warranted.

Medical researchers have been making tremendous strides, and it is the purpose of the *Health Reference Series* to stay current with the most recent advances. Each decision to update a volume is made on an individual basis. Some of the considerations include how much new information is available and the feedback we receive from people who use the books. If there is a topic you would like to see added to the update list, or an area of medical concern you feel has not been adequately addressed, please write to:

Editor
Health Reference Series
Omnigraphics, Inc.
155 W. Congress, Suite 200
Detroit, MI 48226
E-mail: editorial@omnigraphics.com

Part One

Introduction to Sexually Transmitted Diseases (STDs)

Chapter 1

Overview of Sexual Health and the Reproductive System

Chapter Contents

Section 1.1—Female Reproductive System 4
Section 1.2—Male Reproductive System 11

Section 1.1

Female Reproductive System

About Human Reproduction

All living things reproduce. Reproduction—the process by which organisms make more organisms like themselves—is one of the things that sets living things apart from nonliving matter. But even though the reproductive system is essential to keeping a species alive, unlike other body systems, it's not essential to keeping an individual alive.

In the human reproductive process, two kinds of sex cells, or gametes, are involved. The male gamete, or sperm, and the female gamete, the egg or ovum, meet in the female's reproductive system to create a new individual.

Both the male and female reproductive systems are essential for reproduction. The female needs a male to fertilize her egg, even though it is she who carries offspring through pregnancy and childbirth.

Humans, like other organisms, pass certain characteristics of themselves to the next generation through their genes, the special carriers of human traits. The genes that parents pass along are what make their children similar to others in their family, but also what make each child unique. These genes come from the male's sperm and the female's egg.

Most species have two sexes: Male and female. Each sex has its own unique reproductive system. They are different in shape and structure, but both are specifically designed to produce, nourish, and transport either the egg or sperm.

Components of the Female Reproductive System

Unlike the male, the human female has a reproductive system located entirely in the pelvis. The external part of the female reproductive organs is called the vulva, which means covering. Located between the legs, the vulva covers the opening to the vagina and other reproductive organs located inside the body.

The fleshy area located just above the top of the vaginal opening is called the mons pubis. Two pairs of skin flaps called the labia (which mean lips) surround the vaginal opening. The clitoris, a small sensory organ, is located toward the front of the vulva where the folds of the labia join. Between the labia are openings to the urethra (the canal that carries urine from the bladder to the outside of the body) and vagina. Once girls become sexually mature, the outer labia and the mons pubis are covered by pubic hair.

A female's internal reproductive organs are the vagina, uterus, fallopian tubes, and ovaries.

The vagina is a muscular, hollow tube that extends from the vaginal opening to the uterus. The vagina is about 3 to 5 inches (8 to 12 centimeters) long in a grown woman. Because it has muscular walls, it can expand and contract. This ability to become wider or narrower allows the vagina to accommodate something as slim as a tampon and as wide as a baby. The vagina's muscular walls are lined with mucous membranes, which keep it protected and moist.

The vagina serves three purposes:

1. It's where the penis is inserted during sexual intercourse.

2. It's the pathway that a baby takes out of a woman's body during childbirth, called the birth canal.

3. It provides the route for the menstrual blood (the period) to leave the body from the uterus.

A thin sheet of tissue with one or more holes in it called the hymen partially covers the opening of the vagina. Hymens are often different from female to female. Most women find their hymens have stretched or torn after their first sexual experience, and the hymen may bleed a little (this usually causes little, if any, pain). Some women who have had sex don't have much of a change in their hymens, though.

The vagina connects with the uterus, or womb, at the cervix (which means neck). The cervix has strong, thick walls. The opening of the cervix is very small (no wider than a straw), which is why a tampon can never get lost inside a girl's body. During childbirth, the cervix can expand to allow a baby to pass.

The uterus is shaped like an upside-down pear, with a thick lining and muscular walls—in fact, the uterus contains some of the strongest muscles in the female body. These muscles are able to expand

and contract to accommodate a growing fetus and then help push the baby out during labor. When a woman isn't pregnant, the uterus is only about three inches (seven and a half centimeters) long and two inches (five centimeters) wide.

At the upper corners of the uterus, the fallopian tubes connect the uterus to the ovaries. The ovaries are two oval-shaped organs that lie to the upper right and left of the uterus. They produce, store, and release eggs into the fallopian tubes in the process called ovulation. Each ovary measures about one and a half to two inches (four to five centimeters) in a grown woman.

There are two fallopian tubes, each attached to a side of the uterus. The fallopian tubes are about 4 inches (10 centimeters) long and about as wide as a piece of spaghetti. Within each tube is a tiny passageway no wider than a sewing needle. At the other end of each fallopian tube is a fringed area that looks like a funnel. This fringed area wraps around the ovary but doesn't completely attach to it. When an egg pops out of an ovary, it enters the fallopian tube. Once the egg is in the fallopian tube, tiny hairs in the tube's lining help push it down the narrow passageway toward the uterus.

The ovaries are also part of the endocrine system because they produce female sex hormones such as estrogen and progesterone.

What the Female Reproductive System Does

The female reproductive system enables a woman to:

- produce eggs (ova);
- have sexual intercourse;
- protect and nourish the fertilized egg until it is fully developed;
- give birth.

Sexual reproduction couldn't happen without the sexual organs called the gonads. Although most people think of the gonads as the male testicles, both sexes actually have gonads: In females the gonads are the ovaries. The female gonads produce female gametes (eggs); the male gonads produce male gametes (sperm). After an egg is fertilized by the sperm, the fertilized egg is called the zygote.

When a baby girl is born, her ovaries contain hundreds of thousands of eggs, which remain inactive until puberty begins. At puberty, the pituitary gland, located in the central part of the brain, starts making hormones that stimulate the ovaries to produce female sex hormones, including estrogen. The secretion of these hormones causes a girl to develop into a sexually mature woman.

Toward the end of puberty, girls begin to release eggs as part of a monthly period called the menstrual cycle. Approximately once a month, during ovulation, an ovary sends a tiny egg into one of the fallopian tubes.

Unless the egg is fertilized by a sperm while in the fallopian tube, the egg dries up and leaves the body about two weeks later through the uterus—this is menstruation. Blood and tissues from the inner lining of the uterus combine to form the menstrual flow, which in most girls lasts from three to five days. A girl's first period is called menarche.

It's common for women and girls to experience some discomfort in the days leading to their periods. Premenstrual syndrome (PMS) includes both physical and emotional symptoms that many girls and women get right before their periods, such as acne, bloating, fatigue, backaches, sore breasts, headaches, constipation, diarrhea, food cravings, depression, irritability, or difficulty concentrating or handling stress. PMS is usually at its worst during the seven days before a girl's period starts and disappears once it begins.

Many girls also experience abdominal cramps during the first few days of their periods caused by prostaglandins, chemicals in the body that make the smooth muscle in the uterus contract. These involuntary contractions can be either dull or sharp and intense.

It can take up to two years from menarche for a girl's body to develop a regular menstrual cycle. During that time, her body is adjusting to the hormones puberty brings. On average, the monthly cycle for an adult woman is 28 days, but the range is from 23 to 35 days.

Fertilization

If a female and male have sex within several days of the female's ovulation, fertilization can occur. When the male ejaculates (when semen leaves a male's penis), between 0.05 and 0.2 fluid ounces (1.5 to 6.0 mL) of semen is deposited into the vagina. Between 75 and 900 million sperm are in this small amount of semen, and they "swim" up from the vagina through the cervix and uterus to meet the egg in the fallopian tube. It takes only one sperm to fertilize the egg.

About a week after the sperm fertilizes the egg, the fertilized egg (zygote) has become a multicelled blastocyst. A blastocyst is about the size of a pinhead, and it's a hollow ball of cells with fluid inside. The blastocyst burrows itself into the lining of the uterus, called the endometrium. The hormone estrogen causes the endometrium to become

7

thick and rich with blood. Progesterone, another hormone released by the ovaries, keeps the endometrium thick with blood so that the blastocyst can attach to the uterus and absorb nutrients from it. This process is called implantation.

As cells from the blastocyst take in nourishment, another stage of development, the embryonic stage, begins. The inner cells form a flattened circular shape called the embryonic disk, which will develop into a baby. The outer cells become thin membranes that form around the baby. The cells multiply thousands of times and move to new positions to eventually become the embryo.

After approximately eight weeks, the embryo is about the size of an adult's thumb, but almost all of its parts—the brain and nerves, the heart and blood, the stomach and intestines, and the muscles and skin—have formed.

During the fetal stage, which lasts from nine weeks after fertilization to birth, development continues as cells multiply, move, and change. The fetus floats in amniotic fluid inside the amniotic sac. The fetus receives oxygen and nourishment from the mother's blood via the placenta, a disk-like structure that sticks to the inner lining of the uterus and connects to the fetus via the umbilical cord. The amniotic fluid and membrane cushion the fetus against bumps and jolts to the mother's body.

Pregnancy lasts an average of 280 days—about 9 months. When the baby is ready for birth, its head presses on the cervix, which begins to relax and widen to get ready for the baby to pass into and through the vagina. The mucus that has formed a plug in the cervix loosens, and with amniotic fluid, comes out through the vagina when the mother's water breaks.

When the contractions of labor begin, the walls of the uterus contract as they are stimulated by the pituitary hormone oxytocin. The contractions cause the cervix to widen and begin to open. After several hours of this widening, the cervix is dilated (opened) enough for the baby to come through. The baby is pushed out of the uterus, through the cervix, and along the birth canal. The baby's head usually comes first; the umbilical cord comes out with the baby and is cut after the baby is delivered.

The last stage of the birth process involves the delivery of the placenta, which at that point is called the afterbirth. After it has separated from the inner lining of the uterus, contractions of the uterus push it out, along with its membranes and fluids.

Problems of the Female Reproductive System

Some girls might experience reproductive system problems, such as [the following]:

Problems of the Vulva and Vagina

Vulvovaginitis is an inflammation of the vulva and vagina. It may be caused by irritating substances (such as laundry soaps or bubble baths) or poor personal hygiene (such as wiping from back to front after a bowel movement). Symptoms include redness and itching in the vaginal and vulvar areas and sometimes vaginal discharge. Vulvovaginitis also can be caused by an overgrowth of *Candida*, a fungus normally present in the vagina.

Nonmenstrual vaginal bleeding is most commonly due to the presence of a vaginal foreign body, often wadded-up toilet paper. It may also be due to urethral prolapse, in which the mucous membranes of the urethra protrude into the vagina and form a tiny, doughnut-shaped mass of tissue that bleeds easily. It also can be due to a straddle injury (such as when falling onto a gymnastics beam or bicycle frame) or vaginal trauma from sexual abuse.

Labial adhesions, the sticking together or adherence of the labia in the midline, usually appear in infants and young girls. Although there are usually no symptoms associated with this condition, labial adhesions can lead to an increased risk of urinary tract infection. Sometimes topical estrogen cream is used to help separate the labia.

Problems of the Ovaries and Fallopian Tubes

Ectopic pregnancy occurs when a fertilized egg, or zygote, doesn't travel into the uterus, but instead grows rapidly in the fallopian tube. A woman with this condition can develop severe abdominal pain and should see a doctor because surgery may be necessary.

Endometriosis occurs when tissue normally found only in the uterus starts to grow outside the uterus—in the ovaries, fallopian tubes, or other parts of the pelvic cavity. It can cause abnormal bleeding, painful periods, and general pelvic pain.

Ovarian tumors, although they're rare, can occur. Girls with ovarian tumors may have abdominal pain and masses that can be felt in the abdomen. Surgery may be needed to remove the tumor.

Ovarian cysts are noncancerous sacs filled with fluid or semisolid material. Although they are common and generally harmless, they can become a problem if they grow very large. Large cysts may push on surrounding organs, causing abdominal pain. In most cases, cysts will disappear on their own and treatment is unnecessary. If the cysts are painful, a doctor may prescribe birth control pills to alter their growth or they may be removed by a surgeon.

9

Polycystic ovary syndrome is a hormone disorder in which too many male hormones (androgens) are produced by the ovaries. This condition causes the ovaries to become enlarged and develop many fluid-filled sacs, or cysts. It often first appears during the teen years. Depending on the type and severity of the condition, it may be treated with drugs to regulate hormone balance and menstruation.

Ovarian torsion, or the twisting of the ovary, can occur when an ovary becomes twisted because of a disease or a developmental abnormality. The torsion blocks blood from flowing through the blood vessels that supply and nourish the ovaries. The most common symptom is lower abdominal pain. Surgery is usually necessary to correct it.

Menstrual Problems

A variety of menstrual problems can affect girls, including [the following]:

- Dysmenorrhea is when a girl has painful periods.

- Menorrhagia is when a girl has a very heavy period with excess bleeding.

- Oligomenorrhea is when a girl misses or has infrequent periods, even though she's been menstruating for a while and isn't pregnant.

- Amenorrhea is when a girl has not started her period by the time she is 16 years old or 3 years after starting puberty, has not developed signs of puberty by age 14, or has had normal periods but has stopped menstruating for some reason other than pregnancy.

Infections of the Female Reproductive System

- **Sexually transmitted infections (STIs):** These include infections and diseases such as pelvic inflammatory disease (PID), human immunodeficiency virus/acquired immunodeficiency syndrome (HIV/AIDS), human papillomavirus (HPV, or genital warts), syphilis, chlamydia, gonorrhea, and genital herpes (HSV [herpes simplex virus]). Most are spread from one person to another by sexual contact.

- **Toxic shock syndrome:** This uncommon illness is caused by toxins released into the body during a type of bacterial infection that is more likely to develop if a tampon is left in too long. It can produce high fever, diarrhea, vomiting, and shock.

If you think your daughter may have symptoms of a problem with her reproductive system or if you have questions about her growth and development, talk to your doctor—many problems with the female reproductive system can be treated.

Section 1.2

Male Reproductive System

"Male Reproductive System," May 2010, reprinted with permission from www.kidshealth.org. This information was provided by KidsHealth®, one of the largest resources online for medically reviewed health information written for parents, kids, and teens. For more articles like this, visit www.KidsHealth.org, or www.TeensHealth.org. Copyright © 1995–2012 The Nemours Foundation. All rights reserved.

Reproduction

All living things reproduce. Reproduction—the process by which organisms make more organisms like themselves—is one of the things that sets living things apart from nonliving things. But even though the reproductive system is essential to keeping a species alive, unlike other body systems it's not essential to keeping an individual alive.

In the human reproductive process, two kinds of sex cells, or gametes, are involved. The male gamete, or sperm, and the female gamete, the egg or ovum, meet in the female's reproductive system to create a new individual. Both the male and female reproductive systems are essential for reproduction.

Humans, like other organisms, pass certain characteristics of themselves to the next generation through their genes, the special carriers of human traits. The genes parents pass along to their offspring are what make kids similar to others in their family, but they're also what make each child unique. These genes come from the father's sperm and the mother's egg, which are produced by the male and female reproductive systems.

Understanding the male reproductive system, what it does, and the problems that can affect it can help you better understand your son's reproductive health.

About the Male Reproductive System

Most species have two sexes: Male and female. Each sex has its own unique reproductive system. They are different in shape and structure, but both are specifically designed to produce, nourish, and transport either the egg or sperm.

Unlike the female, whose sex organs are located entirely within the pelvis, the male has reproductive organs, or genitals, that are both inside and outside the pelvis. The male genitals include:

- the testicles;
- the duct system, which is made up of the epididymis and the vas deferens;
- the accessory glands, which include the seminal vesicles and prostate gland;
- the penis.

In a guy who has reached sexual maturity, the two testicles, or testes, produce and store millions of tiny sperm cells. The testicles are oval-shaped and grow to be about two inches (five centimeters) in length and one inch (three centimeters) in diameter. The testicles are also part of the endocrine system because they produce hormones, including testosterone. Testosterone is a major part of puberty in boys, and as a guy makes his way through puberty, his testicles produce more and more of it. Testosterone is the hormone that causes boys to develop deeper voices, bigger muscles, and body and facial hair, and it also stimulates the production of sperm.

Alongside the testicles are the epididymis and the vas deferens, which make up the duct system of the male reproductive organs. The vas deferens is a muscular tube that passes upward alongside the testicles and transports the sperm-containing fluid called semen. The epididymis is a set of coiled tubes (one for each testicle) that connects to the vas deferens.

The epididymis and the testicles hang in a pouch-like structure outside the pelvis called the scrotum. This bag of skin helps to regulate the temperature of testicles, which need to be kept cooler than body temperature to produce sperm. The scrotum changes size to maintain the right temperature. When the body is cold, the scrotum shrinks and becomes tighter to hold in body heat. When it's warm, the scrotum becomes larger and more floppy to get rid of extra heat. This happens without a guy ever having to think about it. The brain and the nervous system give the scrotum the cue to change size.

12

The accessory glands, including the seminal vesicles and the prostate gland, provide fluids that lubricate the duct system and nourish the sperm. The seminal vesicles are sac-like structures attached to the vas deferens to the side of the bladder. The prostate gland, which produces some of the parts of semen, surrounds the ejaculatory ducts at the base of the urethra, just below the bladder. The urethra is the channel that carries the semen to the outside of the body through the penis. The urethra is also part of the urinary system because it is also the channel through which urine passes as it leaves the bladder and exits the body.

The penis is actually made up of two parts: The shaft and the glans. The shaft is the main part of the penis and the glans is the tip (sometimes called the head). At the end of the glans is a small slit or opening, which is where semen and urine exit the body through the urethra. The inside of the penis is made of a spongy tissue that can expand and contract.

All boys are born with a foreskin, a fold of skin at the end of the penis covering the glans. Some boys are circumcised, which means that a doctor or clergy member cuts away the foreskin. Circumcision is usually performed during a baby boy's first few days of life. Although circumcision is not medically necessary, parents who choose to have their children circumcised often do so based on religious beliefs, concerns about hygiene, or cultural or social reasons. Boys who have circumcised penises and those who don't are no different: All penises work and feel the same, regardless of whether the foreskin has been removed.

What the Male Reproductive System Does

The male sex organs work together to produce and release semen into the reproductive system of the female during sexual intercourse. The male reproductive system also produces sex hormones, which help a boy develop into a sexually mature man during puberty.

When a baby boy is born, he has all the parts of his reproductive system in place, but it isn't until puberty that he is able to reproduce. When puberty begins, usually between the ages of 10 and 14, the pituitary gland—which is located near the brain—secretes hormones that stimulate the testicles to produce testosterone. The production of testosterone brings about many physical changes. Although the timing of these changes is different for every guy, the stages of puberty generally follow a set sequence.

- During the first stage of male puberty, the scrotum and testes grow larger.

- Next, the penis becomes longer, and the seminal vesicles and prostate gland grow.

- Hair begins to appear in the pubic area and later it grows on the face and underarms. During this time, a male's voice also deepens.

- Boys also undergo a growth spurt during puberty as they reach their adult height and weight.

Sperm

A male who has reached puberty will produce millions of sperm cells every day. Each sperm is extremely small: Only 1/600 of an inch (0.05 millimeters long). Sperm develop in the testicles within a system of tiny tubes called the seminiferous tubules. At birth, these tubules contain simple round cells, but during puberty, testosterone and other hormones cause these cells to transform into sperm cells. The cells divide and change until they have a head and short tail, like tadpoles. The head contains genetic material (genes). The sperm use their tails to push themselves into the epididymis, where they complete their development. It takes sperm about four to six weeks to travel through the epididymis.

The sperm then move to the vas deferens, or sperm duct. The seminal vesicles and prostate gland produce a whitish fluid called seminal fluid, which mixes with sperm to form semen when a male is sexually stimulated. The penis, which usually hangs limp, becomes hard when a male is sexually excited. Tissues in the penis fill with blood and it becomes stiff and erect (an erection). The rigidity of the erect penis makes it easier to insert into the female's vagina during sexual intercourse. When the erect penis is stimulated, muscles around the reproductive organs contract and force the semen through the duct system and urethra. Semen is pushed out of the male's body through his urethra—this process is called ejaculation. Each time a guy ejaculates, it can contain up to 500 million sperm.

When the male ejaculates during intercourse, semen is deposited into the female's vagina. From the vagina the sperm make their way up through the cervix and move through the uterus with help from uterine contractions. If a mature egg is in one of the female's fallopian tubes, a single sperm may penetrate it, and fertilization, or conception, occurs.

This fertilized egg is now called a zygote and contains 46 chromosomes—half from the egg and half from the sperm. The genetic material from the male and female has combined so that a new individual can be created. The zygote divides again and again as it grows in the female's uterus, maturing over the course of the pregnancy into an embryo, a fetus, and finally a newborn baby.

Things That Can Go Wrong with the Male Reproductive System

Boys may sometimes experience reproductive system problems, including [the following]:

Disorders of the Scrotum, Testicles, or Epididymis

Conditions affecting the scrotal contents may involve the testicles, epididymis, or the scrotum itself.

- **Testicular trauma:** Even a mild injury to the testicles can cause severe pain, bruising, or swelling. Most testicular injuries occur when the testicles are struck, hit, kicked, or crushed, usually during sports or due to other trauma. Testicular torsion, when one of the testicles twists around, cutting off its blood supply, is also a problem that some teen males experience, although it's not common. Surgery is needed to untwist the cord and save the testicle.

- **Varicocele:** This is a varicose vein (an abnormally swollen vein) in the network of veins that run from the testicles. Varicoceles commonly develop while a boy is going through puberty. A varicocele is usually not harmful, although it can damage the testicle or decrease sperm production. Take your son to see his doctor if he is concerned about changes in his testicles.

- **Testicular cancer:** This is one of the most common cancers in men younger than 40. It occurs when cells in the testicle divide abnormally and form a tumor. Testicular cancer can spread to other parts of the body, but if it's detected early, the cure rate is excellent. Teen boys should be encouraged to learn to perform testicular self-examinations.

- **Epididymitis:** Epididymitis is inflammation of the epididymis, the coiled tubes that connect the testes with the vas deferens. It is usually caused by an infection, such as the sexually transmitted disease chlamydia, and results in pain and swelling next to one of the testicles.

- **Hydrocele:** A hydrocele occurs when fluid collects in the membranes surrounding the testes. Hydroceles may cause swelling in the scrotum around the testicle but are generally painless. In some cases, surgery may be needed to correct the condition.

- **Inguinal hernia:** When a portion of the intestines pushes through an abnormal opening or weakening of the abdominal wall and into the groin or scrotum, it is known as an inguinal hernia. The hernia may look like a bulge or swelling in the groin area. It can be corrected with surgery.

Disorders of the Penis

Disorders affecting the penis include [the following]:

- **Inflammation of the penis:** Symptoms of penile inflammation include redness, itching, swelling, and pain. Balanitis occurs when the glans (the head of the penis) becomes inflamed. Posthitis is foreskin inflammation, which is usually due to a yeast or bacterial infection.

- **Hypospadias:** This is a disorder in which the urethra opens on the underside of the penis, not at the tip.

- **Phimosis:** This is a tightness of the foreskin of the penis and is common in newborns and young children. It usually resolves itself without treatment. If it interferes with urination, circumcision (removal of the foreskin) may be recommended.

- **Paraphimosis:** This may develop when the foreskin of a boy's uncircumcised penis is retracted (pulled down to expose the glans) and becomes trapped so it can't be returned to the unretracted position. As a result, blood flow to the head of the penis may be impaired, and your son may experience pain and swelling. A doctor may use lubricant to make a small incision so the foreskin can be pulled forward. If that doesn't work, circumcision may be recommended.

- **Ambiguous genitalia:** This occurs when a child is born with genitals that aren't clearly male or female. In most boys born with this disorder, the penis may be very small or nonexistent, but testicular tissue is present. In a small number of cases, the child may have both testicular and ovarian tissue.

- **Micropenis:** This is a disorder in which the penis, although normally formed, is well below the average size, as determined by standard measurements.

If your son has symptoms of a problem with his reproductive system or he has questions about growth and sexual development, talk with your doctor—many problems with the male reproductive system can be treated.

16

Chapter 2

What Is an STD?

What is a sexually transmitted disease (STD)?

It is an infection passed from person to person through intimate sexual contact. STDs are also called sexually transmitted infections, or STIs.

How many people have STDs and who is infected?

In the United States about 19 million new infections are thought to occur each year. These infections affect men and women of all backgrounds and economic levels. But almost half of new infections are among young people ages 15 to 24. Women are also severely affected by STDs. They have more frequent and more serious health problems from STDs than men. African-American women have especially high rates of infection.

How do you get an STD?

You can get an STD by having intimate sexual contact with someone who already has the infection. You can't tell if a person is infected because many STDs have no symptoms. But STDs can still be passed from person to person even if there are no symptoms. STDs are spread during vaginal, anal, or oral sex or during genital touching. So it's

"Sexually Transmitted Infections Fact Sheet," by the Office on Women's Health (www.womenshealth.gov), part of the U.S. Department of Health and Human Services, November 16, 2009.

possible to get some STDs without having intercourse. Not all STDs are spread the same way.

Can STDs cause health problems?

Yes. Each STD causes different health problems. But overall, untreated STDs can cause cancer, pelvic inflammatory disease, infertility, pregnancy problems, widespread infection to other parts of the body, organ damage, and even death.

Having an STD also can put you at greater risk of getting HIV [human immunodeficiency virus]. For one, not stopping risky sexual behavior can lead to infection with other STDs, including HIV. Also, infection with some STDs makes it easier for you to get HIV if you are exposed.

What are the symptoms of STDs?

Many STDs have only mild or no symptoms at all. When symptoms do develop, they often are mistaken for something else, such as urinary tract infection or yeast infection. This is why screening for STDs is so important. The STDs listed in the following text are among the most common or harmful to women.

Bacterial vaginosis (BV): Most women have no symptoms. Women with symptoms may have the following:

- Vaginal itching

- Pain when urinating

- Discharge with a fishy odor

Chlamydia: Most women have no symptoms. Women with symptoms may have the following:

- Abnormal vaginal discharge

- Burning when urinating

- Bleeding between periods

Infections that are not treated, even if there are no symptoms, can lead to the following:

- Lower abdominal pain

- Low back pain

- Nausea

- Fever
- Pain during sex

Genital herpes: Some people may have no symptoms. During an outbreak, the symptoms are clear:

- Small red bumps, blisters, or open sores where the virus entered the body, such as on the penis, vagina, or mouth
- Vaginal discharge
- Fever
- Headache
- Muscle aches
- Pain when urinating
- Itching, burning, or swollen glands in genital area
- Pain in legs, buttocks, or genital area

Symptoms may go away and then come back. Sores heal after two to four weeks.

Gonorrhea: Symptoms are often mild, but most women have no symptoms. If symptoms are present, they most often appear within 10 days of becoming infected. Symptoms include the following:

- Pain or burning when urinating
- Yellowish and sometimes bloody vaginal discharge
- Bleeding between periods
- Pain during sex
- Heavy bleeding during periods

Infection that occurs in the throat, eye, or anus also might have symptoms in these parts of the body.

Hepatitis B: Some women have no symptoms. Women with symptoms may have the following:

- Low-grade fever
- Headache and muscle aches
- Tiredness
- Loss of appetite

- Upset stomach or vomiting

- Diarrhea

- Dark-colored urine and pale bowel movements

- Stomach pain

- Skin and whites of eyes turning yellow

HIV/AIDS [acquired immunodeficiency syndrome]: Some women may have no symptoms for 10 years or more. About half of people with HIV get flu-like symptoms about three to six weeks after becoming infected. Symptoms people can have for months or even years before the onset of AIDS include the following:

- Fevers and night sweats

- Feeling very tired

- Quick weight loss

- Headache

- Enlarged lymph nodes

- Diarrhea, vomiting, and upset stomach

- Mouth, genital, or anal sores

- Dry cough

- Rash or flaky skin

- Short-term memory loss

   Women also might have these signs of HIV:

- Vaginal yeast infections and other vaginal infections, including STDs

- Pelvic inflammatory disease (PID) that does not get better with treatment

- Menstrual cycle changes

Human papillomavirus (HPV): Some women have no symptoms. Women with symptoms may have the following:

- Visible warts in the genital area, including the thighs: Warts can be raised or flat, alone or in groups, small or large, and sometimes they are cauliflower-shaped.

- Growths on the cervix and vagina: They are often invisible.

Pubic lice (sometimes called crabs): Symptoms include the following:

- Itching in the genital area
- Finding lice or lice eggs

Syphilis: Syphilis progresses in stages. Symptoms of the primary stage are a single, painless sore appearing 10 to 90 days after infection. It can appear in the genital area, mouth, or other parts of the body. The sore goes away on its own.

If the infection is not treated, it moves to the secondary stage. This stage starts three to six weeks after the sore appears. Symptoms of the secondary stage are the following:

- Skin rash with rough, red or reddish-brown spots on the hands and feet that usually does not itch and clears on its own
- Fever
- Sore throat and swollen glands
- Patchy hair loss
- Headaches and muscle aches
- Weight loss
- Tiredness

In the latent stage, symptoms go away, but can come back. Without treatment, the infection may or may not move to the late stage. In the late stage, symptoms are related to damage to internal organs, such as the brain, nerves, eyes, heart, blood vessels, liver, bones, and joints. Some people may die.

Trichomoniasis (sometimes called trich): Many women do not have symptoms. Symptoms usually appear 5 to 28 days after exposure and can include the following:

- Yellow, green, or gray vaginal discharge (often foamy) with a strong odor
- Discomfort during sex and when urinating
- Itching or discomfort in the genital area
- Lower abdominal pain (rarely)

How do you get tested for STDs?

There is no one test for all STDs. Ask your doctor about getting tested for STDs. She or he can tell you what test(s) you might need and how it is done. Testing for STDs is also called STD screening. Testing (or screening) for STDs can involve the following:

- Pelvic and physical exam by a doctor who looks for signs of infection, such as warts, rashes, or discharge

- Blood sample

- Urine sample

- Fluid or tissue sample in which a swab is used to collect a sample that can be looked at under a microscope or sent to a lab for testing

These methods are used for many kinds of tests. So if you have a pelvic exam and Pap test, for example, don't assume that you have been tested for STDs. Pap testing is mainly used to look for cell changes that could be cancer or precancer. Although a Pap test sample also can be used to perform tests for HPV, doing so isn't routine. And a Pap test does not test for other STDs. If you want to be tested for STDs, including HPV, you must ask.

You can get tested for STDs at your doctor's office or a clinic. But not all doctors offer the same tests. So it's important to discuss your sexual health history to find out what tests you need and where you can go to get tested.

Who needs to get tested for STDs?

If you are sexually active, talk to your doctor about STD screening. Which tests you might need and how often depend mainly on your sexual history and your partner's. Talking to your doctor about your sex life might seem too personal to share. But being open and honest is the only way your doctor can help take care of you. Also, don't assume you don't need to be tested for STDs if you have sex only with women. Talk to your doctor to find out what tests make sense for you.

How are STDs treated?

The treatment depends on the type of STD. For some STDs, treatment may involve taking medicine or getting a shot. For other STDs that can't be cured, like herpes, treatment can help to relieve the symptoms.

Only use medicines prescribed or suggested by your doctor. There are products sold over the Internet that falsely claim to prevent or treat STDs, such as herpes, chlamydia, human papillomavirus, and HIV. Some of these drugs claim to work better than the drugs your doctor will give you. But this is not true, and the safety of these products is not known.

What can I do to keep from getting an STD?

You can lower your risk of getting an STD with the following steps. The steps work best when used together. No single strategy can protect you from every single type of STD.

- Don't have sex. The surest way to keep from getting any STD is to practice abstinence. This means not having vaginal, oral, or anal sex. Keep in mind that some STDs, like genital herpes, can be spread without having intercourse.

- Be faithful. Having a sexual relationship with one partner who has been tested for STDs and is not infected is another way to lower your risk of getting infected. Be faithful to each other. This means you only have sex with each other and no one else.

- Use condoms correctly and every time you have sex. Use condoms for all types of sexual contact, even if intercourse does not take place. Use condoms from the very start to the very end of each sex act, and with every sex partner. A male latex condom offers the best protection. You can use a male polyurethane condom if you or your partner has a latex allergy. For vaginal sex, use a male latex condom or a female condom if your partner won't wear a condom. For anal sex, use a male latex condom. For oral sex, use a male latex condom. A dental dam might also offer some protection from some STDs.

- Know that some methods of birth control, like birth control pills, shots, implants, or diaphragms, will not protect you from STDs. If you use one of these methods, be sure to also use a condom correctly every time you have sex.

- Talk with your sex partner(s) about STDs and using condoms before having sex. It's up to you to set the ground rules and to make sure you are protected.

- Don't assume you're at low risk for STDs if you have sex only with women. Some common STDs are spread easily by skin-to-skin contact. Also, most women who have sex with women have had sex with men, too. So a woman can get an STD from a male partner and then pass it to a female partner.

• Talk frankly with your doctor and your sex partner(s) about any STDs you or your partner has or has had. Talk about symptoms, such as sores or discharge. Try not to be embarrassed. Your doctor is there to help you with any and all health problems. Also, being open with your doctor and partner will help you protect your health and the health of others.

• Have a yearly pelvic exam. Ask your doctor if you should be tested for STDs and how often you should be retested. Testing for many STDs is simple and often can be done during your checkup. The sooner an STD is found, the easier it is to treat.

• Avoid using drugs or drinking too much alcohol. These activities may lead to risky sexual behavior, such as not wearing a condom.

How do STDs affect pregnant women and their babies?

STDs can cause many of the same health problems in pregnant women as women who are not pregnant. But having an STD also can threaten the pregnancy and unborn baby's health. Having an STD during pregnancy can cause early labor, a woman's water to break early, and infection in the uterus after the birth.

Some STDs can be passed from a pregnant woman to the baby before and during the baby's birth. Some STDs, like syphilis, cross the placenta and infect the baby while it is in the uterus. Other STDs, like gonorrhea, chlamydia, hepatitis B, and genital herpes, can be passed from the mother to the baby during delivery as the baby passes through the birth canal. HIV can cross the placenta during pregnancy and infect the baby during the birth process.

The harmful effects to babies may include the following:

• Low birth weight

• Eye infection

• Pneumonia

• Infection in the baby's blood

• Brain damage

• Lack of coordination in body movements

• Blindness

- Deafness

- Acute hepatitis

- Meningitis

- Chronic liver disease

- Cirrhosis

- Stillbirth

Some of these problems can be prevented if the mother receives routine prenatal care, which includes screening tests for STDs starting early in pregnancy and repeated close to delivery, if needed. Other problems can be treated if the infection is found at birth.

What can pregnant women do to prevent problems from STDs?

Pregnant women should be screened at their first prenatal visit for STDs, including the following:

- Chlamydia

- Gonorrhea

- Hepatitis B

- HIV

- Syphilis

In addition, some experts recommend that women who have had a premature delivery in the past be screened and treated for bacterial vaginosis (BV) at the first prenatal visit. Even if a woman has been tested for STDs in the past, she should be tested again when she becomes pregnant.

Chlamydia, gonorrhea, syphilis, trichomoniasis, and BV can be treated and cured with antibiotics during pregnancy. Viral STDs, such as genital herpes and HIV, have no cure. But antiviral medication may be appropriate for some pregnant woman with herpes to reduce symptoms. For women who have active genital herpes lesions at the onset of labor, a cesarean delivery (C-section) can lower the risk of passing the infection to the newborn. For women who are HIV positive, taking antiviral medicines during pregnancy can lower the risk of giving HIV to the newborn to less than two percent. C-section is also an option for some women with HIV. Women who test negative for hepatitis B may receive the hepatitis B vaccine during pregnancy.

Do STDs affect breastfeeding?

If you have HIV, do not breastfeed. You can pass the virus to your baby. Talk with your doctor, nurse, or a lactation consultant about the risk of passing the STD to your baby while breastfeeding. If you have chlamydia or gonorrhea, you can keep breastfeeding. If you have syphilis or herpes, you can keep breastfeeding as long as the sores are covered. Syphilis and herpes are spread through contact with sores and can be dangerous to your newborn. If you have sores on your nipple or areola, stop breastfeeding on that breast. Pump or hand express your milk from that breast until the sore clears. Pumping will help keep up your milk supply and prevent your breast from getting engorged or overly full. You can store your milk to give to your baby in a bottle for another feeding. But if parts of your breast pump that contact the milk also touch the sore(s) while pumping, you should throw the milk away.

If you are being treated for an STD, ask your doctor about the possible effects of the drug on your breastfeeding baby. Most treatments for STDs are safe to use while breastfeeding.

Is there any research being done on STDs?

Yes. Research on STDs is a public health priority. Research is focused on prevention, diagnosis, and treatment.

With prevention, researchers are looking at strategies such as vaccines and topical microbicides. One large study is testing a herpes vaccine for women. Topical microbicides could play a big role in protecting women from getting STDs. But so far, they have been difficult to design. They are gels or creams that would be put into the vagina to kill or stop the STD before it could infect someone. Researchers are also looking at the reasons some people are at higher risk of STDs and ways to lower these risks.

Early and fast diagnosis of STDs means treatment can start right away. Early treatment helps to limit the effects of an STD and keep it from spreading to others. Researchers are looking at quick, easy, and better ways to test for STDs, including vaginal swabs women can use to collect a sample for testing. They also are studying the reasons why many STDs have no symptoms, which can delay diagnosis.

Research also is underway to develop new ways to treat STDs. For instance, more and more people are becoming infected with types of gonorrhea that do not respond well to drugs. So scientists are working to develop new antibiotics to treat these drug-resistant types. An example of treatment research success is the life-prolonging effects of new drugs used to treat HIV.

Chapter 3

Trends in STD Infection in the United States

STD Trends in the United States

This text summarizes 2010 national data on gonorrhea, chlamydia, and syphilis. The data are based on state and local STD case reports from a variety of private and public sources, the majority of which come from non-STD clinic settings, such as private physician offices and health maintenance organizations.

Trends

STDs are one of the most critical health challenges facing the nation today. CDC estimates that there are 19 million new infections every year in the United States.

STDs cost the U.S. health care system $17 billion every year—and cost individuals even more in immediate and life-long health consequences.

CDC's surveillance report includes data on the three STDs that physicians are required to report to local or state public health authorities—gonorrhea, chlamydia, and syphilis—which represent only a fraction of the true burden of STDs. Some common STDs, like human papillomavirus (HPV) and genital herpes, are not required to be reported.

This chapter contains text excerpted from "STD Trends in the United States: 2010 National Data for Gonorrhea, Chlamydia, and Syphilis," by the Centers for Disease Control and Prevention (CDC, www.cdc.gov), November 17, 2011, and text excerpted from "Basic Statistics," by the Division of HIV/AIDS Prevention, CDC, August 11, 2011.

The latest CDC data show troubling trends in three treatable STDs:

- **Gonorrhea:** While reported rates are at historically low levels, cases increased slightly from last year and more than 300,000 cases were reported in 2010. There are also signs from other CDC surveillance systems that the disease may become resistant to the only available treatment option.

- **Chlamydia:** Case reports have been increasing steadily over the past 20 years, and in 2010, 1.3 million chlamydia cases were reported. While the increase is due to expanded screening efforts, and not to an actual increase in the number of people with chlamydia, a majority of infections still go undiagnosed. Less than half of sexually active young women are screened annually as recommended by CDC.

- **Syphilis:** The overall syphilis rate decreased for the first time in a decade, and is down 1.6 percent since 2009. However, the rate among young black men has increased dramatically over the past five years (134 percent). Other CDC data also show a significant increase in syphilis among young black men who have sex with men (MSM), suggesting that new infections among MSM are driving the increase in young black men. The finding is particularly concerning as there has also been a sharp increase in HIV [human immunodeficiency virus] infections among this population.

Young People and STDs

Young people represent 25 percent of the sexually experienced population in the United States, but account for nearly half of new STDs. The long-lasting health effects are particularly serious for young people:

- Untreated gonorrhea and chlamydia can silently steal a young woman's chance to have her own children later in life. Each year, untreated STDs cause at least 24,000 women in the United States to become infertile.

- Untreated syphilis can lead to serious long-term complications, including brain, cardiovascular, and organ damage. Syphilis in pregnant women can also result in congenital syphilis (syphilis among infants), which can cause stillbirth, death soon after birth, and physical deformity and neurological complications in children who survive. Untreated syphilis in pregnant women results in infant death in up to 40 percent of cases.

- Studies suggest that people with gonorrhea, chlamydia, or syphilis are at increased risk for HIV. Given the increase in both syphilis and HIV among young black gay and bisexual men, it is particularly urgent to diagnose and treat both diseases.

Race, Age, and Sexual Orientation

STDs affect people of all races, ages, and sexual orientations, though some individuals experience greater challenges in protecting their health. When individual risk behaviors are combined with barriers to quality health information and STD prevention services, the risk of infection increases. While everyone should have the opportunity to make choices that allow them to live healthy lives regardless of their income, education, or racial/ethnic background, the reality is that if an individual lacks resources or has difficult living conditions, the journey to health and wellness can be harder. Even with similar levels of individual risk, African Americans and Latinos sometimes face barriers that contribute to increased rates of STDs and are more affected by these diseases than whites.

Basic Statistics on HIV/AIDS

HIV Prevalence Estimate

Prevalence is the number of people living with HIV [human immunodeficiency virus] infection at the end of a given year.

At the end of 2008, an estimated 1,178,350 persons aged 13 and older were living with HIV infection in the United States. Of those, 20% had undiagnosed HIV infections.

HIV Incidence Estimate

Incidence is the number of new HIV infections that occur during a given year. CDC estimates that approximately 50,000 people are newly infected with HIV each year in the United States. In 2009 (the most recent year that data are available), there were an estimated 48,100 new HIV infections. Most (61%) of these new infections occurred in gay and bisexual men. Black/African American men and women were also strongly affected and were estimated to have an HIV incidence rate than was seven times as high as the incidence rate among whites.

Diagnoses of HIV Infection

In 2009, the estimated number of diagnoses of HIV infection in the 40 states and 5 U.S.-dependent areas with confidential name-based

HIV infection reporting was 42,959. Of these, 42,011 were in the 40 states and 948 were in the 5 dependent areas. In the 40 states, diagnoses of HIV infection among adults and adolescents totaled 41,845 with 31,872 diagnoses in males and 9,973 diagnoses in females. Among children under age 13 years, there were an estimated 166 diagnoses of HIV infection in 2009.

Estimated numbers resulted from statistical adjustment that accounted for delays in reporting to the health department (but not for incomplete reporting) and missing risk factor information, where appropriate.

Because totals for the estimated numbers were calculated independently of the values for the subpopulations, the subpopulation values may not equal the totals.

Diagnoses of HIV infection by age: Table 3.1 identifies the estimated number of diagnoses of HIV infection in the 40 states with confidential name-based HIV infection reporting in 2009 and the distribution of ages at time of diagnosis.

Diagnoses of HIV infection by race/ethnicity: CDC tracks diagnoses of HIV infection information on seven racial and ethnic groups: American Indian/Alaska Native; Asian; Black/African American; Hispanic/Latino; Native Hawaiian/Other Pacific Islander; White; and Multiple Races.

Table 3.1. Estimated Number of Diagnoses of HIV Infection by Age

Age (Years)	Estimated Number of Diagnoses of HIV Infection, 2009
Under 13	166
Ages 13–14	21
Ages 15–19	2,036
Ages 20–24	6,237
Ages 25–29	5,951
Ages 30–34	5,020
Ages 35–39	5,232
Ages 40–44	5,519
Ages 45–49	4,865
Ages 50–54	3,323
Ages 55–59	2,004
Ages 60–64	900
Ages 65 or older	736

Table 3.2. Race, Ethnicity, and Diagnoses of HIV Infection

Race or Ethnicity	Estimated Number of Diagnoses of HIV Infection, 2009
American Indian/Alaska Native	189
Asian	470
Black/African American	21,652
Hispanic/Latino	7,347
Native Hawaiian/Other Pacific Islander	34
White	11,803
Multiple Races	516

Table 3.3. Types of Transmission and HIV Diagnoses

Transmission Category	Estimated Number of Diagnoses of HIV Infection, 2009		
	Adult and Adolescent Males	Adult and Adolescent Females	Total
Male-to-male sexual contact	23,846	—	23,846
Injection drug use	2,449	1,483	3,932
Male-to-male sexual contact and injection drug use	1,131	—	1,131
Heterosexual contact*	4,399	8,461	12,860
Other**	47	29	76

Notes: * Heterosexual contact with a person known to have, or to be at high risk for, HIV infection. ** Includes hemophilia, blood transfusion, perinatal exposure, and risk not reported or not identified.

Table 3.2 identifies the estimated number of diagnoses of HIV infection in the 40 states with confidential name-based HIV infection reporting, by race or ethnicity, in 2009.

Diagnoses of HIV Infection by transmission category: Six common transmission categories are male-to-male sexual contact, injection drug use, male-to-male sexual contact and injection drug use, heterosexual contact, mother-to-child (perinatal) transmission, and other (includes blood transfusions and unknown cause).

Table 3.3 illustrates the distribution of the estimated number of diagnoses of HIV infection among adults and adolescents in the 40 states with confidential name-based HIV infection reporting, by transmission category.

Persons Living with a Diagnosis of HIV Infection

At the end of 2008, the estimated number of persons living with a diagnosis of HIV infection in the 40 states and 5 U.S.-dependent areas with confidential name-based HIV infection reporting was 682,668. In the 40 states only, this included 660,062 adults and adolescents, and 3,022 children under age 13 years.

Data include persons with a diagnosis of HIV infection regardless of the stage of disease at diagnosis. Estimated numbers resulted from statistical adjustment that accounted for delays in reporting to the health department (but not for incomplete reporting) and missing risk factor information, where appropriate.

Because of delays in reporting of deaths, data are only available through the end of 2008. The exclusion of data from the most recent year allows at least 18 months for deaths to be reported and for these persons to be removed from calculations of persons living with a diagnosis of HIV infection.

Totals include persons of unknown race/ethnicity. Because totals for the estimated numbers were calculated independently of the values for the subpopulations, the subpopulation values may not equal the totals.

Deaths of Persons with a Diagnosis of HIV Infection

In 2008, the estimated number of deaths of persons with a diagnosis of HIV infection in the 40 states and 5 U.S.-dependent areas with confidential name-based HIV infection reporting was 17,374. In the 40 states only, this included 16,762 adults and adolescents, and 7 children under age 13 years at death.

Deaths of persons with a diagnosis of HIV infection may be due to any cause.

Data include persons with a diagnosis of HIV infection regardless of the stage of disease at diagnosis. Estimated numbers resulted from statistical adjustment that accounted for delays in reporting to the health department (but not for incomplete reporting) and missing risk factor information, where appropriate. Because of delays in reporting of deaths, data are only available through the end of 2008. The exclusion of data from the most recent year allows at least 18 months for deaths of persons with a diagnosis of HIV infection to be reported.

Totals include persons of unknown race/ethnicity. Because totals for the estimated numbers were calculated independently of the values for the subpopulations, the subpopulation values may not equal the totals.

AIDS Diagnoses

In 2009, the estimated number of persons diagnosed with AIDS [acquired immunodeficiency syndrome] in the United States and 5 U.S.-dependent areas was 34,993. Of these, 34,247 were diagnosed in the 50 states and the District of Columbia and 747 were diagnosed in the dependent areas. In the 50 states and the District of Columbia, 25,587 AIDS diagnoses were among adult and adolescent males, 8,647 were among adult and adolescent females, and 13 diagnoses were among children under age 13 years.

The cumulative estimated number of AIDS diagnoses through 2009 in the United States and dependent areas was 1,142,714. Of these, 1,108,611 were diagnosed in the 50 states and the District of Columbia and 34,103 were diagnosed in the dependent areas. In the 50 states and the District of Columbia, 878,366 cumulative AIDS diagnoses were among adult and adolescent males, 220,795 were among adult and adolescent females, and 9,448 were among children under age 13 years.

Estimated numbers resulted from statistical adjustment that accounted for delays in reporting to the health department (but not for incomplete reporting) and missing risk factor information, where appropriate.

Cumulative totals include persons of unknown race/ethnicity. Because totals for the estimated numbers were calculated independently of the values for the subpopulations, the subpopulation values may not equal the totals.

Persons Living with an AIDS Diagnosis

At the end of 2008, the estimated number of persons living with an AIDS diagnosis in the United States and dependent areas was 490,696. In the 50 states and the District of Columbia, this included 479,161 adults and adolescents, and 707 children under age 13 years at the end of the year.

Estimated numbers resulted from statistical adjustment that accounted for delays in reporting to the health department (but not for incomplete reporting) and missing risk factor information, where appropriate.

Because of delays in reporting of deaths, data are only available through the end of 2008. The exclusion of data from the most recent year allows at least 18 months for deaths to be reported and for these persons to be removed from calculations of persons living with an AIDS diagnosis.

Totals include persons of unknown race/ethnicity. Because totals for the estimated numbers were calculated independently of the values for the subpopulations, the subpopulation values may not equal the totals.

Deaths of Persons with an AIDS Diagnosis

In 2008, the estimated number of deaths of persons with an AIDS diagnosis in the United States and dependent areas was 16,605. In the 50 states and the District of Columbia, this included 16,084 adults and adolescents, and 4 children under age 13 years.

The cumulative estimated number of deaths of persons with an AIDS diagnosis in the United States and dependent areas, through 2008, was 617,025. In the 50 states and the District of Columbia, this included 589,547 adults and adolescents, and 4,949 children under age 13 years at death.

Deaths of persons with an AIDS diagnosis may be due to any cause.

Estimated numbers resulted from statistical adjustment that accounted for delays in reporting to the health department (but not for incomplete reporting) and missing risk factor information, where appropriate. Because of delays in reporting of deaths, data are only available through the end of 2008. The exclusion of data from the most recent year allows at least 18 months for deaths of persons with an AIDS diagnosis to be reported.

Totals include persons of unknown race/ethnicity. Because totals for the estimated numbers were calculated independently of the values for the subpopulations, the subpopulation values may not equal the totals.

Chapter 4

Trends in STD Infection Worldwide

Chapter Contents

Section 4.1—Trends in STDs Other Than HIV/AIDS 36

Section 4.2—The Global HIV/AIDS Epidemic 41

Section 4.1

Trends in STDs Other Than HIV/AIDS

"Sexually Transmitted Infections." Geneva, World Health Organization, August 2011 (Fact sheet no. 110 http://www.who.int/mediacentre/factsheets/fs110/en/index.html, accessed 16 April 2012). © World Health Organization. Reprinted with permission.

Key Facts

- 448 million new infections of curable sexually transmitted (syphilis, gonorrhea, chlamydia, and trichomoniasis) infections occur yearly.

- Some sexually transmitted infections exist without symptoms.

- In pregnant women with untreated early syphilis, 25% of pregnancies result in stillbirth and 14% in neonatal death.

- Sexually transmitted infections are the main preventable cause of infertility, particularly in women.

- WHO (World Health Organization) recommends a syndromic approach to diagnosis and management of sexually transmitted infections.

Sexually Transmitted Infections (STIs) Are a Public Health Issue

According to 2005 WHO estimates, 448 million new cases of curable STIs (syphilis, gonorrhea, chlamydia, and trichomoniasis) occur annually throughout the world in adults aged 15–49 years. This does not include HIV [human immunodeficiency virus] and other STIs which continue to adversely affect the lives of individuals and communities worldwide. In developing countries, STIs and their complications rank in the top five disease categories for which adults seek health care.

Infections and Transmission

STIs are infections that are spread primarily through person-to-person sexual contact. There are more than 30 different sexually transmissible bacteria, viruses, and parasites. Several, in particular HIV and syphilis, can also be transmitted from mother to child during pregnancy and childbirth, and through blood products and tissue transfer.

STIs are caused by bacteria, viruses, and parasites. Some of the most common infections are in the following text.

Common Bacterial Infections

- *Neisseria gonorrhoeae* (causes gonorrhea or gonococcal infection)
- *Chlamydia trachomatis* (causes chlamydial infections)
- *Treponema pallidum* (causes syphilis)
- *Haemophilus ducreyi* (causes chancroid)
- *Klebsiella granulomatis* (previously known as *Calymmatobacterium granulomatis*; causes granuloma inguinale or donovanosis)

Common Viral Infections

- Human immunodeficiency virus (causes AIDS [acquired immunodeficiency syndrome])
- Herpes simplex virus type 2 (causes genital herpes)
- Human papillomavirus (causes genital warts and certain subtypes lead to cervical cancer in women)
- Hepatitis B virus (causes hepatitis and chronic cases may lead to cancer of the liver)
- Cytomegalovirus (causes inflammation in a number of organs including the brain, the eye, and the bowel)

Parasites

- *Trichomonas vaginalis* (causes vaginal trichomoniasis)
- *Candida albicans* (causes vulvovaginitis in women; inflammation of the glans penis and foreskin [balano-posthitis] in men)

STIs without Symptoms

Some STIs exist without symptoms. For example, up to 70% of women and a significant proportion of men with gonococcal and/or chlamydial infections experience no symptoms at all. Both symptomatic and asymptomatic infections can lead to the development of serious complications, discussed in the following text.

STIs Adversely Affect the Health of Women

Untreated STIs can have critical implications for reproductive, maternal, and newborn health. STIs are the main preventable cause of infertility, particularly in women.

For example, 10–40% of women with untreated chlamydial infection develop symptomatic pelvic inflammatory disease. Post-infection tubal damage is responsible for 30–40% of cases of female infertility. Furthermore, women who have had pelvic inflammatory disease are 6–10 times more likely to develop an ectopic (tubal) pregnancy than those who have not, and 40–50% of ectopic pregnancies can be attributed to previous pelvic inflammatory disease.

Infection with certain types of the human papillomavirus can lead to the development of genital cancers, particularly cervical cancer in women.

STIs and Adverse Outcomes of Pregnancy

Untreated STIs are associated with congenital and perinatal infections in neonates, particularly in regions where rates of infection remain high.

In pregnant women with untreated early syphilis, 25% of pregnancies result in stillbirth and 14% in neonatal death—an overall perinatal mortality of about 40%.

Up to 35% of pregnancies among women with untreated gonococcal infection result in spontaneous abortions and premature deliveries, and up to 10% in perinatal deaths. In the absence of prophylaxis, 30–50% of infants born to mothers with untreated gonorrhea and up to 30% of infants born to mothers with untreated chlamydial infection will develop a serious eye infection (ophthalmia neonatorum), which can lead to blindness if not treated early. Worldwide, 1000–4000 newborn babies become blind every year because of this condition.

STIs and HIV

The presence of untreated STIs (both those which cause ulcers or those which do not) increase the risk of both acquisition and transmission of HIV by a factor of up to 10. Prompt treatment for STIs is thus important to reduce the risk of HIV infection. Controlling STIs is important for preventing HIV infection, particularly in people with high-risk sexual behaviors.

STI Syndromes

Although many different pathogens cause STIs, some display similar or overlapping signs (what the individual or the health-care provider sees on examination) and symptoms (what the patient feels such as pain or irritation). Some of these signs and symptoms are easily recognizable and consistent, giving what is known as a syndrome that signals the presence of one or a number of pathogens. For example, a discharge from the urethra in men can be caused by gonorrhea alone, chlamydia alone, or both together.

The main syndromes of common STIs are:

- urethral discharge;

- genital ulcers;

- inguinal swellings (bubo, which is a swelling in the groin);

- scrotal swelling;

- vaginal discharge;

- lower abdominal pain;

- neonatal eye infections (conjunctivitis of the newborn).

STI Syndromic Approach to Patient Management

The traditional method of diagnosing STIs is by laboratory tests. However, these are often unavailable or too expensive. Since 1990 WHO has recommended a syndromic approach to diagnosis and management of STIs in patients presenting with consistently recognized signs and symptoms of particular STIs.

The syndromic approach uses flowcharts to guide diagnosis and treatment is more accurate than diagnosis based on clinical tests alone, even in experienced hands. The syndromic approach is a scientific approach and offers accessible and immediate treatment that is effective. It is also more cost-effective for some syndromes than use of laboratory tests.

The pathogens causing any particular syndrome need to be determined locally and flowcharts adapted accordingly. Furthermore, regular monitoring of the organisms causing each syndrome should be conducted on a regular basis to validate the treatment recommendations.

Prevention

The most effective means to avoid becoming infected with or transmitting a sexually transmitted infection is to abstain from sexual intercourse (i.e., oral, vaginal, or anal sex) or to have sexual intercourse only within a long-term, mutually monogamous relationship with an uninfected partner. Male latex condoms, when used consistently and correctly, are highly effective in reducing the transmission of HIV and other sexually transmitted infections, including gonorrhea, chlamydial infection, and trichomoniasis.

WHO Response

The control of STIs is a priority for WHO. The World Health Assembly endorsed the global strategy for the prevention and control of STIs in May 2006.

More recently, the United Nations Secretary-General Global Strategy for Women's and Children's Health highlighted the need for a comprehensive, integrated package of essential interventions and services. The Strategy urges partners to ensure that women and children have access to a universal package of guaranteed benefits, including family-planning information and services, antenatal, newborn, and postnatal care, emergency obstetric and newborn care, and the prevention of HIV and other sexually transmitted infections. Such a package could accelerate the response towards meeting the lagging health-related Millennium Development Goals.

Section 4.2

The Global HIV/AIDS Epidemic

Excerpted from *Global HIV/AIDS Response: Epidemic update and health sector progress toward Universal Access—Progress Report 2011.* Geneva, World Health Organization, November 2011 (http://www.who.int/hiv/pub/progress_report2011/en/). © World Health Organization. Reprinted with permission.

At the end of 2010, an estimated 34 million people (31,600,000–35,200,000) were living with HIV [human immunodeficiency virus] globally, including 3.4 million [3,000,000–3,800,000] children less than 15 years. There was 2.7 million [2,400,000–2,900,000] new HIV infections in 2010, including 390,000 [340,000–450,000] among children less than 15 years.

Globally, the annual number of people newly infected with HIV continues to decline, although there is stark regional variation. In sub-Saharan Africa, where most of the people newly infected with HIV live, an estimated 1.9 million [1,700,000–2,100,000] people became infected in 2010. This was 16% fewer than the estimated 2.2 million [2,100,000–2,400,000] people newly infected with HIV in 2001 and 27% fewer than the annual number of people newly infected between 1996 and 1998, when the incidence of HIV in sub-Saharan Africa peaked overall.

The annual number of people dying from AIDS [acquired immunodeficiency syndrome]-related causes worldwide is steadily decreasing from a peak of 2.2 million [2,100,000–2,500,000] in 2005 to an estimated 1.8 million [1,600,000–1,900,000] in 2010. The number of people dying from AIDS-related causes began to decline in 2005–2006 in sub-Saharan Africa, South and South-East Asia, and the Caribbean and has continued subsequently.

In 2010, an estimated 250,000 [220,000–290,000] children less than 15 died from AIDS-related causes, 20% fewer than in 2005.

Not all regions and countries fit the overall trends, however. The annual number of people newly infected with HIV has risen in the Middle East and North Africa from 43,000 [31,000–57,000] in 2001 to 59,000 [40,000–73,000] in 2010. After slowing drastically in the early

41

2000s, the incidence of HIV infection in Eastern Europe and Central Asia has been accelerating again since 2008.

The trends in AIDS-related deaths also differ. In Eastern Europe and Central Asia, the number of people dying from AIDS-related causes increased more than 10-fold between 2001 and 2010 (from about 7800 [6000–11,000] to 90,000 [74,000–110,000]). In the same period, the number of people dying from AIDS-related caused increased by 60% in the Middle East and North Africa (from 22,000 [9700–38,000] to 35,000 [25,000–42,000]) and more than doubled in East Asia (from 24,000 [16,000–45,000] to 56,000 [40,000–76,000]).

Introducing antiretroviral therapy has averted 2.5 million deaths in low- and middle-income countries globally since 1995. Sub-Saharan Africa accounts for the vast majority of the averted deaths: About 1.8 million.

Providing antiretroviral prophylaxis to pregnant women living with HIV has prevented more than 350,000 children from acquiring HIV infection since 1995. Eighty-six percent of the children who avoided infection live in sub-Saharan Africa, the region with the highest prevalence of HIV infection among women of reproductive age.

Chapter 5

Women and STDs

Chapter Contents

Section 5.1—Ten Ways STDs Impact Women
        Differently Than Men 44

Section 5.2—STDs in Women 46

Section 5.3—STDs in Women Who Have Sex
        with Women 49

Section 5.1

Ten Ways STDs Impact Women Differently Than Men

"10 Ways STDs Impact Women Differently from Men," by the Centers for Disease Control and Prevention (CDC, www.cdc.gov), April 2011.

Sexually transmitted diseases (STDs) remain a major public health challenge in the United States, especially among women, who disproportionately bear the long-term consequences of STDs. For example, each year untreated STDs cause infertility in at least 24,000 women in the United States, and untreated syphilis in pregnant women results in infant death in up to 40 percent of cases. Testing and treatment are keys to reducing disease and infertility associated with undiagnosed STDs.

Why are women so severely affected by STDs? In the following text are ways STDs impact women differently from men.

1. A woman's anatomy can place her at a unique risk for STD infection, compared to a man.

The lining of the vagina is thinner and more delicate than the skin on a penis, so it's easier for bacteria and viruses to penetrate. Also, the vagina is a good environment (moist) for bacteria to grow.

2. Women are less likely to have symptoms of common STDs—such as chlamydia and gonorrhea—compared to men.

If symptoms do occur, they can go away even though the infection may remain.

3. Women are more likely to confuse symptoms of an STD for something else.

Women often have normal discharge or think that burning/itching is related to a yeast infection. Men usually notice symptoms like discharge because it is unusual

4. Women may not see symptoms as easily as men.

Genital ulcers (like from herpes or syphilis) can occur in the vagina and may not be easily visible, whereas men may be more likely to notice sores on their penis.

5. STDs can lead to serious health complications and affect a woman's future reproductive plans.

- Untreated STDs can lead to pelvic inflammatory disease, which can result in infertility and ectopic pregnancy.

- Chlamydia (one of the most common STDs) results in few complications in men.

- Women who are pregnant can pass STDs to their babies. Genital herpes, syphilis, and HIV [human immunodeficiency virus] can be passed to babies during pregnancy and at delivery. The harmful effects of STDs in babies may include stillbirth (a baby that is born dead), low birth weight (less than five pounds), brain damage, blindness, and deafness.

7. Human papillomavirus (HPV) is the most common sexually transmitted infection in women and is the main cause of cervical cancer.

While HPV is also very common in men, most do not develop any serious health problems.

However, there is also good news about women and STDs.

8. Women typically see their doctor more often than men.

Women should use this time with their doctor as an opportunity to ask for STD testing, and not assume STD testing is part of their annual exam. Although the Pap test screens for cervical cancer, it is not a good test for other types of cancer or STDs.

9. There is a vaccine to prevent HPV.

Available treatments for other STDs can prevent serious health consequences, such as infertility, if diagnosed and treated early.

10. There are resources available for women to learn more about actions they can take to protect themselves

and their partners from STDs, and where to receive testing and treatment.

- Healthcare providers—A doctor or physician can provide patient-specific information about STD prevention, protection, and tests.

- 800-CDC-INFO (800-232-4636)—Operators can provide information about local STD testing sites and put callers in touch with trained professionals to answer questions about STDs.

- FindSTDTest.org—This website provides users with locations for HIV and STD testing and STD vaccines around the United States.

- www.cdc.gov/std—CDC's website includes comprehensive information about STDs, including fact sheets on STDs and Pregnancy (www.cdc.gov/std/pregnancy) and STDs and Infertility (www.cdc.gov/std/infertility).

Section 5.2

STDs in Women

Excerpted from "STDs in Women and Infants," by the Centers for Disease Control and Prevention (CDC, www.cdc.gov), November 22, 2010.

Public Health Impact

Women and infants disproportionately bear the long-term consequences of STDs. Women infected with *C. trachomatis* [chlamydia] or *N. gonorrhoeae* [gonorrhea] can develop PID [pelvic inflammatory disease], which, in turn, can lead to reproductive system morbidity such as ectopic pregnancy and tubal factor infertility. An estimated 10%–20% of women with chlamydia or gonorrhea may develop PID if they do not receive adequate treatment. Among women with PID, tubal scarring can cause involuntary infertility in 20% of women, ectopic pregnancy in 9%, and chronic pelvic pain in 18%.

About 80%–90% of chlamydial infections and 50% of gonococcal infections in women are asymptomatic. These infections are detected primarily through screening. The vague symptoms associated with PID cause 85% of women to delay seeking medical care, thereby increasing the risk for infertility and ectopic pregnancy. Data from a randomized controlled trial of chlamydia screening in a managed care setting suggest that such screening programs can reduce the incidence of PID by as much as 60%.

HPV [human papillomavirus] infections are highly prevalent in the United States, especially among young sexually active women. Although most HPV infections in women resolve within one year, they are a major concern because persistent infection with specific types of the virus are causally related to cervical cancer; these types also cause Papanicolaou (Pap) smear abnormalities. Other types cause genital warts, low-grade Pap smear abnormalities, and, rarely, recurrent respiratory papillomatosis in infants born to infected mothers.

Direct Impact on Pregnancy

Chlamydia and gonorrhea can result in adverse outcomes of pregnancy, including neonatal ophthalmia and in the case of chlamydia, neonatal pneumonia. Although topical prophylaxis of infants at delivery is effective for prevention of gonococcal ophthalmia neonatorum, prevention of neonatal pneumonia requires prenatal detection and treatment.

Genital infections with HSV are extremely common, can cause painful outbreaks, and can have serious consequences for pregnant women.

When a woman has a syphilis infection during pregnancy, she can transmit the infection to the fetus in utero. This transmittal can result in fetal death or an infant born with physical and mental developmental disabilities. Most cases of congenital syphilis are easily preventable if women are screened for syphilis and treated early during prenatal care.

Chlamydia—United States

During 2008–2009, the rate of chlamydial infections in women increased from 579.4 to 592.2 cases per 100,000 females. Chlamydia rates exceeded gonorrhea rates among women in all states.

Gonorrhea—United States

Like chlamydia, gonorrhea is often asymptomatic in women. Thus, gonorrhea screening is an important strategy for the identification of gonorrhea among women. Large-scale screening programs for gonorrhea in women began in the 1970s. After an initial increase in cases detected through screening, gonorrhea rates for both women and men declined steadily throughout the 1980s and early 1990s and then reached a plateau. The gonorrhea rate for women (105.5 cases per 100,000 females) decreased in 2009 for the second time in two years.

Although the gonorrhea rate in men has historically been higher than the rate in women, the gonorrhea rate among women has been slightly higher than the rate among men for eight consecutive years.

Congenital Syphilis

Trends in congenital syphilis usually follow trends in P&S [primary and secondary] syphilis among women, with a lag of one to two years. The rate of P&S syphilis among women declined 95.4% (from 17.3 to 0.8 cases per 100,000 females) during 1990–2004. The rate of congenital syphilis declined by 92.4% (from a peak of 107.3 cases to 8.2 cases per 100,000 live births) during 1991–2005. However, the rate in women has increased since 2004, and the rate of congenital syphilis has likewise increased since 2005.

The rate of P&S syphilis among women was 1.4 cases per 100,000 women in 2009, and the rate of congenital syphilis was 10.0 cases per 100,000 live births in 2009. The highest rates of P&S syphilis among women and congenital syphilis were observed in the South.

Although most cases of congenital syphilis occur among infants whose mothers have had some prenatal care, late or limited prenatal care has been associated with congenital syphilis. Failure of health care providers to adhere to maternal syphilis screening recommendations also contributes to the occurrence of congenital syphilis.

Pelvic Inflammatory Disease

Accurate estimates of PID and tubal factor infertility resulting from chlamydial and gonococcal infections are difficult to obtain, in part because definitive diagnoses of these conditions can be complex. Hospitalizations for PID declined steadily throughout the 1980s and early 1990s, but remained relatively constant from 2000 through 2007, the most recent year for which data are available.

The estimated number of initial visits to physicians' offices for PID generally declined during 2000–2009.

Racial disparities in diagnosed PID have been observed in both ambulatory and hospitalized settings. Disease rates were two to three times higher among black women than among white women. These disparities are consistent with the marked racial disparities observed for chlamydia and gonorrhea. However, because of the subjective methods by which PID is diagnosed, racial disparity data should be interpreted with caution.

Ectopic Pregnancy

Evidence suggests that health care practices associated with clinical management of ectopic pregnancy changed in the late 1980s and early 1990s. Before that time, treatment of ectopic pregnancy usually required admission to a hospital. Hospitalization statistics were therefore useful for monitoring trends in ectopic pregnancy. During 1997–2006, hospitalizations for ectopic pregnancy remained generally stable. As of the publication date of this report, 2008 data were not available. The data that are available suggest that nearly half of all ectopic pregnancies are treated on an outpatient basis.

Section 5.3

STDs in Women Who Have Sex with Women

"Lesbian and Bisexual Health Fact Sheet," by the Office on Women's Health (www.womenshealth.gov), part of the U.S. Department of Health and Human Services, February 17, 2011.

Women who have sex with women are at risk for sexually transmitted infections (STIs). Lesbian and bisexual women can transmit STIs to each other through the following:

- Skin-to-skin contact

- Mucosa contact (e.g., mouth to vagina)

- Vaginal fluids

- Menstrual blood

- Sharing sex toys

Some STIs are more common among lesbians and bisexual women and may be passed easily from woman to woman (such as bacterial vaginosis). Other STIs are much less likely to be passed from woman to woman through sex (such as HIV). When lesbians get these less common STIs, it may be because they also have had sex with men, especially when they were younger. It is also important to remember that some of the less common STIs may not be passed between women during sex, but through sharing needles used to inject drugs. Bisexual women may be more likely to get infected with STIs that are less common for lesbians, since bisexuals have typically had sex with men in the past or are presently having sex with a man.

Common STIs that can be passed between women include the following:

Bacterial vaginosis (BV): BV is more common in lesbian and bisexual women than in other women. The reason for this is unknown. BV often occurs in both members of lesbian couples.

The vagina normally has a balance of mostly "good" bacteria and fewer "harmful" bacteria. BV develops when the balance changes. With BV, there is an increase in harmful bacteria and a decrease in good bacteria.

Sometimes BV causes no symptoms. But over one half of women with BV have vaginal itching or discharge with a fishy odor. BV can be treated with antibiotics.

Chlamydia: Chlamydia is caused by bacteria. It's spread through vaginal, oral, or anal sex. It can damage the reproductive organs, such as the uterus, ovaries, and fallopian tubes. The symptoms of chlamydia are often mild—in fact, it's known as a "silent infection." Because the symptoms are mild, you can pass it to someone else without even knowing you have it.

Chlamydia can be treated with antibiotics. Infections that are not treated, even if there are no symptoms, can lead to the following:

- Lower abdominal pain
- Lower back pain
- Nausea
- Fever
- Pain during sex
- Bleeding between periods

Genital herpes: Genital herpes is an STI caused by the herpes simplex viruses type 1 (HSV-1) or type 2 (HSV-2). Most genital herpes is caused by HSV-2. HSV-1 can cause genital herpes. But it more commonly causes infections of the mouth and lips, called fever blisters or cold sores. You can spread oral herpes to the genitals through oral sex.

Most people have few or no symptoms from a genital herpes infection. When symptoms do occur, they usually appear as one or more blisters on or around the genitals or rectum. The blisters break, leaving tender sores that may take up to four weeks to heal. Another outbreak can appear weeks or months later. But it almost always is less severe and shorter than the first outbreak.

Although the infection can stay in the body forever, the outbreaks tend to become less severe and occur less often over time. You can pass genital herpes to someone else even when you have no symptoms.

There is no cure for herpes. Drugs can be used to shorten and prevent outbreaks or reduce the spread of the virus to others.

Human papillomavirus (HPV): HPV can cause genital warts. If left untreated, HPV can cause abnormal changes on the cervix that can lead to cancer. Most people don't know they're infected with HPV because they don't have symptoms. Usually the virus goes away on its own without causing harm. But not always. The Pap test checks for abnormal cell growths caused by HPV that can lead to cancer in women. If you are age 30 or older, your doctor may also do an HPV test with your Pap test. This is a DNA test that detects most of the high-risk types of HPV. It helps with cervical cancer screening. If you're younger than 30 years old and have had an abnormal Pap test result, your doctor may give you an HPV test. This test will show if HPV caused the abnormal cells on your cervix.

Both men and women can spread the virus to others whether or not they have any symptoms. Lesbians and bisexual women can transmit HPV through direct genital skin-to-skin contact, touching, or sex toys used with other women. Lesbians who have had sex with men are also at risk of HPV infection. This is why regular Pap tests are just as important for lesbian and bisexual women as they are for heterosexual women.

There is no treatment for HPV, but a healthy immune (body defense) system can usually fight off HPV infection. Two vaccines (Cervarix and Gardasil) can protect girls and young women against the types of HPV that cause most cervical cancers. The vaccines work best when given before a person's first sexual contact, when she could be exposed to HPV. Both vaccines are recommended for 11- and 12-year-old-girls. But the vaccines also can be used in girls as young as 9 and in women through age 26 who did not get any or all of the shots when they were younger. These vaccines are given in a series of three shots. It is best

51

to use the same vaccine brand for all three doses. Ask your doctor which brand vaccine is best for you. Gardasil also has benefits for men in preventing genital warts and anal cancer caused by HPV. It is approved for use in boys as young as 9 and for young men through age 26. The vaccine does not replace the need to wear condoms to lower your risk of getting other types of HPV and other sexually transmitted infections. If you do get HPV, there are treatments for diseases caused by it. Genital warts can be removed with medicine you apply yourself or treatments performed by your doctor. Cervical and other cancers caused by HPV are most treatable when found early. There are many options for cancer treatment.

Pubic lice: Also known as crabs, pubic lice are small parasites that live in the genital areas and other areas with coarse hair. Pubic lice are spread through direct contact with the genital area. They can also be spread through sheets, towels, or clothes. Pubic lice can be treated with creams or shampoos you can buy at the drug store.

Trichomoniasis (trich): Trichomoniasis is caused by a parasite that can be spread during sex. You can also get trichomoniasis from contact with damp, moist objects, such as towels or wet clothes. Symptoms include the following:

- Yellow, green, or gray vaginal discharge (often foamy) with a strong odor
- Discomfort during sex and when urinating
- Irritation and itching of the genital area
- Lower abdominal pain (in rare cases)

Trichomoniasis can be treated with antibiotics.

Less common STIs that may affect lesbians and bisexual women include the following:

Gonorrhea: Gonorrhea is a common STI but is not commonly passed during woman-to-woman sex. However, it could be since it does live in vaginal fluid. It is caused by a type of bacteria that can grow in warm, moist areas of the reproductive tract, like the cervix, uterus, and fallopian tubes in women. It can grow in the urethra in men and women. It can also grow in the mouth, throat, eyes, and anus. Even when women have symptoms, they are often mild and are sometimes thought to be from a bladder or other vaginal infection.

Symptoms include the following:

- Pain or burning when urinating

- Yellowish and sometimes bloody vaginal discharge

- Bleeding between menstrual periods

Gonorrhea can be treated with antibiotics.

Hepatitis B: Hepatitis B is a liver disease caused by a virus. It is spread through bodily fluids, including blood, semen, and vaginal fluid. People can get hepatitis B through sexual contact, by sharing needles with an infected person, or through mother-to-child transmission at birth. Some women have no symptoms if they get infected with the virus.

Women with symptoms may have the following:

- Mild fever

- Headache and muscle aches

- Tiredness

- Loss of appetite

- Nausea or vomiting

- Diarrhea

- Dark-colored urine and pale bowel movements

- Stomach pain

- Yellow skin and whites of eyes

There is a vaccine that can protect you from hepatitis B.

HIV/AIDS (human immunodeficiency virus/acquired immunodeficiency syndrome): HIV is spread through body fluids, such as blood, vaginal fluid, semen, and breast milk. It is primarily spread through sex with men or by sharing needles. Women who have sex with women can spread HIV, but this is rare. Some women with HIV may have no symptoms for 10 years or more.

Women with HIV symptoms may have the following:

- Extreme fatigue (tiredness)

- Rapid weight loss

- Frequent low-grade fevers and night sweats

- Frequent yeast infections (in the mouth)

- Vaginal yeast infections

- Other STIs

- Pelvic inflammatory disease (an infection of the uterus, ovaries, or fallopian tubes)

- Menstrual cycle changes

- Red, brown, or purplish blotches on or under the skin or inside the mouth, nose, or eyelids

AIDS is the final stage of HIV infection. HIV infection turns to AIDS when you have one or more opportunistic infections, certain cancers, or a very low CD4 cell count.

Syphilis: Syphilis is an STI caused by bacteria. It's passed through direct contact with a syphilis sore during vaginal, anal, or oral sex. Untreated syphilis can infect other parts of the body. It is easily treated with antibiotics. Syphilis is very rare among lesbians. But, you should talk to your doctor if you have any sores that don't heal.

Chapter 6

Men and STDs

Chapter Contents

Section 6.1—HPV in Men 56

Section 6.2—HIV/AIDS in Men 62

Section 6.3—STDs in Men Who Have Sex with Men 64

Section 6.1

HPV in Men

"HPV and Men—Fact Sheet," by the Centers for Disease Control and
Prevention (CDC, www.cdc.gov), December 19, 2011.

What is genital human papillomavirus (HPV)?

Genital human papillomavirus (HPV) is a common virus. Most sexually active people in the United States will have HPV at some time
in their lives. There are more than 40 types of HPV that are passed
on through sexual contact. These types can infect the genital areas of
men, including the skin on and around the penis or anus. They can
also infect the mouth and throat.

How do men get HPV?

HPV is passed on through genital contact—most often during
vaginal and anal sex. HPV may also be passed on during oral sex.
Since HPV usually causes no symptoms, most men and women can
get HPV—and pass it on—without realizing it. People can have HPV
even if years have passed since they had sex. Even men with only one
lifetime sex partner can get HPV.

What are the health problems caused by HPV in men?

Most men who get HPV (of any type) never develop any symptoms or
health problems. But some types of HPV can cause genital warts. Other
types can cause cancers of the penis, anus, or oropharynx (back of the
throat, including base of the tongue and tonsils.) The types of HPV that can
cause genital warts are not the same as the types that can cause cancer.

Note: Anal cancer is not the same as colorectal cancer. Colorectal
cancer is more common than anal cancer, and is not caused by HPV.

How common are HPV-related health problems in men?

About 1% of sexually active men in the United States have genital
warts at any one time.

Cancers of the penis, anus, and oropharynx are uncommon, and only a subset of these cancers is actually related to HPV. Each year in the United States there are about:

- 400 men who get HPV-related cancer of the penis;
- 1,500 men who get HPV-related cancer of the anus;
- 5,600 men who get cancers of the oropharynx (back of throat), but many of these cancers are related to tobacco and alcohol use, not HPV.

Some men are more likely to develop HPV-related diseases than others:

- Gay and bisexual men (who have sex with other men) are about 17 times more likely to develop anal cancer than men who only have sex with women.
- Men with weakened immune systems, including those who have HIV (human immunodeficiency virus), are more likely than other men to develop anal cancer. Men with HIV are also more likely to get severe cases of genital warts that are harder to treat.

What are the signs and symptoms?

Most men who get HPV never develop any symptoms or health problems. But for those who do develop health problems, these are some of the signs and symptoms.

Genital Warts

- One or more growths on the penis, testicles, groin, thighs, or in/around the anus may appear.
- Warts may be single, grouped, raised, flat, or cauliflower-shaped. They usually do not hurt.
- Warts may appear within weeks or months after sexual contact with an infected person.

Anal Cancer

- Sometimes there are no signs or symptoms.
- Symptoms of anal cancer include anal bleeding, pain, itching, or discharge.
- Swollen lymph nodes in the anal or groin area may occur.

- Changes in bowel habits or the shape of your stool may occur.

Penile Cancer

- First signs of penile cancer include changes in color, skin thickening, or a build-up of tissue on the penis.

- Later signs of penile cancer include a growth or sore on the penis. It is usually painless, but in some cases, the sore may be painful and bleed.

Cancers of the Oropharynx

- Sore throat or ear pain that doesn't go away is a sign of cancer of the oropharynx.

- Other symptoms include constant coughing, pain or trouble swallowing or breathing, weight loss, hoarseness or voice changes that last more than two weeks, or a lump or mass in the neck.

Is there a test for HPV in men?

Currently, there is no HPV test recommended for men. The only approved HPV tests on the market are for screening women for cervical cancer. They are not useful for screening for HPV-related cancers or genital warts in men.

- Screening for anal cancer is not routinely recommended for men. This is because more research is needed to find out if it can actually prevent anal cancer. However, some experts do recommend yearly anal cancer screening (anal Pap tests) for gay, bisexual, and HIV-positive men—since anal cancer is more common in these men.

- There is no approved test to find genital warts for men or women. However, most of the time, you can see genital warts. If you think you may have genital warts, you should see a health care provider.

- There is no test for men to check one's overall HPV status. But HPV usually goes away on its own, without causing health problems. So an HPV infection that is found today will most likely not be there a year or two from now.

- Screening tests are not available for penile cancer.

You can check for any abnormalities on your penis, scrotum, or around the anus. See your doctor if you find warts, blisters, sores, ulcers, white patches, or other abnormal areas on your penis—even if they do not hurt.

Is there a treatment or cure for HPV?

There is no treatment or cure for HPV. But there are ways to treat the health problems caused by HPV in men.

Genital warts can be treated with medicine, removed (surgery), or frozen off. Some of these treatments involve a visit to the doctor. Others can be done at home by the patient himself. No one treatment is better than another. But warts often come back within a few months after treatment—so several treatments may be needed. Treating genital warts may not necessarily lower a man's chances of passing HPV on to his sex partner. If warts are not treated, they may go away on their own, stay the same, or grow (in size or number). They will not turn into cancer.

Cancers of the penis, anus, and oropharynx can be treated with surgery, radiation therapy, and chemotherapy. Often, two or more of these treatments are used together. Patients should decide with their doctors which treatments are best for them.

Are there ways to lower my chances of getting HPV?

A safe and effective HPV vaccine (Gardasil) can protect boys and men against the HPV types that cause most genital warts and anal cancers. It is given in three shots over six months.

Condoms (if used with every sex act, from start to finish) may lower your chances of passing HPV to a partner or developing HPV-related diseases. But HPV can infect areas that are not covered by a condom—so condoms may not fully protect against HPV.

Because HPV is so common and usually invisible, the only sure way to prevent it is not to have sexual contact. Even people with only one lifetime sex partner can get HPV, if their partner was infected with HPV.

I heard about a new HPV vaccine—can it help me?

If you are 26 or younger, there is an HPV vaccine that can help protect you against the types of HPV that most commonly cause problems in men. The HPV vaccine (Gardasil) works by preventing four common HPV types, two that cause most genital warts and two that cause cancers, including anal cancer. It protects against new HPV infections; it does not cure existing HPV infections or disease (like genital warts). It is most effective when given before a person's first sexual contact (i.e., when s/he may be exposed to HPV).

CDC recommends the HPV vaccine for all boys ages 11 or 12, and for males through age 21, who have not already received all three doses. The vaccine is also recommended for gay and bisexual men (or any man who has sex with men), and men with compromised immune systems (including HIV) through age 26, if they did not get fully vaccinated when they were younger. The vaccine is safe for all men through age 26, but it is most effective when given at younger ages.

The HPV vaccine is very safe and effective, with no serious side effects. The most common side effect is soreness in the arm. Studies show that the vaccine can protect men against genital warts and anal cancers. It is likely that this vaccine also protects men from other HPV-related cancers, like cancers of the penis and oropharynx (back of throat, including base of tongue and tonsils), but there are no vaccine studies that have evaluated these outcomes.

I just found out that my partner has HPV. What does it mean for my health?

Partners usually share HPV. If you have been with your partner for a long time, you probably have HPV already. Most sexually active adults will have HPV at some time in their lives. Although HPV is common, the health problems caused by HPV are much less common.

Condoms may lower your chances of getting HPV or developing HPV-related diseases, if used with every sex act, from start to finish. You may want to consider talking to your doctor about being vaccinated against HPV if you are 26 years or younger. But not having sex is the only sure way to avoid HPV.

If your partner has genital warts, you should avoid having sex until the warts are gone or removed. You can check for any abnormalities on your penis, such as genital warts. Also, you may want to get checked by a health care provider for genital warts and other sexually transmitted disease (STDs).

What does it mean for our relationship?

A person can have HPV for many years before it is found or causes health problems. So there is no way to know if your partner gave you HPV, or if you gave HPV to your partner. HPV should not be seen as a sign that you or your partner is having sex outside of your relationship.

I just found out I have genital warts. What does it mean for me and my partner?

Having genital warts may be hard to cope with, but they are not a threat to your health. People with genital warts can still lead normal, healthy lives.

Because genital warts may be easily passed on to sex partners, you should inform them about having genital warts and avoid sexual activity until the warts are gone or removed. There are ways to protect your partner.

You and your partner may benefit from getting screened for other STDs.

If used with every sex act, male latex condoms may lower your chances of passing genital warts. But HPV can infect areas that are not covered by a condom—so condoms may not fully protect against HPV.

It is important that sex partners discuss their health and risk for STDs. However, it is not clear if there is any health benefit to informing future sex partners about a past diagnosis of genital warts because it is not known how long a person remains contagious after warts are gone.

Section 6.2

HIV/AIDS in Men

Excerpted from Centers for Disease Control and Prevention. *HIV Surveillance Report*, 2009; vol. 21. http://www.cdc.gov/hiv/topics//surveillance/resources/reports/. Published February 2011. Accessed July 16, 2012.

Diagnoses of HIV Infection

From 2006 through 2009, the estimated number and the estimated rate of annual diagnoses of HIV infection in the 40 states with confidential name-based HIV [human immunodeficiency virus] infection reporting remained stable. In 2009, the estimated rate of diagnoses of HIV infection in the 40 states was 17.4 per 100,000 population.

From 2006 through 2009, the rate among males remained stable. In 2009, males accounted for 76% of all diagnoses of HIV infection among adults and adolescents. The rate among adult and adolescent males was 32.7.

From 2006 through 2009, among adult and adolescent males, the annual number of diagnosed HIV infections attributed to male-to-male sexual contact increased. The numbers of infections attributed to injection drug use and those attributed to male-to-male sexual contact and injection drug use decreased. The number of infections attributed to heterosexual contact remained stable. In 2009, the diagnosed infections attributed to male-to-male sexual contact (57%) and the infections attributed to heterosexual contact (31%) accounted for approximately 87% of diagnosed HIV infections in the 40 states.

AIDS Diagnoses

From 2006 through 2009, the estimated number and the estimated rate of annual AIDS [acquired immunodeficiency syndrome] diagnoses in the United States decreased. In 2009, the estimated rate of AIDS diagnoses in the United States was 11.2 per 100,000 population.

From 2006 through 2009, the rates among adult and adolescent males and females decreased. Adult and adolescent males accounted for 75% of all AIDS diagnoses made during 2009. The rate among adults and adolescents in 2009 was 20.6 among males.

From 2006 through 2009, among adult and adolescent males, the annual numbers of AIDS diagnoses with infection attributed to injection drug use or to male-to-male sexual contact and injection drug use decreased. The numbers of AIDS diagnoses with infection attributed to male-to-male sexual contact or to heterosexual contact remained stable.

Deaths

Deaths of Persons with a Diagnosis of HIV Infection

From 2006 through 2008, the annual estimated number and rate of deaths of persons with a diagnosis of HIV infection in the 40 states with confidential name-based HIV infection reporting remained stable. Readers should use caution when interpreting trend data on the estimated number of deaths because the estimates for the most recent year are most subject to uncertainty. In 2008, the estimated rate of deaths of persons with a diagnosis of HIV infection was 7.0 per 100,000 population. Deaths of persons with a diagnosis of HIV infection may be due to any cause (i.e., may or may not be related to HIV infection).

From 2006 through 2008, among adult and adolescent males, the rate of deaths remained stable. Among males with diagnosed HIV infection attributed to male-to-male sexual contact and those with infection attributed to heterosexual contact, deaths increased. Deaths of males with diagnosed HIV infection attributed to injection drug use and those with infection attributed to male-to-male sexual contact and injection drug use decreased.

Deaths of Persons with an AIDS Diagnosis

During 2006–2008 in the United States, the annual estimated number of deaths among persons with an AIDS diagnosis decreased 5%. The annual estimated rate of deaths per 100,000 population decreased 7%. Readers should use caution when interpreting trend data on the estimated number of deaths because the estimates for the most recent year are most subject to uncertainty. In 2008, the estimated rate of deaths of persons with an AIDS diagnosis was 5.3 per 100,000 population. Deaths of persons with an AIDS diagnosis may be due to any cause.

From 2006 through 2008, among adult and adolescent males, the overall rate of deaths decreased. The numbers of deaths of males with an AIDS diagnosis with infection attributed to injection drug use or to male-to-male sexual contact and injection drug use also decreased. The numbers of deaths of males with infection attributed to male-to-male sexual contact or to heterosexual contact remained stable.

Section 6.3

STDs in Men Who Have Sex with Men

Excerpted from "STDs in Men Who Have Sex with Men,"
by the Centers for Disease Control and Prevention
(CDC, www.cdc.gov), November 22, 2010.

Notifiable disease surveillance data on syphilis and data from GISP [Gonococcal Isolate Surveillance Project] suggest that some STDs in MSM [men who have sex with men], including men who have sex with both women and men, are increasing. Because STDs and the behaviors associated with acquiring them increase the likelihood of acquiring and transmitting HIV [human immunodeficiency virus] infection, the rise in STDs among MSM may be associated with an increase in HIV diagnoses among MSM.

With the exception of reported syphilis cases, most nationally notifiable STD surveillance data do not include information on sexual behaviors; therefore, data on national trends in STDs among MSM in the United States are not currently available. Furthermore, testing strategies are often suboptimal for detecting STDs in MSM. Testing for gonorrhea and chlamydia in MSM largely focuses on detecting urethral infections, which are more likely to be symptomatic than pharyngeal or rectal infections. Data from enhanced surveillance projects are presented to provide information on STDs in MSM.

Monitoring Trends in Prevalence of STDs among MSM Who Visit STD Clinics

In 2005, SSuN [STD Surveillance Network] was established to improve the capacity of national, state, and local STD programs to detect, monitor, and respond rapidly to trends in STDs through enhanced collection, reporting, analysis, visualization, and interpretation of disease information. SSuN currently includes 12 collaborating local and state health departments. In 2009, a total of 42 STD clinics at these 12 sites collected enhanced behavioral and demographic information on patients who presented for care to these clinics. During 1999–2008, similar enhanced surveillance data were collected in eight STD clinics, including three community-based gay men's health clinics, through the MSM Prevalence Monitoring Project.

For data reported in this text, MSM were defined as men who either reported having sex with another man in the three months before STD testing or who self-reported as gay/homosexual or bisexual. MSW [men having sex with women] were defined as men who reported having sex with women only within the three months before STD testing or who did not report the sex of their sex partner, but reported that they considered themselves straight/heterosexual.

Gonorrhea and Chlamydial Infection

In 2009, the proportion of MSM who tested positive for gonorrhea and chlamydia at SSuN STD clinics varied by city. A larger proportion of MSM who visited SSuN STD clinics tested positive for gonorrhea than tested positive for chlamydia in all cities except New Orleans (where the proportions were equal) and Birmingham (where the proportion for chlamydia was higher).

Across the participating sites, about the same number of MSM were tested for gonorrhea (17,007) and chlamydia (16,615). The median site-specific gonorrhea prevalence was 14.9% (range by site: 6.5%–27.9%). The median site-specific chlamydia prevalence was 11.2% (range by site: 4.5%–18.5%). For this report, a person who tested positive for gonorrhea or chlamydia more than one time was counted only once.

Co-Infection with Syphilis and HIV

In 2009, the proportion of MSM who presented to SSuN clinics with P&S [primary and secondary] syphilis infection who also were infected with HIV ranged from 30% in Birmingham to 74% in Baltimore. The median site-specific proportion was 44.4%. P&S syphilis was identified by provider diagnosis and HIV was identified by laboratory report, self-report, or provider diagnosis.

Nationally Notifiable Syphilis Surveillance Data

P&S syphilis increased in the United States during 2005–2009, with a 59.3% increase in the number of P&S syphilis cases among men and a 66.7% increase among women. In 2009, the rate of reported P&S syphilis among men (7.8 cases per 100,000 males) was 5.6 times higher than the rate among women (1.4 cases per 100,000 females). Higher rates were observed in men than in women for all racial and ethnic groups.

In 2009, MSM accounted for 62% of all P&S syphilis cases in the United States. MSM accounted for more cases than MSW or women in all racial and ethnic groups.

Gonococcal Isolate Surveillance Project

GISP is a national sentinel surveillance system designed to monitor trends in antimicrobial susceptibilities of strains of *N. gonorrhoeae* in the United States. GISP also reports the percentage of *N. gonorrhoeae* isolates obtained from MSM. Overall, the proportion of isolates from MSM in selected STD clinics from GISP sentinel sites has increased steadily, from 4.6% in 1990 to 25.3% in 2009. The proportion of isolates from MSM varies geographically, with the largest proportion reported from the West Coast.

Chapter 7

STDs in Children

Chapter Contents

Section 7.1—Child Sexual Abuse and STDs.................................. 68
Section 7.2—Child Abuse Survivors Have Higher
          Risk for STDs in Adulthood 71

Section 7.1

Child Sexual Abuse and STDs

Excerpted from "STDs and Child Sexual Abuse,"
by the U.S. Department of Justice (www.ncjrs.gov), December 2002.
Reviewed by David A. Cooke, MD, FACP, July 10, 2012.

Sexually transmitted diseases (STDs) comprise a wide range of infections and conditions that are transmitted mainly by sexual activity. The classic STDs, gonorrhea and syphilis, are now being overshadowed by a new set of STDs that are not only more common, but are also more difficult to diagnose and treat.

These new STDs include infections caused by *Chlamydia trachomatis* (chlamydia), human papillomavirus (HPV), bacterial vaginosis (BV), and human immunodeficiency virus (HIV). Rapid application of new technology to the diagnosis of STDs has led to a growing array of diagnostic laboratory tests that require critical evaluation by clinicians and a critical review by law enforcement.

Accurate information about STDs in victims of sexual abuse has been hindered by a variety of factors:

• The prevalence of sexually transmitted infections may vary regionally and among different populations within the same region.

• Few studies have attempted to differentiate between infections existing prior to sexual abuse and those that result from abuse. The presence of a preexisting infection in adults is usually related to prior sexual activity. In children, however, preexisting infections may be related to prolonged colonization after perinatal acquisition (acquisition immediately before and after birth), inadvertent nonsexual spread, prior peer sexual activity, or prior sexual abuse.

• The incubation periods for STDs range from a few days for gonorrhea to several months for HPV. The incubation periods and the timing of an examination after an episode of abuse are critically important in detecting infections.

When presented with a child with an STD, law enforcement officials must attempt to determine absolutely if the infection was associated with sexual contact and, for the purposes of prosecution, whether appropriate diagnostic methods were used. The following facts should be kept in mind:

- STDs may be transmitted during sexual assault.

- Multiple episodes of abuse increase the risk of STD infection, probably by increasing the number of contacts with an infected individual, and rates of infection also vary by the type of assault. For example, vaginal or rectal penetration is more likely to lead to detectable STD infection than fondling.

- Sexual assault is a violent crime that affects children of all ages, including infants.

The majority of children who are sexually abused will have no physical complaints related either to trauma or STD infection. Most sexually abused children do not indicate that they have genital pain or problems.

- In children the isolation of a sexually transmitted organism may be the first indication that abuse has occurred. In most cases, the site of infection is consistent with a child's history of assault.

- Although the presence of a sexually transmissible agent in a child over the age of one month is suggestive of sexual abuse, exceptions do exist. Rectal and genital chlamydia infections in young children may be due to a persistent perinatally acquired infection, which may last for up to three years.

The incidence and prevalence of sexual abuse in children are difficult to estimate.

- Most sexual abuse in childhood escapes detection.

- Patterns of childhood sexual abuse appear to depend on the sex and age of the victim.

- Between 80 and 90 percent of sexually abused children are female (average age is seven to eight years).

- Between 75 and 85 percent of sexually abused children were abused by a male assailant, an adult or minor known to the child. This individual is most likely a family member such as the father, stepfather, mother's boyfriend, or an uncle or other male

69

relative. Victims of unknown assailants tend to be older than children who are sexually abused by someone they know and are usually only subjected to a single episode of abuse.

- Sexual abuse by family members or acquaintances usually involves multiple episodes over periods ranging from one week to years.

- Most victims describe a single type of sexual activity, but over 20 percent have experienced more than one type of forced sexual act. Vaginal penetration has been reported to occur in approximately one-half and anal penetration in one-third of female victims of sexual abuse.

- Over 50 percent of male victims of sexual abuse have experienced anal penetration.

- Other types of sexual activity, including oral-genital contact and fondling, occur in 20 to 50 percent of victims of sexual abuse.

- Children who are sexually abused by known assailants usually experience less physical trauma, including genital trauma, than victims of assaults by strangers because such trauma might arouse suspicion that abuse is occurring.

Section 7.2

Child Abuse Survivors Have Higher Risk for STDs in Adulthood

"Child Abuse Survivors Have Higher Risk for STDs in Adulthood Than Non-abused Adults," by the National Institute of Mental Health (NIMH, www.nimh.nih.gov), part of the National Institutes of Health, April 10, 2009.

A history of child abuse or neglect can increase the risk for STDs in adulthood, according to a study partly funded by NIMH. The researchers reported their findings in the April 2009 supplemental issue of the *American Journal of Public Health*.

Background

Helen W. Wilson, PhD, Rosalind Franklin University of Medicine and Science, and Cathy S. Widom, PhD, John Jay College of the City University of New York, built on their previous work tracking adults who experienced physical or sexual abuse or neglect before age 11.

Based on information obtained from a series of interviews and assessments completed over time, the researchers examined the prevalence of sexually transmitted diseases (STDs) in 754 participants, 328 of whom served as non-abused or neglected controls, with an average age of 41. The researchers also received significant funding from the Eunice Kennedy Shriver National Institute of Child Health and Human Development (NICHD).

Results of the Study

The researchers found that people who had experienced abuse or neglect 30 years prior to the study were more likely than controls to have had an STD. In some cases, abuse survivors were three times as likely to have had more than one type of STD. Childhood sexual abuse appeared to increase risk for STDs in women but not in men. Any kind of childhood abuse increased overall risk for STDs among white participants, but not black.

Significance

This study was the first to show an increased risk of STDs in childhood abuse or neglect survivors tracked over time. The findings emphasize the importance of having supportive family relationships during childhood, and also suggest that screening and early intervention may help diagnose or even prevent STDs in child abuse survivors.

What's Next?

According to the researchers, further study is needed to explore the underlying mechanisms of how childhood maltreatment affects a person's risk for STDs. Understanding the early life experiences and factors that can influence adult health may lead to better methods of screening, identifying, or preventing certain illnesses.

References

Wilson HW, Widom CS. Sexually Transmitted Diseases Among Adults Who Had Been Abused and Neglected as Children: A 30-Year Prospective Study. *Am J Public Health*. 2009 Apr;99 Suppl 1:S197–203.

Chapter 8

STDs in Adolescents and Young Adults

The share of adolescents engaging in sexual activity has declined over the past few decades. Despite the growing attention to prevention and health education, recent data indicate that the rates of unintended pregnancy and sexually transmitted infections (STI) remain higher for young adults than older adults and higher than the rates in most developed nations. This text provides key data on sexual activity, pregnancy, contraceptive use, prevalence of STIs [sexually transmitted infections] among teenagers and young adults, and access to reproductive health services.

Sexual Activity

- Nearly half (46%) of all high school students report ever having had sexual intercourse in 2009, a decline from 54% in 1991. Males are no more likely than females to report having had sex (46%).[1]

"Fact Sheet: Sexual Health of Adolescents and Young Adults in the United States," (#3040-05), The Henry J. Kaiser Family Foundation, January 2011. This information was reprinted with permission from the Henry J. Kaiser Family Foundation. The Kaiser Family Foundation, a leader in health policy analysis, health journalism, and communication, is dedicated to filling the need for trusted, independent information on the major health issues facing our nation and its people. The Foundation is a non-profit private operating foundation, based in Menlo Park, California.

- There are racial/ethnic differences in sexual activity rates among teens. Black high school students are more likely to have had intercourse (65%) compared to White (42%) and Hispanic students (49%). More Black high school students (15%) and Latino students (7%) initiated sex before age 13 compared to White students (4%).[1]

- Twenty-six percent of female teens and 29% of male teens have had more than one sexual partner. The percentage of high school students who report having had four or more sexual partners declined from 18% in 1995 to 15% in 2009.[2]

- Almost one-quarter (22%) of sexually active high school students reported using alcohol or drugs during their most recent sexual encounter, with males having a higher percentage (26%) compared to females (17%), and White males (28%) higher than Black males (21%).[1]

- One in 10 high school students reported having experienced dating violence. Seven percent of students have been physically forced to have sexual intercourse, with females (11%) more likely than males (5%) to report this experience.[1]

- In 2006–2008 it was found that 7% of females ages 18–24 reported that their first sexual intercourse was nonvoluntary. This was more likely to be the case for female teens whose partner was three or more years older (13% nonvoluntary, 19% "really didn't want it to happen at that time").[2]

- "Sexting" is the exchange of explicit sexual messages or images by mobile phone. Ten percent of 14- to 24-year-olds report having shared a naked photo or video of themselves via digital communication such as the internet or text messaging.[3]

Pregnancy

- The United States continues to have among the highest teen pregnancy, birth, and abortion rates in the developed world.[4]

- The pregnancy rate among female teens ages 15–19 in 2006 was 71.5 per 1,000, a drop of 41% since the peak in 1990.[5] Following a long-term decline, the teen birth rate increased slightly between 2005 and 2007. Since then, it has resumed a decreasing trend, and by 2009 dropped to 39.1 per 1,000 females.[6]

- Although birth rates have fallen for teens of all races and ethnicities, the rates for African American, Hispanic, and Native American teens are over twice the rates of White and Asian American youth.

- The vast majority of teen pregnancies are unplanned. These pregnancies comprise a fifth of total unintended pregnancies annually in the United States.[7] Approximately 18% of women having abortions in the United States are teens and 33% are between the ages of 20 and 24.[8]

- Today, 34 states require some level of parental involvement in a minor's decision to have an abortion, up from 18 states in 1991. Twenty states require parental consent, ten require parental notification, and four require both.[9]

Contraception

- One study found that 53% of female and 45% of male adolescents talked about contraception or STIs with their partner before their first time having sex.[10]

- In a nationally representative survey of 14- to 17-year-olds, 80% of boys and 69% of girls said they had used a condom at last sexual intercourse.[11]

- Only 20% of currently sexually active high school students report that they or their partner used birth control pills to prevent pregnancy at last sexual intercourse. White students (27%) were more likely to use birth control pills compared to African American (8%) and Hispanic (11%).[1]

- Twenty-one percent of teen females and 13% of teen males did not use contraception at first intercourse.[2] Research has shown that those who reported condom use at their sexual debut were more likely than those who did not to engage in subsequent protective behaviors.[12]

- Emergency contraception (EC) can prevent pregnancy when taken within a few days of unprotected intercourse. EC is available with a prescription for minors, and over-the-counter for those aged 18 and older. In 2006–2008, 11% of sexually experienced female teens had used Plan B, the first major method of EC in the United States.[2]

Sexually Transmitted Infections (STIs) and HIV/AIDS

- Compared to older adults, sexually active teens and young adults are at higher risk for acquiring STIs, due to a combination of behavioral, biological, and cultural factors. Though they make up 25% of the sexually active population, they account for nearly half of new STI cases.[13]

- HPV [human papillomavirus] is the most common STI among teens. The CDC [Centers for Disease Control and Prevention] estimates that 35% of 14- to 19-year-olds are infected with HPV.[13] Currently, there are two vaccines (Gardasil and Cervarix) that protect against strains of HPV associated with cervical cancer and genital warts. The CDC recommends that all girls and women up to age 26 receive a vaccination.[14]

- Girls and women 15–19 years old had the largest number of reported cases of chlamydia and gonorrhea in 2009 of any age group. Females are at greater risk of acquiring infection, and the consequences include pelvic inflammatory disease, pregnancy complications, and infertility.[15]

- STI screening rates vary among youth. One study estimates that 37% of young men and 70% young women had an STI test in the past year.[16]

- Over 61,000 young people, ages 13–29, were estimated to be living with HIV [human immunodeficiency virus] in the United States in 2007.[17] This age group accounts for 31% of new HIV infections. Most young people with HIV/AIDS [acquired immunodeficiency syndrome] were infected by sexual contact.[18]

- In 2009, 30% of young adults ages 19–29 reported that they had been tested for HIV in the past 12 months.[19] In 2009, 87% of high school students reported that they had been taught about AIDS or HIV infection in school.[1]

Access to Services

- Health insurance coverage and the ability to pay for services affect teen access to reproductive health care. Approximately 33% of young adults 19–25 years old were uninsured and 13% were covered by Medicaid in 2009. Six in 10 (59%) young adults lives in a low-income household (below 200% of the federal poverty level).[20]

- The new health reform law requires private insurance plans that offer dependent coverage to children to extend that coverage to young adults up to age 26.

- The Federal Title X program provides confidential contraceptive services and STD screening and treatment for low-income teens and young adults by funding approximately 4,500 clinics, public health departments, and hospitals, available in 75% of U.S. counties.[21]

- Currently, Medicaid funds 71% of family planning services in the United States.[22] Family planning is a mandatory service under Medicaid and states are not permitted to charge cost-sharing for family planning services.

- Confidentiality affects youth access to health services. Twenty-one states and DC [District of Columbia] have policies that explicitly allow minors to consent to contraceptive services, 25 allow consent in certain circumstances, and 4 have no explicit policy.[23]

References

1. CDC. Youth Risk Behavior Surveillance System: US, 2009. *MMWR*, 57(SS-4). 2010.

2. Abma JC. "Teenagers in the United States: Sexual Activity, Contraceptive Use, and Childbearing" National Survey of Family Growth 2006–2008. National Center for Health Stats, Vital Health Stats, 2010.

3. AP/MTV Digital Abuse Study, 2009 (www.athinline.org).

4. Guttmacher Institute. Teen Pregnancy and Lessons Learned, 2002. Singh S. Adolescent Pregnancy and Childbearing: Levels and Trends in Developed Countries. *Family Planning Perspectives* 2000;32(1):14–23.

5. CDC, 2010 Teen Pregnancy Data.

6. CDC. *National Vital Statistics Reports,* 2007 56(7), "Births: Preliminary Data for 2009," 59(3)2010.

7. Finer LB et al. Disparities in Rates of Unintended Pregnancies in the US: *Perspectives on Sexual and Reproductive Health,* 2006, 38(2):90–96.

8. Guttmacher Inst. Characteristics of U.S. Abortion Patients, 2008. May 2010.

9. Guttmacher Inst. Parental Involvement in Minors' Abortions. *State Policies in Brief,* 2010.

10. Ryan, S. "Adolescents' Discussions About Contraception or STDs with Partners Before First Sex" *PSRH,* 39(3):149–157, 2007.

11. Reece, M. "Condom Use Rates in a National Probability Sample of Males and Females Ages 14 to 94 in the United States" *Journal of Sexual Medicine,* 7 (5), 266–276. 2010.

12. Shafii T. Association Between Condom Use at Sexual Debut and Subsequent Sexual Trajectories: A Longitudinal Study Using Biomarkers. *AJPH,* 97(6). 2007.

13. CDC. *Sexually Transmitted Disease Surveillance.* 2009.

14. CDC. "FDA Licensure of Bivalent HPV for Use in Females and Updated HPV Vaccination Recommendations from the ACIP," *MMWR,* May 28, 2010.

15. CDC. *STDs,* 2009.

16. Cunningham, S. "Relationships Between Perceived STD-Related Stigma STD-Related Shame and STD Screening Among a Household Sample of Adolescents" *PSRH,* 2009.

17. Calculation based on CDC, *HIV/AIDS Surveillance Report,* 2010.

18. CDC. *HIV/AIDS Surveillance in Adolescents and Young Adults,* 2007.

19. Kaiser Family Foundation Survey, March 2009.

20. KFF unpublished analysis of Urban Institute tabs of 2009 ASEC supplement to CPS, 2010.

21. USDHHS Office of Population Affairs: Family Planning (www .hhs.gov).

22. Guttmacher Inst. "Next Steps for America's Family Planning Program: Leveraging the Potential of Medicaid and Title X in an Evolving Health Care System", 2009.

23. Guttmacher Inst. Minors' Access to Contraceptive Services. *State Policies in Brief.* 2010.

Chapter 9

STDs in Older Adults

Like most people, you probably have heard a lot about STDs like HIV and AIDS. You may have thought that these diseases weren't your problem and that only younger people have to worry about them. But anyone at any age can get HIV/AIDS.

HIV (short for human immunodeficiency virus) is a virus that damages the immune system—the system your body uses to fight off diseases. HIV infection leads to a much more serious disease called AIDS (acquired immunodeficiency syndrome). When the HIV infection gets in your body, your immune system can be made weaker. This puts you in danger of getting other life-threatening diseases, infections, and cancers. When that happens, you have AIDS. AIDS is the last stage of HIV infection. If you think you may have HIV, it is very important to get tested. Today there are drugs that can help your body keep the HIV in check and fight against AIDS.

Symptoms of HIV/AIDS

Many people have no symptoms when they first become infected with HIV. It can take as little as a few weeks for minor, flu-like symptoms to show up, or more than 10 years for more serious symptoms to appear. Signs of HIV include headache, cough, diarrhea, swollen glands, lack of energy, loss of appetite, weight loss, fevers and sweats, repeated

"HIV, AIDS, and Older People," by the National Institute on Aging (NIA, www.nia.nih.gov), part of the National Institutes of Health, October 27, 2011.

yeast infections, skin rashes, pelvic and abdominal cramps, sores in the mouth or on certain parts of the body, or short-term memory loss.

How Do People Get HIV and AIDS?

Anyone, at any age, can get HIV and AIDS. HIV usually comes from having unprotected sex or sharing needles with an infected person, or through contact with HIV-infected blood. No matter your age, you may be at risk if the following are true:

- You are sexually active and do not use a latex or polyurethane condom. You can get HIV/AIDS from having sex with someone who has HIV. The virus passes from the infected person to his or her partner in blood, semen, and vaginal fluid. During sex, HIV can get into your body through any opening, such as a tear or cut in the lining of the vagina, vulva, penis, rectum, or mouth. Latex condoms can help prevent an infected person from transferring the HIV virus to you. (Natural condoms do not protect against HIV/AIDS as well as the latex and polyurethane types do.)

- You do not know your partner's drug and sexual history. What you don't know can hurt you. Even though it may be hard to do, it's very important to ask your partner about his or her sexual history and drug use. Here are some questions to ask: Has your partner been tested for HIV/AIDS? Has he or she had a number of different sex partners? Has your partner ever had unprotected sex with someone who has shared needles? Has he or she injected drugs or shared needles with someone else? Drug users are not the only people who might share needles. For example, people with diabetes who inject insulin or draw blood to test glucose levels might share needles.

- You have had a blood transfusion or operation in a developing country at any time.

- You had a blood transfusion in the United States between 1978 and 1985.

HIV/AIDS in Older People

A growing number of older people now have HIV/AIDS. Almost one fourth of all people with HIV/AIDS in this country are age 50 and older. This is because doctors are finding HIV more often than ever before in older people and because improved treatments are helping people with the disease live longer.

But there may even be many more cases than we know about. Why? One reason may be that doctors do not always test older people for HIV/AIDS and so may miss some cases during routine check-ups. Another may be that older people often mistake signs of HIV/AIDS for the aches and pains of normal aging, so they are less likely than younger people to get tested for the disease. Also, they may be ashamed or afraid of being tested. People age 50 and older may have the virus for years before being tested. By the time they are diagnosed with HIV/AIDS, the virus may be in the late stages.

The number of HIV/AIDS cases among older people is growing every year because of the following:

- Older Americans know less about HIV/AIDS than younger people do. They do not always know how it spreads or the importance of using condoms, not sharing needles, getting tested for HIV, and talking about it with their doctor.

- Healthcare workers and educators often do not talk with middle-aged and older people about HIV/AIDS prevention.

- Older people are less likely than younger people are to talk about their sex lives or drug use with their doctors.

- Doctors may not ask older patients about their sex lives or drug use or talk to them about risky behaviors.

Anyone facing a serious disease like HIV/AIDS may become very depressed. This is a special problem for older people, who may not have a strong network of friends or family who can help. At the same time, they also may be coping with other diseases common to aging such as high blood pressure, diabetes, or heart problems. As the HIV/AIDS gets worse, many will need help getting around and caring for themselves. Older people with HIV/AIDS need support and understanding from their doctors, family, and friends.

HIV/AIDS can affect older people in yet another way. Many younger people who are infected turn to their parents and grandparents for financial support and nursing care. Older people who are not themselves infected by the virus may find they have to care for their own children with HIV/AIDS and then sometimes for their orphaned or HIV-infected grandchildren. Taking care of others can be mentally, physically, and financially draining. This is especially true for older caregivers. The problem becomes even worse when older caregivers have AIDS or other serious health problems. Remember, it is important to get tested for HIV/AIDS early. Early treatment increases the chances of living longer.

81

HIV/AIDS in People of Color and Women

The number of HIV/AIDS cases is rising in people of color across the country. More than half of all people with HIV/AIDS are African American or Hispanic.

The number of cases of HIV/AIDS for women has also been growing over the past few years. The rise in the number of cases in women of color age 50 and older has been especially steep. Most got the virus from sex with infected partners. Many others got HIV through shared needles. Because women may live longer than men, and because of the rising divorce rate, many widowed, divorced, and separated women are dating these days. Like older men, many older women may be at risk because they do not know how HIV/AIDS is spread. Women who no longer worry about getting pregnant may be less likely to use a condom and to practice safe sex. Also, vaginal dryness and thinning often occur as women age. When that happens, sexual activity can lead to small cuts and tears that raise the risk for HIV/AIDS.

Treatment and Prevention

There is no cure for HIV/AIDS. But if you become infected, there are drugs that help keep the HIV virus in check and slow the spread of HIV in the body. Doctors are now using a combination of drugs called HAART (highly active antiretroviral therapy) to treat HIV/AIDS. Although it is not a cure, HAART is greatly reducing the number of deaths from AIDS in this country.

Remember, there are things you can do to keep from getting HIV/AIDS. Practice the steps below to lower your risk:

- If you are having sex, make sure your partner has been tested and is free of HIV. Use male or female condoms (latex or polyure-thane) during sexual intercourse.

- Do not share needles or any other equipment used to inject drugs.

- Get tested if you or your partner had a blood transfusion between 1978 and 1985.

- Get tested if you or your partner has had an operation or blood transfusion in a developing country at any time.

Chapter 10

Racial Disparities in STD Rates

Chapter Contents

Section 10.1—Overview of STD Racial Disparities..................... 84

Section 10.2—African Americans Disproportionately
    Affected by STDs 89

Section 10.3—Latinos Bear a Disproportionate
    Burden of the HIV Epidemic 93

Section 10.1

Overview of STD
Racial Disparities

Excerpted from "STDs in Racial and Ethnic Minorities,"
by the Centers for Disease Control and Prevention (CDC,
www.cdc.gov), November 22, 2010.

Surveillance data show higher rates of reported STDs among some racial or ethnic minority groups when compared with rates among whites. Race and ethnicity in the United States are risk markers that correlate with other more fundamental determinants of health status, such as poverty, access to quality health care, health care-seeking behavior, illicit drug use, and living in communities with high prevalence of STDs. Acknowledging the disparity in STD rates by race or ethnicity is one of the first steps in empowering affected communities to organize and focus on this problem.

Surveillance data are based on cases of STDs reported to state and local health departments. In many state and local health jurisdictions, reporting from public sources (e.g., STD clinics) is thought to be more complete than reporting from private sources. Because minority populations may use public clinics more than whites, differences in rates between minorities and whites may be increased by this reporting bias. However, prevalence data from population-based surveys confirm the existence of marked STD disparities in some minority populations.

- Chlamydia: In 2009, 26.0% of chlamydia case reports were missing race or ethnicity data, ranging by state from 0.1% to 59.5%.

- Gonorrhea: In 2009, 20.1% of gonorrhea case reports were missing information on race or ethnicity data, ranging by state from 0.0% to 41.8%.

- Syphilis: In 2009, 2.0% of syphilis case reports were missing information on race or ethnicity data, ranging from 0.0% to 19.7% among states with 10 or more cases of P&S [primary and secondary] syphilis.

Chlamydia

Chlamydia rates based on reported cases increased during 2008–2009 among blacks, whites, and Hispanics. Among Asians/Pacific Islanders and American Indians/Alaska Natives, rates decreased slightly. During 2005–2009, chlamydia rates increased by 26.3% among blacks, 3.9% among American Indians/Alaska Natives, 13.4% among Hispanics, 0.4% among Asians/Pacific Islanders, and 17.9% among whites.

Blacks

In 2009, about 48% of all reported chlamydia cases occurred among blacks. Overall, the rate of chlamydia among blacks in the United States was more than eight times that among whites. The rate of chlamydia among black women was nearly eight times higher than the rate among white women (2,095.5 and 270.2 per 100,000 women, respectively). The chlamydia rate among black men was almost 12 times as high as the rate among white men (970.0 and 84.0 cases per 100,000 men, respectively).

American Indians/Alaska Natives

In 2009, the chlamydia rate among American Indians/Alaska Natives was 776.5 cases per 100,000 population, a decrease of 1.5% from the 2008 rate of 788.3. Overall, the rate of chlamydia among American Indians/Alaska Natives in the United States was more than four times that among whites.

Asians/Pacific Islanders

In 2009, the chlamydia rate among Asians/Pacific Islanders was 149.0 cases per 100,000 population, a slight decrease from the 2008 rate of 149.3. The overall rate among Asians/Pacific Islanders was lower than the rate among whites.

Hispanics

In 2009, the chlamydia rate among Hispanics was 504.2 cases per 100,000 population, which is a small increase from the 2008 rate of 494.8 cases and nearly three times higher than the rate among whites (178.8).

Gonorrhea

During 2008–2009, gonorrhea rates decreased 12.0% in whites, 10.6% in blacks, 9.6% in Hispanics, and 8.1% in Asians/Pacific Islanders. The gonorrhea rate in American Indians/Alaska Natives increased 5.5%.

Blacks

In 2009, about 71% of all reported cases of gonorrhea occurred among blacks. The rate of gonorrhea among blacks in 2009 was 556.4 cases per 100,000 population, which was 20.5 times higher than the rate among whites. This disparity has changed little in recent years (17.6 times higher in 2005 and 20.1 times higher in 2008). This disparity was larger for black men (25.8 times higher) than for black women (17.0 times higher).

As in 2008, the disparity in gonorrhea rates for blacks in 2009 was larger in the Midwest and Northeast (28.4 and 26.7 times higher, respectively) than in the South or the West (16.2 and 13.9 times higher, respectively).

Considering all racial, ethnic, and age categories, gonorrhea rates were highest for blacks aged 15–19 and 20–24 years in 2009. Black women aged 15–19 years had a gonorrhea rate of 2,613.8 cases per 100,000 women. This rate was 16.7 times higher than the rate among white women in the same age group (156.7).

Black men aged 15–19 years had a gonorrhea rate of 1,316.4 cases per 100,000 men, which was 38.3 times higher than the rate among white men in the same age group (34.4). Among men and women aged 20–24 years, the gonorrhea rate among blacks was 17.8 times higher than the rate among whites (2,356.7 and 132.2, respectively).

American Indians/Alaska Natives

In 2009, the gonorrhea rate among American Indians/Alaska Natives was 113.3 cases per 100,000 population, which was 4.2 times higher than the rate among whites. This disparity was similar to that in recent years (3.7 times higher in 2005). The disparity between gonorrhea rates for American Indians/Alaska Natives and whites was larger for American Indian/Alaska Native women (4.5 times higher) than for American Indian/Alaska Native men (3.6 times higher).

In 2009, the disparity in gonorrhea rates for American Indians/ Alaska Natives was slightly larger in the West and Midwest (4.7 times higher in both regions) than in the Northeast or South (3.5 and 3.0 times higher, respectively).

Asians/Pacific Islanders

In 2009, the gonorrhea rate among Asians/Pacific Islanders was 18.1 cases per 100,000 population, which was lower than the rate among whites. This difference is larger for Asian/Pacific Islander women than for Asian/Pacific Islander men. In 2009, rates among Asians/Pacific Islanders were again lower than rates among whites in all four regions of the United States.

Hispanics

In 2009, the gonorrhea rate among Hispanics was 58.6 cases per 100,000 population, which was higher than the rate among whites. This disparity was similar to that in recent years and was higher for Hispanic men than for Hispanic women. The disparity in gonorrhea rates for Hispanics was larger in the Northeast (4.1 times higher) than in the South (2.2 times higher), the Midwest (1.9 times higher), or the West (1.7 times higher).

Primary and Secondary Syphilis

The syphilis epidemic in the late 1980s occurred primarily among men who have sex with women only (MSW) and minority populations. During the 1990s, the rate of P&S syphilis declined among all racial and ethnic groups. During 2005–2009, the rate increased among all racial and ethnic groups except American Indians/Alaska Natives.

Blacks

During 2008–2009, the rate of P&S syphilis among blacks increased 11.6% (from 17.2 to 19.2 cases per 100,000 population). In 2009, 52.4% of all cases reported to CDC were among blacks and 30.4% of all cases were among whites.

Compared with whites, the overall 2009 rate for blacks was 9.1 times higher, while the 2008 rate was 7.8 times higher. In 2009, the rate of P&S syphilis among black men was 8 times higher than the rate among white men; the rate among black women was more than 20 times higher than the rate among white women.

In some age groups, particularly black men and women aged 15–19 years and 20–24 years, disparities have increased markedly in recent years as rates of disease have increased. During 2005–2009, rates among men aged 15–19 years increased the most among black men (167%). During the same period, rates among black men aged 20–24 years increased 212% (from 30.2 to 94.2 cases per 100,000 population); this increase was the highest reported regardless of age, sex, or race/ethnicity. The 2009 rate among men aged 15–19 years was 26 times higher for blacks than for whites.

Among black women aged 15–24 years, rates increased more than twofold during 2005–2009. In 2009, rates were 29 times higher for black women aged 15–19 years than for white women of the same age.

Recent trends in syphilis rates in young black men are of particular concern given data indicating high HIV incidence in this population.

American Indians/Alaska Natives

During 2008–2009, the rate of P&S syphilis among American Indians/Alaska Natives increased 4.3% (from 2.3 to 2.4 cases per 100,000 population). In 2009, 0.4% of all cases reported to CDC were among American Indians/Alaska Natives. Compared with whites, the 2009 rate of P&S syphilis for American Indians/Alaska Natives was 1.1 times higher.

Asians/Pacific Islanders

During 2008–2009, the rate of P&S syphilis among Asians/Pacific Islanders increased 6.7% (from 1.5 to 1.6 cases per 100,000 population). In 2009, 1.6% of all cases reported to CDC were among Asians/Pacific Islanders. Compared with whites, the 2009 rate of P&S syphilis for Asians/Pacific Islanders was 0.8 times higher.

Hispanics

During 2008–2009, the rate of P&S syphilis among Hispanics decreased 2.2% (from 4.6 to 4.5 cases per 100,000 population). In 2009, 15.1% of all cases reported to CDC were among Hispanics. Compared with whites, the 2009 rate of P&S syphilis for Hispanics was 2.1 times higher.

Congenital Syphilis

In 2009, the rate of congenital syphilis (which is based on the mother's race/ethnicity) was 34.9 cases per 100,000 live births among blacks and 12.0 cases per 100,000 live births among Hispanics. These rates are 12.9 and 4.4 times higher, respectively, than the rate among whites (2.7 cases per 100,000 live births).

Section 10.2

African Americans Disproportionately Affected by STDs

Excerpted from "African Americans and Sexually
Transmitted Diseases," by the Centers for Disease Control and
Prevention (CDC, www.cdc.gov), April 2011.

Sexually transmitted diseases (STDs) pose a serious and widespread health threat in the United States. Though most STDs can be easily diagnosed and treated, many have no noticeable symptoms, and infected individuals may not seek testing or treatment. As a result, many infections go undetected. Without treatment, individuals with STDs are at risk of serious health problems, such as infertility. Also, individuals who are already infected with STDs are at least two to five times more likely than those who are uninfected to acquire HIV infection.

STDs affect people of all races, ages, and sexual orientations, though some individuals experience greater challenges in protecting their health. STDs take an especially heavy toll on African Americans, particularly young African-American women and men. For example, blacks represent just 14 percent of the U.S. population, yet account for approximately half of all reported chlamydia and syphilis cases and almost three quarters of all reported gonorrhea cases.

STDs among African Americans

Despite recent success in the prevention and control of STDs, some Americans are at greater risk of infection than others.

When risk behaviors are combined with barriers to quality health information and STD prevention services, the risk of infection increases. To ensure that individuals have the opportunity to make healthy decisions, it is essential to address both the individual and social dynamics that contribute to their risk for STDs.

While everyone should have the opportunity to make choices that allow them to live healthy lives regardless of their income, education, or racial/ethnic background, the reality is that inadequate resources and challenging living conditions make the journey to health and wellness harder for some, and can lead to circumstances that increase a person's risk for STDs. African Americans sometimes face barriers that contribute to increased rates of STDs:

- A person's social environment can determine the availability of healthy sexual partners. Because STD prevalence is already higher in African-American communities than in others, even the individual in this community who has only one sex partner can be at increased risk of infection, and individuals within these communities face a greater chance of infection with each sexual encounter.

- People who struggle financially may end up in circumstances that increase their risk for STDs. For example, those who can't afford the basic necessities may have trouble accessing and affording quality health care, making it difficult to receive STD testing and other prevention services. Recent data show that nearly one fifth of African Americans do not have health insurance and a quarter of African-American families live in poverty.

- Higher rates of incarceration among African-American men have led to imbalanced ratios of men to women in black communities, which can help fuel the spread of STDs.

- The quality and consistency of STD care can also be affected by the fact that African Americans tend to use medical care services and treatments less than whites, which research suggests may be partly related to mistrust of the medical system. Mistrust can also negatively affect communication between health care providers and African-American patients, as can lack of cultural competence among health care providers. In addition, research shows that the legacy effects of social discrimination can impact the quality of STD care many African Americans experience.

Chlamydia

It is estimated that 2.8 million new chlamydia cases occur in the United States each year, but more than half remain undiagnosed and unreported. Still, chlamydia remains the most commonly reported infectious disease in the United States. It affects blacks, who account for nearly half of the more than 1.2 million reported chlamydia cases (48 percent or 593,428 cases), more than other racial/ethnic groups of the United States. See Figure 10.1. Women bear a heavier chlamydia burden than men, which is especially concerning, given that untreated chlamydia can lead to infertility in women. Because chlamydia is so common and can cause infertility, CDC recommends annual screening for sexually active young women.

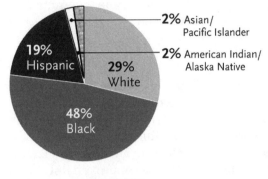

Total Cases: **1,218,155**

Figure 10.1. Reported chlamydia cases by race/ethnicity, 2009.

Gonorrhea

Reported gonorrhea cases have declined steadily in recent years. There was a 10 percent overall decrease in 2009, which puts gonorrhea rates at their lowest level since CDC began tracking the disease in 1941. While gonorrhea rates are declining for all races and ethnicities, since 2006, the decrease has been smaller for blacks (15 percent) than for Hispanics (21 percent) or whites (25 percent). See Figure 10.2

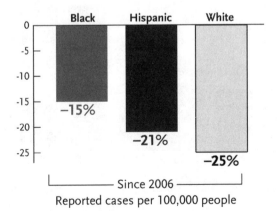

Figure 10.2. Gonorrhea declining at slower pace among minorities.

Like chlamydia, gonorrhea is substantially underdiagnosed and underreported. It is estimated that about twice as many new gonorrhea infections occur each year than are actually reported to CDC. Also like chlamydia, undiagnosed and untreated gonorrhea can lead to infertility in women. CDC recommends annual gonorrhea testing for high-risk sexually active women.

Syphilis

Syphilis has been on the rise since 2001. New reports show that more than half of all reported primary and secondary (P&S) syphilis cases (the early and most infectious stages of the disease) are among blacks (7,278 cases). In 2009, the P&S rate for black women was more than 20 times higher than the rate for white women, and the congenital syphilis rate for black infants was approximately 13 times higher than the rate for white infants. Moreover, P&S syphilis cases among black men 15 to 24 years of age continue to increase significantly; over the last five years, syphilis cases increased more than 150% among young black men. See Figure 10.3.

The majority of P&S syphilis cases occur among men who have sex with men (62 percent of all reported cases). CDC recommends that sexually active men who have sex with men be tested at least annually for syphilis. This is especially important because research shows that people with syphilis are at an increased risk of acquiring HIV.

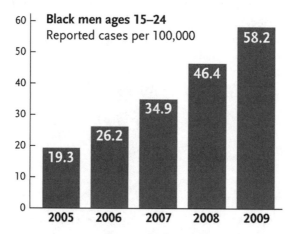

Figure 10.3. Syphilis rate rising sharply among young black men.

Section 10.3

Latinos Bear a Disproportionate Burden of the HIV Epidemic

"HIV and AIDS Among Latinos," by the Centers for Disease Control and Prevention (CDC, www.cdc.gov), October 2011.

HIV [human immunodeficiency virus] is a serious health threat to Latino communities in the United States. Because there is no single Latino culture in the United States, the factors driving the epidemic in this population are as diverse as the communities themselves. While prevention efforts have helped to maintain stability in the overall level of new HIV infections among Latinos for more than a decade, this population continues to be affected by HIV at far too high a level.

Although the number of new infections among Latinos has been lower than that of whites and blacks, Latinos bear a disproportionate burden of the HIV epidemic. See Figures 10.4 and 10.5.

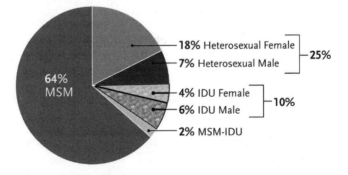

Figure 10.4. *Estimated new HIV infections among Hispanics, 2009, by transmission category.*

- Hispanics represent approximately 16 percent of the U.S. population and the latest CDC estimates show that they account for more than 17 percent of people living with HIV in the United States (205,400 persons), and an estimated 20 percent of new infections each year (9,400 infections).

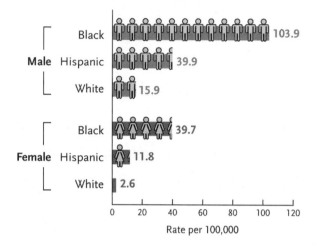

Figure 10.5. *Estimated rate of new HIV infections, 2009, by gender and race/ethnicity.*

- Approximately one in 36 Hispanic men will be diagnosed with HIV during their lifetime, as will one in 106 Hispanic women.

- Men account for more than three quarters (79 percent) of new infections among Hispanics. Women account for 21 percent.

- The rate of new HIV infections among Hispanic men is almost three times that among white men, with gay and bisexual men particularly affected.

- Most new infections among Hispanic men (81 percent) occur among men who have sex with men (MSM).

- In a study of 21 major U.S. cities in 2008, approximately 18 percent of Hispanic MSM were infected. Among those who were HIV-infected, nearly half (46 percent) were unaware that they were infected.

- The rate of new HIV infections among Hispanic women is more than four times that of white women.

- AIDS [acquired immunodeficiency syndrome] continues to claim the lives of too many Latino men and women. Since the beginning of the epidemic, more than 89,000 Hispanics with AIDS have died.

Complex Factors Increase Risk

Socioeconomic factors: The social and economic realities of some Latinos' lives can increase HIV risk, including poverty, discrimination, and lack of access to healthcare. Language barriers may also affect the quality of care.

Stigma: The stigma associated with HIV and homosexuality may help to spread HIV in Latino communities. In some communities, the cultural value of machismo may create reluctance to acknowledge sensitive, yet risky behaviors, such as male-to-male sexual contact and substance abuse. Fear of disclosing risk behavior or sexual orientation may prevent Latinos from seeking testing, treatment and prevention services, and support from friends and family. As a result, too many Latinos lack critical information about how to prevent infection.

Cultural factors: There is no single Latino culture in the United States. Research shows that Latinos born in different countries have different behavioral risk factors for HIV. For example, data suggest that Hispanics born in Puerto Rico are more likely than other Hispanics to contract HIV as a result of injection drug use or high-risk heterosexual contact. By contrast, sexual contact with other men is the primary cause of HIV infection among men born in places such as Mexico and the United States.

High prevalence of sexually transmitted diseases (STDs) and higher rates of HIV: Data show that the burden of STDs among Latinos is high. Because STDs can place individuals at higher risk for HIV infection, high STD prevalence may contribute to higher HIV incidence among Latino men and women. Additionally, disproportionate rates of HIV among Latinos and the current high prevalence of HIV in Latino communities increases the likelihood that Latinos will encounter an HIV-infected sex or drug-injecting partner, placing them at greater risk.

Chapter 11

STDs in People in Correctional Facilities

Multiple studies and surveillance projects have demonstrated a high prevalence of STDs [sexually transmitted diseases] in persons entering jails and juvenile corrections facilities. Prevalence rates for chlamydia and gonorrhea in these settings are consistently among the highest observed in any venue. Screening for chlamydia, gonorrhea, and syphilis at intake offers an opportunity to identify infections, prevent complications, and reduce transmission in the general community.

For example, data from one study in a location with high syphilis incidence suggested that screening and treatment of female inmates for syphilis may reduce syphilis in the general community. In some locations, a substantial proportion of all early syphilis cases are reported from corrections facilities.

In 2009, STD screening data from corrections facilities were reported in 37 states and Puerto Rico for chlamydia, 36 states and Puerto Rico for gonorrhea, and 19 states for syphilis. Line-listed (i.e., case-specific) data for chlamydia and gonorrhea are provided to CDC through the Infertility Prevention Project (IPP). Aggregate syphilis data are reported to CDC by local and state STD prevention programs. The findings presented in this text are based on 50,968 chlamydia tests of women, 129,548 chlamydia tests of men, 42,124 gonorrhea tests of women, and 114,984 gonorrhea tests of men.

"STDs in Persons Entering Correctional Facilities," by the Centers for Disease Control and Prevention (CDC, www.cdc.gov), November 22, 2010.

Chlamydia

Overall, chlamydia positivity was higher in women than in men for all age groups.

- Males in juvenile corrections facilities—Among males aged 12–18 years entering 123 juvenile corrections facilities, the overall chlamydia positivity was 6.6%. Chlamydia positivity increased from 1.2% for adolescent males aged 12 years to 10.1% for those aged 18 years.

- Females in juvenile corrections facilities—Among females aged 12–18 years entering 83 juvenile corrections facilities, the overall chlamydia positivity was 14.8%. Positivity increased from 4.7% for females aged 12 years to 16.2% for those aged 16 years and remained high for women aged 17–18 years.

- Men in adult corrections facilities—Among men entering 59 adult corrections facilities in 2009, positivity in men younger than aged 20 years (10.8%) was higher than the overall prevalence observed in adolescent males entering juvenile facilities (6.6%). Chlamydia positivity decreased with age, from 10.8% for those younger than aged 20 years to 1.8% for those older than 34 years. Overall positivity among adult men entering corrections facilities in 2009 was 6.6%.

- Women in adult corrections facilities—Among women entering 31 adult corrections facilities in 2009, positivity was 7.2%. Chlamydia positivity decreased with age, from 16.6% for those younger than aged 20 years to 2.3% for those older than aged 34 years. Overall chlamydia positivity in women entering adult corrections facilities (7.2%) was substantially lower than that in adolescent females entering juvenile corrections facilities (14.8%). However, chlamydia positivity among women younger than aged 20 years entering adult corrections facilities was higher than that among women entering juvenile corrections facilities.

Gonorrhea

Overall, gonorrhea positivity in women was uniformly higher than in men for all age groups.

- Males in juvenile corrections facilities—The overall gonorrhea positivity for adolescent males entering 118 juvenile corrections facilities in 2009 was 1.0%. Positivity increased with age, from 0.1% for those aged 12 years to 1.4% for those aged 18 years.

- Females in juvenile corrections facilities—The overall gonorrhea positivity for adolescent females entering 71 juvenile corrections facilities in 2009 was 3.9%. Positivity increased with age, from 1.8% for those aged 12 years to 4.4% for those aged 16 years and remained high for women aged 17–18 years.

- Men in adult corrections facilities—The overall gonorrhea positivity for men entering 57 adult corrections facilities in 2009 was 1.2%. Positivity was highest in men younger than aged 20 years (2.2%) and declined with age to 0.4% in men older than aged 34 years. Men younger than aged 20 years entering adult facilities had higher gonorrhea positivity than males entering juvenile corrections facilities.

- Women in adult corrections facilities—Among women entering 29 adult corrections facilities in 2009, overall gonorrhea positivity was 1.6%. Positivity decreased with age, from 3.1% among those younger than aged 20 years to 0.7% among those older than aged 34 years. Women younger than aged 20 years entering adult facilities had lower gonorrhea positivity than females entering juvenile corrections facilities.

Syphilis

In 2008, reports of P&S syphilis from correctional facilities accounted for 7% of P&S syphilis among men who have sex with women only (MSW), 5% among women, and 1% among men who have sex with men (MSM). In 2009, reports of P&S syphilis from correctional facilities accounted for 5% of P&S syphilis among MSW, 4% among women, and 1% among MSM.

Chapter 12

Recent STD Research Findings

Sexually Transmitted Diseases

Sexually transmitted diseases are an important global health priority because of their devastating impact on women and infants and their inter-relationships with HIV/AIDS [human immunodeficiency virus/acquired immunodeficiency syndrome]. STDs and HIV are linked by biological interactions and because both infections occur in the same populations. Infection with certain STDs can increase the risk of getting and transmitting HIV as well as alter the way the disease progresses. In addition, STDs can cause long-term health problems, particularly in women and infants. Some of the health complications that arise from STDs include pelvic inflammatory disease, infertility, tubal or ectopic pregnancy, cervical cancer, and perinatal or congenital infections in infants born to infected mothers.

Basic Research

The ultimate objective of research supported by the National Institute of Allergy and Infectious Diseases (NIAID) is to develop effective

This chapter contains text excerpted from the following documents by the National Institute of Allergy and Infectious Diseases (NIAID, www.niaid.nih .gov), part of the National Institutes of Health: "Sexually Transmitted Diseases (STDs)," updated March 5, 2012; "Basic Research," updated March 31, 2011; "Diagnostics," updated April 13, 2009; "Treatment," updated April 13, 2009; and "Prevention," updated March 8, 2011.

prevention and treatment approaches to control STDs. To develop these strategies, basic research is necessary toward understanding the structure, function, growth, pathogenesis, and evolution of STD bacterial, viral, parasitic, protozoan, and fungal agents. Another important aspect of basic research is to examine the impact of STDs in various populations.

NIAID's work in genomic sequencing further accelerates STD biological research and discovery. NIAID has collected genomic data on STD pathogens and made it available to qualified researchers through public databases. Recent advances include the genomic sequencing of pathogens responsible for trichomoniasis, chlamydia, gonorrhea, and human genital ulcer disease (chancroid). The sequencing of genomes allows researchers to read and decipher genetic data that may aid in the development of novel diagnostics, topical medications, and vaccines.

Diagnostics

Early and rapid diagnosis of STDs increases the chance to limit effects of the disease. Left untreated, STDs, such as gonorrhea, syphilis, chlamydia, genital herpes, and human papillomavirus, can lead to devastating and sometimes long-term complications. These complications include blindness, bone deformities, brain damage, cancer, heart disease, infertility, birth defects, mental retardation, and even death.

Healthcare providers diagnose STDs through physical examination, blood tests, or swabbed cultures. Diagnosis of STDs by self-obtained vaginal swabs was the focus of an NIAID-supported workshop. However, many people infected by an STD have little or no symptoms of the infection. NIAID scientists are conducting immunology studies to address why many STDs in people are asymptomatic. These studies may also uncover how an infection's mutation contributes to STD drug resistance and the processes associated with repeat infection and coinfection (for example, syphilis and HIV/AIDS).

Treatment

There are many different kinds of STDs, and the types of treatment are as varied as their symptoms. NIAID supports the development and licensure of vaccines, topical microbicides, and drug treatments, such as antibiotics and antifungals, for the microbes that cause STDs. No STD is harmless. Even the curable ones can cause serious consequences if left untreated. HIV is of particular concern as biological evidence demonstrates the increased likelihood of acquiring and transmitting HIV when STDs are present.

Today, scientists at NIAID are testing new vaccines for STDs, such as herpes, and new ways to treat drug-resistant STDs, such as gonorrhea, in animal models and clinical trials. Research findings may lead to faster, safer, and more effective treatments.

Prevention

A cornerstone of public health is disease prevention. Tools to prevent STDs, such as vaccines, topical microbicides, and behavioral interventions, are a vital part of protecting the public against infectious diseases. Gardasil, a vaccine against the four most common strains of human papillomavirus (HPV), is an exciting accomplishment in the field of STDs. However, the work to develop safe and effective vaccines against other STDs continues. Most notably are the ongoing clinical trials to evaluate an investigational vaccine to prevent genital herpes.

Barrier methods—such as latex condoms and topical microbicides (a substance applied to the vagina or rectum that kills or disables the microbes that cause STDs)—offer highly effective protection against STDs. NIAID-funded researchers are conducting clinical trials to test new topical microbicides and female-barrier methods to prevent STDs. Used correctly and consistently these products may greatly reduce a person's risk of acquiring or transmitting most STDs, including gonorrhea, chlamydia, trichomonas, syphilis, HPV, and HIV/AIDS.

In addition, NIAID-supported researchers are conducting interventional and behavioral studies to identify social and economic conditions and sexual behaviors that may increase a person's vulnerability to STDs. Results of this work may reduce health disparities, especially among youth, women, and underrepresented minorities.

Part Two

Types of STDs

Chapter 13

Common Symptoms of STDs

What are sexually transmitted diseases (STDs)?

Sexually transmitted diseases (STDs) are diseases that are mainly passed from one person to another during sex. There are at least 25 different sexually transmitted diseases with a range of different symptoms. These diseases may be spread through vaginal, anal, and oral sex.

Most sexually transmitted diseases will only affect you if you have sexual contact with someone who has an STD. However there are some infections, for example scabies, which are referred to as STDs because they are most commonly transmitted sexually, but which can also be passed on in other ways.

What are sexually transmitted infections (STIs)?

Sexually transmitted infection (STI) is another name for sexually transmitted disease (STD). The name STI is often preferred because there are a few STDs, such as chlamydia, that can infect a person without causing any actual disease (i.e., unpleasant symptoms). Someone without symptoms may not think of themselves as having a disease, but they may still have an infection that needs treating.

How can you tell if you have a sexually transmitted disease?

You may become aware that you have an STD because of symptoms, or it may be that a sexual partner tells you they have an STD which they might have passed on to you. Some sexually transmitted diseases can be transmitted by an infected person even if they don't have any symptoms. Certain STDs can also be transmitted from a pregnant woman to her unborn child.

If you think you might have been exposed to an STD then you should go to see a doctor. Many sexually transmitted diseases can be easily cured, but if left untreated, they may cause unpleasant symptoms and could lead to long-term damage such as infertility. It is important that anyone diagnosed with an STD informs everyone they have had sex with within the past year (or everyone following the partner they believe may have infected them).

What are common STD symptoms?

STD symptoms vary, but the most common are soreness, unusual lumps or sores, itching, pain when urinating, and/or an unusual discharge from the genitals.

To see pictures of common STDs, please visit www.avert.org/std -pictures.htm.

Which are the most common sexually transmitted diseases?

In the following text are some of the most common STDs and other genital diseases. To find out more about HIV [human immunodeficiency virus], visit www.avert.org/hiv.htm.

Bacterial vaginosis: Bacterial vaginosis (BV) is caused by an imbalance in the normal healthy bacteria found in the vagina. Although it is relatively harmless and may pass unnoticed, it can sometimes produce an abundance of unpleasant fishy smelling discharge.

BV is not strictly an STD as it is not transmitted via sexual intercourse. However, it can be exacerbated by sex and is more frequently found in sexually active women than those who have never had intercourse.

While there is no clear explanation as to why BV occurs, there have been suggestions that the alkaline nature of semen could be one cause, as it may upset the acidic nature of the vaginal bacteria. Another cause can be the use of an intrauterine contraceptive device (coil).

A woman cannot pass BV to a man, but it is important she receives treatment as BV can occasionally travel up into the uterus and fallopian tubes and cause a more serious infection. Treatment for BV consists of applying a cream to the vagina or taking antibiotics.

Chlamydia: Chlamydia is one of the most commonly reported bacterial sexually transmitted diseases. It is caused by the *Chlamydia trachomatis* bacterium. It infects the urethra, rectum, and eyes in both sexes, and the cervix in women. If left untreated, long-term infection can lead to fertility problems in women. Chlamydia is transmitted through genital contact and/or sexual intercourse with someone already infected. Symptoms of chlamydia usually show between one and three weeks after exposure but may not emerge until much later.

Crabs or pubic lice: Crabs or pubic lice are small crab-shaped parasites that burrow into the skin to feed on blood. They live on coarse body hair, predominantly pubic hair, but can also be found in armpit hair, facial hair, and even on eyelashes. The lice are yellow-grey in color and use their crab-like claws to grip hair strands. They can sometimes be spotted moving on the skin.

Crabs are easily passed on during sex, but can also be passed on through sharing clothes, towels, or bedding with someone who has them. Crabs cannot be transmitted via toilet seats or swimming pools.

Symptoms of crabs are usually noticed around five days to seven weeks after infection and include:

- itchy skin;
- inflammation of the affected area;
- sometimes visible lice and eggs;
- spots of blood as lice feed from blood vessels in the skin.

Although there is no effective way to prevent becoming infected during sex, a person who has crabs can reduce the risk to others by washing bedding, towels, and clothes on a hot wash to kill off the parasites.

Treatment for public lice is easy, consisting of special shampoos, lotions, and creams that kill the lice and their eggs. It is not necessary to shave pubic hair as this is unlikely to remove all lice.

Genital warts: Genital warts are caused by some subtypes of human papillomavirus (HPV). They can appear on the skin anywhere in the genital area as small whitish or flesh-colored bumps, or larger, fleshy, cauliflower-like lumps. They are unlikely to cause pain but may itch and can be difficult to spot. Often there are no other symptoms of genital warts, but if a woman has a wart on her cervix she may experience slight bleeding or unusual colored vaginal discharge.

Gonorrhea: Gonorrhea (once known as the clap) is a sexually transmitted infection that can infect the urethra, cervix, rectum, anus, and throat. Symptoms of gonorrhea usually appear between 1 and 14 days after exposure, but it is possible to have no symptoms. Men are more likely to notice symptoms than women. Symptoms can include:

- a burning sensation when urinating;

- a white/yellow discharge from the penis;

- a change in vaginal discharge;

- irritation or discharge from the anus (if the rectum is infected).

Hepatitis: Hepatitis refers to viral infections that cause inflammation of the liver. Several different types of hepatitis virus exist (labeled A to G), with hepatitis A, B, and C being the most common. Hepatitis can occur following excessive and prolonged consumption of alcohol or the use of certain medicines and drugs, but it is most commonly caused by a virus. Read more about the different transmission routes of hepatitis at www.avert.org/hepatitis.htm.

Herpes: Herpes is caused by two strains of the herpes simplex virus, type 1 (HSV-1) and type 2 (HSV-2). HSV-2 is more common and usually manifests itself in the genital and anal area, whereas HSV-1 is more likely to affect the mouth and lips in the form of cold sores. On a global scale, HSV-2 is a very common STD. Symptoms of herpes usually appear two to seven days after first exposure to the virus and last two to four weeks. Both men and women may have multiple symptoms, including:

- itching or tingling sensations in the genital or anal area;

- small fluid-filled blisters that burst leaving small painful sores;

- pain when passing urine over the open sores (especially in women);

- headaches;

- backache;

- flu-like symptoms, including swollen glands or fever.

Once the first outbreak of blisters has gone, the herpes virus hides away in nerve fibers near the infection site, where it remains dormant, causing no symptoms. Symptoms may come back later (particularly during times of stress and illness) but usually in less severe and shorter episodes. Read more about herpes at www.avert.org/herpes .htm.

Molluscum contagiosum: Molluscum contagiosum (MC, also known as water warts) is a common viral infection, which results in a skin disease. Small papules usually appear on exposed skin such as the torso, thighs, genitalia, and anus, around two to eight weeks after initial infection with the virus. The pearl-shaped papules are usually between one to five mm in diameter, are filled with a gungy, white, contagious fluid, and often appear in clusters.

MC can be transmitted through direct skin-to-skin contact and also indirectly through sharing towels, baths, or clothing with someone infected. It is not strictly an STD as it often occurs in children, especially those prone to skin conditions such as eczema. Children are more likely to assist transmission by scratching the infected sites, although it should be noted that the chance of passing on the virus is small.

MC is grouped with STDs because of the risk of transmission through close body contact during sex, which is why it is often screened for in sexual health clinics. The risk of becoming infected with MC can be reduced by:

- using condoms during sex, although this only offers partial protection as MC can be passed on by anal/genital lesions not covered by the condom;
- covering affected areas of skin (where possible) with clothing or sterile dressings;
- not sharing baths, clothing, and towels.

The recommended treatment is often to leave MC to clear up by itself (which usually takes around 6 to 18 months) as medical removal can leave scarring. If requested, the lesions can however be removed by various medical treatments such as cryotherapy (freezing), diathermy (burning), or curettage (cutting or scraping).

In an HIV-positive person, a large outbreak of molluscum contagiosum may indicate that the immune system is critically weak and it is advisable to seek medical attention.

Scabies: Scabies is an intensely itchy, contagious skin infestation of the parasitic mite *Sarcoptes scabiei*. The adult female mite is around 0.4 mm (1/60 of an inch) long and barely visible to the human eye, with the male being half that size. Female mites burrow into the outer layer of the skin (stratum corneum) to lay eggs. Symptoms begin two to six weeks after infection and include:

- burrows that appear as silvery or brown wavy lines up to 15 mm (half an inch) in length (The burrows can appear anywhere, but usually occur on the webbing between fingers and toes, on the genitals, around the anus, or on the buttocks, elbows, or wrists);

- an intensely itchy rash of inflamed pimple-like lumps (papules/ lesions) as an allergic reaction to the mites, their eggs, and feces;

- widespread itching, particularly at night or after baths when the body is warmer, as a reaction to the mites.

Again, scabies it not strictly a sexually transmitted disease, as the scabies mite can be passed on through other forms of prolonged direct skin contact. Scabies has been known to spread rapidly in crowded conditions where there is frequent contact between people, such as in care homes or child care facilities. It is also possible, but much less likely, to acquire the infestation through sharing clothes, towels, or bedding with someone infected. Sexual activity does however carry a particularly high risk of transmission.

There is no effective way to prevent infection apart from avoiding direct skin contact with an infected person. If a person knows they are infected then they can prevent the infestation spreading by washing clothes and bedding on a hot wash to kill the mites (at 50 degrees Celsius/120 Fahrenheit or above). Treatment comes in the form of lotions that can be bought from pharmacies without prescription and applied to the body to kill the parasites. It is recommended that all people in close contact, such as sexual partners or members of the household, should be treated at the same time, even if they are not yet showing any symptoms of infestation.

Syphilis: Syphilis is a bacterial infection caused by *Treponema pallidum*, which used to be known as the pox. It is usually sexually transmitted, but can also be passed from an infected woman to her unborn child. Syphilis progresses through several stages, of which the primary and secondary stages are very infectious. Syphilis symptoms can be difficult to recognize and may take three months to appear after sexual contact with an infected person. They include:

- one or more painless ulcers on the penis, vagina, vulva, cervix, anus, or mouth;

- small lumps in the groin due to swollen glands;
- a non-itchy rash;
- fever or flu-like symptoms.

Left untreated the infection progresses to a latent stage. This may be followed by tertiary syphilis, which can seriously affect organs such as the heart, and can sometimes lead to death.

Thrush: Thrush, also known as candidiasis, is a yeast infection caused by the Candida species of fungus. Thrush is not technically a sexually transmitted infection, as Candida is a common yeast that is found on the skin and genitals of most people, even those who have not had sex. Candida is usually suppressed by the immune system and the natural bacteria found in the body, but there are many things that can upset the balance and allow Candida to grow. Thrush occurs a lot less frequently in men.

The symptoms of a thrush infection are:

- in women, irritation, itching, thick white discharge, redness, soreness, and swelling of the vagina and vulva;
- in men, irritation, discharge from the penis, difficulty pulling back the foreskin usually caused by the swelling of the head of the penis (balanitis).

There are many causes of thrush, but the most common are:

- in women, wearing nylon or Lycra clothes that are too tight (the lack of air circulation can cause Candida to proliferate);
- certain antibiotics or contraceptive pills that alter the pH balance of the vagina;
- a change in the hormonal balance in pregnant women, causing a change in the level of normal bacteria;
- spermicides (found on some condoms) or perfumed toiletries that irritate the vagina or penis;
- douching (washing out the vagina) or using tampons;
- sexual contact (either genital or oral) with someone who carries the Candida yeast.

Treatment for thrush involves applying an anti-fungal cream that contains clotrimazole. If an infection is recurring then fluconazole may

113

be prescribed to be taken orally, unless the patient is pregnant. It may also be suggested to wash the genitals with water to avoid irritation and to wear loose-fitting cotton underwear and clothes.

Trichomoniasis: Trichomoniasis (also known as trich) is caused by the single-celled organism *Trichomonas vaginalis,* which is transmitted through sex. It can infect the vagina and the male and female urethra. Often this STD presents no symptoms, though women are more likely to have symptoms than men. If symptoms do appear, they can include:

- discharge in both men and women (sometimes copious and unpleasant smelling in women);

- discomfort or pain while having sex;

- pain when urinating and inflammation of the urethra.

Women may also experience an inflammation of the vulva and they may develop cystitis (an infection of the urinary system).

Transmission is usually through vaginal, anal, or oral sex with an infected person. The most effective prevention method is to practice safer sex by using condoms.

Treatment for both men and women is a drug called metronidazole which can be taken orally or applied as a gel. It is important for any sexual partners to also be treated as trichomoniasis can be carried and spread without symptoms. If a woman is pregnant then she should seek medical advice before pursuing treatment.

Chapter 14

Chancroid

What is chancroid?

Chancroid is a highly contagious yet curable sexually transmitted disease (STD) caused by the bacteria *Haemophilus ducreyi* [hum-AH-fill-us DOO-cray]. Chancroid causes ulcers, usually of the genitals. Swollen, painful lymph glands, or inguinal buboes [in-GWEEN-al BEW-boes], in the groin area are often associated with chancroid. Left untreated, chancroid may facilitate the transmission of HIV [human immunodeficiency virus].

How common is it?

Chancroid is very common in Africa and is becoming more common in the United States.

How do people get chancroid?

Chancroid is transmitted in two ways:

- Sexual transmission through skin-to-skin contact with open sore(s)

- Non-sexual transmission when pus-like fluid from the ulcer is moved to other parts of the body or to another person

"Chancroid," reprinted with permission from the Illinois Department of Public Health (http://www.idph.state.il.us). © 2012 State of Illinois.

A person is considered to be infectious when ulcers are present. There has been no reported disease in infants born to women with active chancroid at time of delivery.

What are the signs or symptoms of chancroid?

Symptoms usually occur within 4–10 days from exposure. They rarely develop earlier than 3 days or later than 10 days.

The ulcer begins as a tender, elevated bump, or papule, that becomes a pus-filled, open sore with eroded or ragged edges.

The ulcer is soft to the touch (unlike a syphilis chancre that is hard or rubbery). The term soft chancre is frequently used to describe the chancroid sore.

The ulcers can be very painful in men but women are often unaware of them.

Because chancroid is often asymptomatic in women, they may be unaware of the lesion(s).

Painful lymph glands may occur in the groin, usually only on one side; however, they can occur on both sides.

How is chancroid diagnosed?

Diagnosis is made by isolating the bacteria *Hemophilus ducreyi* in a culture from a genital ulcer. The chancre is often confused with syphilis, herpes, or lymphogranuloma venereum; therefore, it is important that your health care provider rule these diseases out.

A Gram stain to identify *H. ducreyi* is possible but can be misleading because of other organisms found in most genital ulcers.

What is the treatment for chancroid?

Chancroid can be treated with antibiotics. Successful treatment cures the infection, resolves symptoms, and prevents transmission to others. Treatment regimens may include the following: azithromycin, ceftriaxone, ciprofloxacin (not recommended for pregnant or nursing females, or people younger than 18 years), and erythromycin base.

A follow-up examination should be conducted three to seven days after treatment begins. If treatment is successful, ulcers usually improve within three to seven days. The time required for complete healing is related to the size of the ulcer. Large ulcers may require two weeks or longer to heal. In severe cases, scarring may result. Partners should be examined and treated regardless of whether symptoms are present.

How can chancroid be prevented?

- Abstinence (not having sex)
- Mutual monogamy [having sex with only one uninfected partner]
- Latex condoms for vaginal, oral, and anal sex

Using latex condoms may protect the penis or vagina from infection, but does not protect other areas such as the scrotum or anal area. Chancroid lesions can occur in genital areas that are covered or protected by a latex condom, but may also occur in areas that are not covered or protected by a condom. Latex condoms, when used consistently and correctly, can reduce the risk of chancroid, genital herpes, syphilis, and genital warts, only when the infected areas are covered or protected by the condom.

If you do get chancroid, avoid contact with the infected area to prevent chance of spreading the infection to other parts of the body.

Why worry?

Chancroid has been well established as a cofactor for HIV transmission. Moreover, persons with HIV may experience slower healing of chancroid, even with treatment, and may need to take medications for a longer period of time. Complications from chancroid include:

- In 50 percent of cases, the lymph node glands in the groin become infected within five to eight days of appearance of initial sores.
- Glands on one side become enlarged, hard, painful, and fuse together to form a bubo (BEW-bo), an inflammation and swelling of one or more lymph nodes with overlying red skin. Surgical drainage of the bubo may be necessary to relieve pain.
- Ruptured buboes are susceptible to secondary bacterial infections.
- In uncircumcised males, new scar tissue may result in phimosis [constriction so the foreskin cannot be retracted over the head of the penis]. Circumcision may be required to correct this.

What should I tell my partner?

You should talk to your partner as soon as you learn you have chancroid. Telling a partner can be hard, but it's important that you talk to your partner as soon as possible so she or he can get treatment.

How do I address the subject with my healthcare provider?

If you have a genital ulcer or painful, swollen lymph nodes, you need to talk to your doctor about whether or not you should be tested. However, it's important to remember that some people, usually women, are asymptomatic. If you are having unprotected sex or discover that your partner is having unprotected sex with another person, you may want to ask your doctor about being tested for STDs.

Chapter 15

Chlamydia

Chapter Contents

Section 15.1—What Is Chlamydia?... 120

Section 15.2—Chlamydia Is the Most Common Cause
of Nongonococcal Urethritis 123

Section 15.3—Chlamydia Treatment... 127

Section 15.1

What Is Chlamydia?

Excerpted from "Chlamydia—CDC Fact Sheet," by the Centers for Disease
Control and Prevention (CDC, www.cdc.gov), updated February 2012.

What is chlamydia?

Chlamydia is a common sexually transmitted disease (STD) caused
by the bacterium, *Chlamydia trachomatis,* which can damage a woman's reproductive organs. Even though symptoms of chlamydia are
usually mild or absent, serious complications that cause irreversible
damage, including infertility, can occur silently before a woman ever
recognizes a problem. Chlamydia also can cause discharge from the
penis of an infected man.

How common is chlamydia?

Chlamydia is the most frequently reported bacterial sexually
transmitted disease in the United States. In 2010, 1,307,893 chlamydial infections were reported to CDC from 50 states and the District
of Columbia. Under-reporting is substantial because most people
with chlamydia are not aware of their infections and do not seek
testing. Also, testing is not often done if patients are treated for their
symptoms. An estimated 2.8 million infections occur annually in the
United States. Women are frequently reinfected if their sex partners
are not treated.

How do people get chlamydia?

Chlamydia can be transmitted during vaginal, anal, or oral sex.
Chlamydia can also be passed from an infected mother to her baby
during vaginal childbirth.

Any sexually active person can be infected with chlamydia. The
greater the number of sex partners, the greater the risk of infection.
Because the cervix (opening to the uterus) of teenage girls and young
women is not fully matured and is probably more susceptible to infection, they are at particularly high risk for infection if sexually active.

Since chlamydia can be transmitted by oral or anal sex, men who have sex with men are also at risk for chlamydial infection.

What are the symptoms of chlamydia?

Chlamydia is known as a "silent" disease because the majority of infected people have no symptoms. If symptoms do occur, they usually appear within one to three weeks after exposure.

In women, the bacteria initially infect the cervix and the urethra (urine canal). Women who have symptoms might have an abnormal vaginal discharge or a burning sensation when urinating. If the infection spreads from the cervix to the fallopian tubes (tubes that carry fertilized eggs from the ovaries to the uterus), some women still have no signs or symptoms; others have lower abdominal pain, low back pain, nausea, fever, pain during intercourse, or bleeding between menstrual periods. Chlamydial infection of the cervix can spread to the rectum.

Men with signs or symptoms might have a discharge from their penis or a burning sensation when urinating. Men might also have burning and itching around the opening of the penis. Pain and swelling in the testicles are uncommon.

Men or women who have receptive anal intercourse may acquire chlamydial infection in the rectum, which can cause rectal pain, discharge, or bleeding. Chlamydia can also be found in the throats of women and men having oral sex with an infected partner.

What complications can result from untreated chlamydia?

If untreated, chlamydial infections can progress to serious reproductive and other health problems with both short-term and long-term consequences. Like the disease itself, the damage that chlamydia causes is often silent.

In women, untreated infection can spread into the uterus or fallopian tubes and cause pelvic inflammatory disease (PID). This happens in about 10 to 15 percent of women with untreated chlamydia. Chlamydia can also cause fallopian tube infection without any symptoms. PID and silent infection in the upper genital tract can cause permanent damage to the fallopian tubes, uterus, and surrounding tissues. The damage can lead to chronic pelvic pain, infertility, and potentially fatal ectopic pregnancy (pregnancy outside the uterus). Chlamydia may also increase the chances of becoming infected with HIV (human immunodeficiency virus), if exposed.

To help prevent the serious consequences of chlamydia, screening at least annually for chlamydia is recommended for all sexually active women age 25 years and younger. An annual screening test also is recommended for older women with risk factors for chlamydia (a new sex partner or multiple sex partners). All pregnant women should have a screening test for chlamydia.

Complications among men are rare. Infection sometimes spreads to the epididymis (the tube that carries sperm from the testis), causing pain, fever, and, rarely, sterility.

Rarely, genital chlamydial infection can cause arthritis that can be accompanied by skin lesions and inflammation of the eye and urethra (Reiter syndrome).

How does chlamydia affect a pregnant woman and her baby?

In pregnant women, there is some evidence that untreated chlamydial infections can lead to premature delivery. Babies who are born to infected mothers can get chlamydial infections in their eyes and respiratory tracts. Chlamydia is a leading cause of early infant pneumonia and conjunctivitis (pink eye) in newborns.

How is chlamydia diagnosed?

There are laboratory tests to diagnose chlamydia. Some can be performed on urine, other tests require that a specimen be collected from a site such as the penis or cervix.

How can chlamydia be prevented?

The surest way to avoid transmission of STDs is to abstain from sexual contact, or to be in a long-term mutually monogamous relationship with a partner who has been tested and is known to be uninfected.

Latex male condoms, when used consistently and correctly, can reduce the risk of transmission of chlamydia.

CDC recommends yearly chlamydia testing of all sexually active women age 25 or younger, older women with risk factors for chlamydial infections (those who have a new sex partner or multiple sex partners), and all pregnant women. An appropriate sexual risk assessment by a health care provider should always be conducted and may indicate more frequent screening for some women.

Any genital symptoms such as an unusual sore, discharge with odor, burning during urination, or bleeding between menstrual cycles could mean an STD infection. If a woman or man has any of these symptoms, they should stop having sex and consult a health care provider immediately. Treating STDs early in women can prevent PID.

Women and men who are told they have an STD and are treated for it should notify all of their recent sex partners (sex partners within the preceding 60 days) so they can see a health care provider and be evaluated for STDs. Sexual activity should not resume until all sex partners have been examined and, if necessary, treated.

Section 15.2

Chlamydia Is the Most Common Cause of Nongonococcal Urethritis

"Non-Gonococcal Urethritis (NGU)," reprinted with permission from the Illinois Department of Public Health (http://www.idph .state.il.us). © 2012 State of Illinois.

What is NGU?

NGU (Non-Gonococcal Urethritis) is an infection of the urethra caused by pathogens (germs) other than gonorrhea.

How common is NGU?

Several types of germs cause NGU, the most common and serious is chlamydia. Chlamydia is very common in both males and females. The diagnosis of NGU is more commonly made in males than in females, mainly due to the anatomical differences. Germs that can cause NGU include but are not limited to:

- *Chlamydia trachomatis* (most common);

- *Ureaplasma urealyticum*;

- *Trichomonas vaginalis* (rare);

- herpes simplex virus (rare);

- *Haemophilus vaginalis*;

- *Mycoplasma genitalium*.

How can I get NGU?

- **Sexually:** Most germs that cause NGU can be passed during sex (vaginal, anal, or oral) that involves direct mucous membrane contact with an infected person.

- **Nonsexual:** These causes of NGU may include: Urinary tract infections, an inflamed prostate gland due to bacteria (bacterial prostatitis), a narrowing or closing of the tube in the penis (urethral stricture), a tightening of the foreskin so that it cannot be pulled back from the head of the penis (phimosis), the result of a process such as inserting a tube into the penis (catheterization).

- **Perinatal:** During birth, infants may be exposed to the germs causing NGU in passage through the birth canal. This may cause the baby to have infections in the eyes (conjunctivitis), ears, and lungs (pneumonia).

What are the signs or symptoms of NGU?

In men (urethral infection) symptoms may include the following:

- Discharge from the penis
- Burning or pain when urinating
- Itching, irritation, or tenderness
- Underwear stain

Symptoms of NGU in women can include:

- discharge from the vagina;
- burning or pain when urinating; and
- abdominal pain or abnormal vaginal bleeding may be an indication that the infection has progressed to pelvic inflammatory disease (PID).

Anal or oral infections may occur in both men and women. Anal infections may result in rectal itching, discharge, or pain during a bowel movement. Oral infections may occur but most (90 percent) of these infections are asymptomatic. Some people might have a sore throat.

How can I find out if I have NGU?

An NGU diagnosis is made when a person has urethritis (inflammation of the urethra), but gonorrhea is ruled out because they have a negative test result.

What can I do to reduce my risk of getting NGU?

- Practice abstinence. Not having sex is the best protection against acquiring NGU and other STDs.

- Use latex condoms, consistently and correctly, from start to finish every time you have sexual intercourse to reduce the risk of transmission of NGU and other STDs.

- Have sex with only one uninfected partner who only has sex with you (mutual monogamy).

- Have regular check-ups if you are sexually active.

- If you have an STD, don't have sex (oral, vaginal, anal) until all partners have been treated.

- Seek prompt, qualified, and appropriate medical intervention, treatment, and follow-up to break the disease cycle.

- Know your partner(s). Careful consideration and open communication between partners may protect all partners involved from infection.

What is the treatment and follow up for NGU?

The main treatments for NGU are the antibiotics azithromycin and doxycycline. Alternative antibiotics are erythromycin and ofloxacin. A woman who is pregnant, or thinks she might be, should tell her doctor. This will ensure that a medicine will be used that will not harm the baby. Take all medications, even if you start to feel better before you finish the bottle. Inform all partners. Abstain from sex until all partners are treated. Return for evaluation by a health care provider if symptoms persist or if symptoms recur after taking all the prescribed medicine.

Why should I worry about NGU?

Left untreated, the germs that cause NGU, especially chlamydia, can lead to serious complications. For men, complications may include:

- epididymitis (inflammation of the epididymis, the elongated, cordlike structure along the posterior border of the testes) which can lead to infertility if left untreated;

- Reiter's syndrome (arthritis);

- conjunctivitis;

- skin lesions;

125

- discharge;

  In women:

- pelvic inflammatory disease (PID) which can result in ectopic (tubal) pregnancy;

- recurrent PID which may lead to infertility;

- chronic pelvic pain;

- urethritis;

- vaginitis;

- mucopurulent cervicitis (MPC);

- spontaneous abortion (miscarriage).

For men or women, infections caused by anal sex may lead to severe proctitis (inflamed rectum).

Infants exposed to the germs causing NGU during passage through the birth canal may develop conjunctivitis (eye infection) and/or pneumonia.

Do I need to talk to my partner about NGU?

Yes. If you have been told that you have NGU, talk to your partner(s), and let them know so they can be tested and treated. The most common cause of NGU is chlamydia, and it is easy to pass from an infected partner to one who is not infected. A man who is diagnosed with NGU should tell his female sex partner(s) and ask her to get tested. He can prevent serious damage to her body by telling her right away. All sex partners of someone diagnosed with NGU should be treated because:

- they may have an infection and not know it;

- it keeps them from passing the infection to others;

- it prevents them from suffering possible medical complications.

Remember: Do not have sex until your partner(s) have been tested and treated.

Should I talk to my health care provider about NGU?

If you are sexually active with more than one person and do not use latex condoms, then you should talk to your health care provider about being tested for STDs and NGU. Not all STDs cause symptoms, and you may have one and not know it.

Section 15.3

Chlamydia Treatment

Excerpted from "Chlamydial Infections," in *Sexually Transmitted Diseases Treatment Guidelines, 2010*, by the Centers for Disease Control and Prevention (CDC, www.cdc.gov), January 28, 2011.

Chlamydial genital infection is the most frequently reported infectious disease in the United States, and prevalence is highest in persons aged 25 years or younger. Several important sequelae can result from *C. trachomatis* infection in women, the most serious of which include PID, ectopic pregnancy, and infertility. Some women who have uncomplicated cervical infection already have subclinical upper-reproductive–tract infection upon diagnosis.

Asymptomatic infection is common among both men and women. To detect chlamydial infections, health-care providers frequently rely on screening tests. Annual screening of all sexually active women aged 25 years or younger is recommended, as is screening of older women with risk factors (e.g., those who have a new sex partner or multiple sex partners). In June 2007, USPSTF [U.S. Preventive Services Task Force] reviewed and updated their chlamydia screening guidance and found that the epidemiology of chlamydial infection in the United States had not changed since the last review (81,271). In issuing recommendations, USPSTF made the decision to alter the age groups used to demonstrate disease incidence (i.e., from persons aged 25 years or younger to those aged 24 years or younger). CDC has not changed its age cutoff, and thus continues to recommend annual chlamydia screening of sexually active women aged 25 years or younger.

Screening programs have been demonstrated to reduce both the prevalence of *C. trachomatis* infection and rates of PID in women. Although evidence is insufficient to recommend routine screening for *C. trachomatis* in sexually active young men because of several factors (including feasibility, efficacy, and cost-effectiveness), the screening of sexually active young men should be considered in clinical settings with a high prevalence of chlamydia (e.g., adolescent clinics, correctional facilities, and STD clinics). Among women, the primary focus of chlamydia screening efforts should be to detect chlamydia and prevent complications, whereas targeted chlamydia screening in men should only be considered when resources permit and do not hinder chlamydia screening efforts in women. An appropriate sexual risk assessment should be conducted for all persons and might indicate more frequent screening for some women or certain men.

Diagnostic Considerations

C. trachomatis urogenital infection in women can be diagnosed by testing urine or by collecting swab specimens from the endocervix or vagina. Diagnosis of *C. trachomatis* urethral infection in men can be made by testing a urethral swab or urine specimen. Rectal *C. trachomatis* infections in persons that engage in receptive anal intercourse can be diagnosed by testing a rectal swab specimen. NAATs [nucleic acid amplification tests], cell culture, direct immunofluorescence, EIA [enzyme-immuno assay], and nucleic acid hybridization tests are available for the detection of *C. trachomatis* on endocervical specimens and urethral swab specimens from men. NAATs are the most sensitive tests for these specimens and are FDA [U.S. Food and Drug Administration]-cleared for use with urine. Some NAATs are cleared for use with vaginal swab specimens, which can be collected by a provider or self-collected by a patient. Self-collected vaginal swab specimens perform at least as well as with other approved specimens using NAATs, and women find this screening strategy highly acceptable. Rectal and oropharyngeal *C. trachomatis* infection in persons engaging in receptive anal or oral intercourse can be diagnosed by testing at the anatomic site of exposure. Most tests, including NAAT and nucleic acid hybridization tests, are not FDA-cleared for use with rectal or oropharyngeal swab specimens, and chlamydia culture is not widely available for this purpose. However, NAATs have demonstrated improved sensitivity and specificity compared with culture for the detection of *C. trachomatis* at rectal sites and at oropharyngeal sites among men. Some laboratories have met CLIA [Clinical Laboratory Improvement Amendment] requirements and have validated NAAT testing on rectal swab specimens for *C. trachomatis*. Recent evidence suggests that the liquid-based cytology specimens collected for Pap smears might be acceptable specimens for NAAT testing, although test sensitivity using these specimens might be lower than those resulting from the use of cervical swab specimens; regardless, certain NAATs have been FDA-cleared for use on liquid-based cytology specimens. Persons who undergo testing and are diagnosed with chlamydia should be tested for other STDs.

Treatment

Treating infected patients prevents sexual transmission of the disease, and treating all sex partners of those testing positive for chlamydia can prevent reinfection of the index patient and infection of other partners. Treating pregnant women usually prevents transmission of *C. trachomatis* to infants during birth. Chlamydia treatment should be provided promptly for all persons testing positive for infection; delays in receiving chlamydia treatment have been associated with complications (e.g., PID) in a limited proportion of chlamydia-infected subjects. Coinfection with *C. trachomatis* frequently occurs among patients who have gonococcal infection; therefore, presumptive treatment of such patients for chlamydia is appropriate. The following recommended treatment regimens and alternative regimens cure infection and usually relieve symptoms: Azithromycin 1 g orally in a single dose or doxycycline 100 mg orally twice a day for seven days. Alternative regimens include erythromycin base 500 mg orally four times a day for seven days, or erythromycin ethylsuccinate 800 mg orally four times a day for seven days, or levofloxacin 500 mg orally once daily for seven days, or ofloxacin 300 mg orally twice a day for seven days.

A meta-analysis of 12 randomized clinical trials of azithromycin versus doxycycline for the treatment of genital chlamydial infection demonstrated that the treatments were equally efficacious, with microbial cure rates of 97% and 98%, respectively. These studies were conducted primarily in populations in which follow-up was encouraged, adherence to a seven-day regimen was effective, and culture or EIA (rather than the more sensitive NAAT) was used for determining microbiological outcome. Azithromycin should always be available to treat patients for whom compliance with multiday dosing is uncertain. The clinical significance and transmissibility of *C. trachomatis* detected at oropharyngeal sites is unclear, and the efficacy of different antibiotic regimens in resolving oropharyngeal chlamydia remains unknown.

In patients who have erratic health-care–seeking behavior, poor treatment compliance, or unpredictable follow-up, azithromycin might be more cost-effective in treating chlamydia because it enables the provision of a single-dose of directly observed therapy. Erythromycin might be less efficacious than either azithromycin or doxycycline, mainly because of the frequent occurrence of gastrointestinal side effects that can lead to noncompliance. Levofloxacin and ofloxacin are effective treatment alternatives but are more expensive and offer no advantage in the dosage regimen. Other quinolones either are not reliably effective against chlamydial infection or have not been evaluated adequately.

To maximize compliance with recommended therapies, medications for chlamydial infections should be dispensed on site, and the first dose should be directly observed. To minimize disease transmission to sex partners, persons treated for chlamydia should be instructed to abstain from sexual intercourse for seven days after single-dose therapy or until completion of a seven-day regimen. To minimize the risk for reinfection, patients also should be instructed to abstain from sexual intercourse until all of their sex partners are treated.

Follow-Up

Except in pregnant women, test-of-cure (i.e., repeat testing three to four weeks after completing therapy) is not advised for persons treated with the recommended or alterative regimens, unless therapeutic compliance is in question, symptoms persist, or reinfection is suspected. Moreover, the validity of chlamydial diagnostic testing at less than 3 weeks after completion of therapy (to identify patients who did not respond to therapy) has not been established. False-negative results might occur in the presence of persistent infections involving limited numbers of chlamydial organisms. In addition, NAAT conducted at less than three weeks after completion of therapy in persons who were treated successfully could yield false-positive results because of the continued presence of nonviable organisms.

A high prevalence of *C. trachomatis* infection has been observed in women and men who were treated for chlamydial infection during the preceding several months. Most post-treatment infections result from reinfection caused by failure of sex partners to receive treatment or the initiation of sexual activity with a new infected partner. Repeat infections confer an elevated risk for PID and other complications. Unlike the test-of-cure, which is not recommended, repeat *C. trachomatis* testing of recently infected women or men should be a priority for providers. Chlamydia-infected women and men should be retested approximately three months after treatment, regardless of whether they believe that their sex partners were treated. If retesting at three months is not possible, clinicians should retest whenever persons next present for medical care in the 12 months following initial treatment.

Management of Sex Partners

Patients should be instructed to refer their sex partners for evaluation, testing, and treatment if they had sexual contact with the patient during the 60 days preceding onset of the patient's symptoms or chlamydia diagnosis. Although the exposure intervals defined for the identification of at-risk sex partners are based on limited evaluation, the most recent sex partner should be evaluated and treated, even if the time of the last sexual contact was more than 60 days before symptom onset or diagnosis.

Among heterosexual patients, if concerns exist that sex partners who are referred to evaluation and treatment will not seek these services (or if other management strategies are impractical or unsuccessful), patient delivery of antibiotic therapy to their partners can be considered. Compared with standard partner referral, this approach, which involves delivering a prescription or the medication itself, has been associated with a trend toward a decrease in rates of persistent or recurrent chlamydia. Patients must also inform their partners of their infection and provide them with written materials about the importance of seeking evaluation for any symptoms suggestive of complications (e.g., testicular pain in men and pelvic or abdominal pain in women). Patient-delivered partner therapy is not routinely recommended for MSM [men who have sex with men] because of a high risk for coexisting infections, especially undiagnosed HIV [human immunodeficiency virus] infection, in their partners.

Patients should be instructed to abstain from sexual intercourse until they and their sex partners have completed treatment. Abstinence should be continued until seven days after a single-dose regimen or after completion of a multiple-dose regimen. Timely treatment of sex partners is essential for decreasing the risk for reinfecting the index patient.

Chapter 16

Donovanosis (Granuloma Inguinale)

Donovanosis (granuloma inguinale) is a sexually transmitted disease that is rarely seen in the United States.

Causes

Donovanosis (granuloma inguinale) is caused by the bacteria *Klebsiella granulomatis*. The disease is commonly found in tropical and subtropical areas such as Southeast India, Guyana, and New Guinea. However, it can sometimes occur in the United States, typically in the Southeast. There are about 100 cases reported per year in the United States.

The disease spreads mostly through vaginal or anal intercourse. Very rarely, it spreads during oral sex.

Men are affected more than twice as often as women. Most infections occur in people ages 20–40. The disease is rarely seen in children or the elderly.

Symptoms

Symptoms can occur 1 to 12 weeks after coming in contact with the bacteria that cause the disease.

- About half of infected men and women have sores in the anal area.

- Small, beefy-red bumps appear on the genitals or around the anus.
- The skin gradually wears away, and the bumps turn into raised, beefy-red, velvety nodules called granulation tissue. They are usually painless, but they bleed easily if injured.
- The disease slowly spreads and destroys genital tissue.
- Tissue damage may spread to the area where the legs meet the torso. This area is called the inguinal folds.
- The genitals and the skin around them lose skin color.

In its early stages, it may be hard to tell the difference between donovanosis and chancroid.

In the later stages, donovanosis may look like advanced genital cancers, lymphogranuloma venereum, and anogenital cutaneous amebiasis.

Exams and Tests

It may be donovanosis if genital sores have been present for a long time and have been spreading.

Tests that may be done include:

- culture of tissue sample (hard to do and not routinely available);
- scrapings or punch biopsy of lesion.

Laboratory tests, such as those used to detect syphilis, are available only on a research basis for diagnosing donovanosis.

Treatment

Antibiotics are used to treat donovanosis. To cure the condition requires long-term treatment. Most treatment courses run three weeks or until the sores have completely healed.

A follow-up examination is important because the disease can reappear after it seems to be cured.

Outlook (Prognosis)

Treating this disease early decreases the chances of tissue damage or scarring. Untreated disease leads to damage of the genital tissue.

Possible Complications

- Genital damage and scarring
- Loss of skin color in genital area
- Permanent genital swelling due to scarring

When to Contact a Medical Professional

Call for an appointment with your health care provider if:

- you have had sexual contact with a person who is known to have donovanosis;
- you develop symptoms of donovanosis.

Prevention

Avoiding all sexual activity is the only absolute way to prevent a sexually transmitted disease such as donovanosis. However, safer sex behaviors may reduce your risk.

The proper use of condoms, either the male or female type, greatly decreases the risk of catching a sexually transmitted disease. You need to wear the condom from the beginning to the end of each sexual activity.

Alternative Names

Granuloma inguinale

References

Ballard RC. Klebsiella granulomatis (Donovanosis, Granuloma Inguinale). In: Mandell GL, Bennett JE, Dolin R, eds. *Principles and Practice of Infectious Diseases*. 7th ed. Philadelphia, Pa: Elsevier Churchill Livingstone; 2009:chap 236.

Eckert LO, Lentz GM. Infections of the lower genital tract: vulva, vagina, cervix, toxic shock syndrome, HIV infections. In: Katz VL, Lentz GM, Lobo RA, Gershenson DM, eds. *Comprehensive Gynecology*. 5th ed. Philadelphia, Pa: Mosby Elsevier; 2007:chap 22.

Workowski KA, Berman SM. Centers for Disease Control and Prevention. Sexually transmitted diseases treatment guidelines 2010. *MMWR* Recomm Rep. 2010 Dec 17:59:1–110.

Chapter 17

Gonorrhea

Chapter Contents

Section 17.1—What Is Gonorrhea? 138

Section 17.2—Gonorrhea Treatment 141

Section 17.3—Antibiotic-Resistant Gonorrhea Infections 144

Section 17.1

What Is Gonorrhea?

"Gonorrhea—CDC Fact Sheet," by the Centers for Disease Control
and Prevention (CDC, www.cdc.gov), April 5, 2011.

What is gonorrhea?

Gonorrhea is a sexually transmitted disease (STD) caused by a bacterium. Gonorrhea can grow easily in the warm, moist areas of the reproductive tract, including the cervix (opening to the womb), uterus (womb), and fallopian tubes (egg canals) in women, and in the urethra (urine canal) in women and men. The bacterium can also grow in the mouth, throat, eyes, and anus.

How common is gonorrhea?

Gonorrhea is a very common infectious disease. CDC estimates that, annually, more than 700,000 people in the United States get new gonorrhea infections and less than half of these infections are reported to CDC. In 2010, 309,341 cases of gonorrhea were reported to CDC.

How do people get gonorrhea?

People get gonorrhea by having sex with someone who has the disease. Having sex means anal, vaginal, or oral sex. Gonorrhea can still be transmitted even if a man does not ejaculate. Gonorrhea can also be spread from an untreated mother to her baby during childbirth.

People who have had gonorrhea and have been treated may get infected again if they have sexual contact with a person infected with gonorrhea.

Who is at risk for gonorrhea?

Any sexually active person can be infected with gonorrhea. It is a very common STD. In the United States, the highest reported rates of infection are among sexually active teenagers, young adults, and African Americans.

What are the symptoms of gonorrhea?

Some men with gonorrhea may have no symptoms at all. However, common symptoms in men include a burning sensation when urinating, or a white, yellow, or green discharge from the penis that usually appears 1 to 14 days after infection. Sometimes men with gonorrhea get painful or swollen testicles.

Most women with gonorrhea do not have any symptoms. Even when a woman has symptoms, they are often mild and can be mistaken for a bladder or vaginal infection. The initial symptoms in women can include a painful or burning sensation when urinating, increased vaginal discharge, or vaginal bleeding between periods. Women with gonorrhea are at risk of developing serious complications from the infection, even if symptoms are not present or are mild.

Symptoms of rectal infection in both men and women may include discharge, anal itching, soreness, bleeding, or painful bowel movements. Rectal infections may also cause no symptoms. Infections in the throat may cause a sore throat, but usually cause no symptoms.

What are the complications of gonorrhea?

Untreated gonorrhea can cause serious and permanent health problems in both women and men.

In women, gonorrhea can spread into the uterus (womb) or fallopian tubes (egg canals) and cause pelvic inflammatory disease (PID). The symptoms may be mild or can be very severe and can include abdominal pain and fever. PID can lead to internal abscesses (pus-filled pockets that are hard to cure) and chronic (long-lasting) pelvic pain. PID can damage the fallopian tubes enough that a woman will be unable to have children. It also can increase her risk of ectopic pregnancy. Ectopic pregnancy is a life-threatening condition in which a fertilized egg grows outside the uterus, usually in a fallopian tube.

In men, gonorrhea can cause a painful condition called epididymitis in the tubes attached to the testicles. In rare cases, this may prevent a man from being able to father children.

If not treated, gonorrhea can also spread to the blood or joints. This condition can be life-threatening.

What about gonorrhea and HIV?

Untreated gonorrhea can increase a person's risk of acquiring or transmitting HIV (human immunodeficiency virus)—the virus that causes AIDS (acquired immunodeficiency syndrome).

How does gonorrhea affect a pregnant woman and her baby?

If a pregnant woman has gonorrhea, she may give the infection to her baby as the baby passes through the birth canal during delivery. This can cause serious health problems for the baby. Treating gonorrhea as soon as it is detected in pregnant women will make these health outcomes less likely. Pregnant women should consult a health care provider for appropriate examination, testing, and treatment, as necessary.

Who should be tested for gonorrhea?

Any sexually active person can be infected with gonorrhea. Anyone with genital symptoms such as discharge, burning during urination, unusual sores, or rash should stop having sex and see a health care provider immediately.

Also, anyone with an oral, anal, or vaginal sex partner who has been recently diagnosed with an STD should see a health care provider for evaluation.

Some people should be tested for gonorrhea even if they do not have symptoms or know of a sex partner who has gonorrhea. Anyone who is sexually active should discuss his or her risk factors with a health care provider and ask whether he or she should be tested for gonorrhea or other STDs.

People who have gonorrhea should also be tested for other STDs.

How is gonorrhea diagnosed?

Most of the time, a urine test can be used to test for gonorrhea. However, if a person has had oral and/or anal sex, swabs may be used to collect samples from the throat and/or rectum. In some cases, a swab may be used to collect a sample from a man's urethra (urine canal) or a woman's cervix (opening to the womb).

What about partners?

If a person has been diagnosed and treated for gonorrhea, he or she should tell all recent anal, vaginal, or oral sex partners so they can see a health care provider and be treated. This will reduce the risk that the sex partners will develop serious complications from gonorrhea and will also reduce the person's risk of becoming reinfected. A person with gonorrhea and all of his or her sex partners must avoid having sex until they have completed their treatment for gonorrhea and until they no longer have symptoms.

How can gonorrhea be prevented?

Latex condoms, when used consistently and correctly, can reduce the risk of getting or giving gonorrhea. The most certain way to avoid gonorrhea is to not have sex or to be in a long-term, mutually monogamous relationship with a partner who has been tested and is known to be uninfected.

Section 17.2

Gonorrhea Treatment

Excerpted from "Gonococcal Infections,"
by the Centers for Disease Control and Prevention
(CDC, www.cdc.gov), January 28, 2011.

In the United States, an estimated 700,000 new *N. gonorrhoeae* infections occur each year. Gonorrhea is the second most commonly reported bacterial STD [sexually transmitted disease]. The majority of urethral infections caused by *N. gonorrhoeae* among men produce symptoms that cause them to seek curative treatment soon enough to prevent serious sequelae, but treatment might not be soon enough to prevent transmission to others. Among women, gonococcal infections might not produce recognizable symptoms until complications (e.g., PID [pelvic inflammatory disease]) have occurred. PID can result in tubal scarring that can lead to infertility or ectopic pregnancy.

Patients infected with *N. gonorrhoeae* frequently are coinfected with *C. trachomatis* [chlamydia]; this finding has led to the recommendation that patients treated for gonococcal infection also be treated routinely with a regimen that is effective against uncomplicated genital *C. trachomatis* infection. Because most gonococci in the United States are susceptible to doxycycline and azithromycin, routine cotreatment might also hinder the development of antimicrobial-resistant *N. gonorrhoeae*. Limited data suggest that dual treatment with azithromycin might enhance treatment efficacy for pharyngeal infection when using oral cephalosporins.

Antimicrobial-Resistant N. gonorrhoeae

Gonorrhea treatment is complicated by the ability of *N. gonorrhoeae* to develop resistance to antimicrobial therapies. Quinolone-resistant *N. gonorrhoeae* strains are now widely disseminated throughout the United States and the world. As of April 2007, quinolones are no longer recommended in the United States for the treatment of gonorrhea and associated conditions, such as PID. Consequently, only one class of antimicrobials, the cephalosporins, is recommended and available for the treatment of gonorrhea in the United States. The CDC website (http://www.cdc.gov/std/gisp) and state health departments can provide the most current information.

To maximize compliance with recommended therapies, medications for gonococcal infections should be dispensed on site. Ceftriaxone in a single injection of 250 mg provides sustained, high bactericidal levels in the blood. Extensive clinical experience indicates that ceftriaxone is safe and effective for the treatment of uncomplicated gonorrhea at all anatomic sites, curing 99.2% of uncomplicated urogenital and anorectal and 98.9% of pharyngeal infections in published clinical trials. A 250-mg dose of ceftriaxone is now recommended over a 125-mg dose given the 1) increasingly wide geographic distribution of isolates demonstrating decreased susceptibility to cephalosporins in vitro, 2) reports of ceftriaxone treatment failures, 3) improved efficacy of ceftriaxone 250 mg in pharyngeal infection (which is often unrecognized), and 4) the utility of having a simple and consistent recommendation for treatment regardless of the anatomic site involved.

A 400-mg oral dose of cefixime does not provide as high, nor as sustained, a bactericidal level as that provided by the 250-mg dose of ceftriaxone. In published clinical trials, the 400-mg dose cured 97.5% of uncomplicated urogenital and anorectal and 92.3% of pharyngeal gonococcal infections. Although cefixime can be administered orally, this advantage is offset by the limited efficacy of cefixime (as well as other oral cephalosporins) for treating gonococcal infections of the pharynx. Providers should inquire about oral sexual exposure and if reported, treat these patients with ceftriaxone because of this drug's well documented efficacy in treating pharyngeal infection.

Single-dose injectable cephalosporin regimens (other than ceftriaxone 250 mg IM [intramuscularly]) that are safe and highly effective against uncomplicated urogenital and anorectal gonococcal infections include ceftizoxime (500 mg, administered IM), cefoxitin (2 g, administered IM with probenecid 1 g orally), and cefotaxime (500 mg, administered IM). None of the injectable cephalosporins offer any advantage over ceftriaxone for urogenital infection, and efficacy for pharyngeal infection is less certain.

Management of Sex Partners

Effective clinical management of patients with treatable STDs requires treatment of the patients' recent sex partners to prevent reinfection and curtail further transmission. Patients should be instructed to refer their sex partners for evaluation and treatment. Sex partners of patients with *N. gonorrhoeae* infection whose last sexual contact with the patient was within 60 days before onset of symptoms or diagnosis of infection in the patient should be evaluated and treated for *N. gonorrhoeae* and *C. trachomatis* infections. If a patient's last sexual intercourse was more than 60 days before onset of symptoms or diagnosis, the patient's most recent sex partner should be treated. Patients should be instructed to abstain from sexual intercourse until therapy is completed and until they and their sex partners no longer have symptoms.

For heterosexual patients with gonorrhea whose partners' treatment cannot be ensured or is unlikely, delivery of antibiotic therapy for gonorrhea (as well as for chlamydia) by the patients to their partners can be considered. Use of this approach should always be accompanied by efforts to educate partners about symptoms and to encourage partners to seek clinical evaluation. For male patients informing female partners, educational materials should include information about the importance of seeking medical evaluation for PID (especially if symptomatic). Possible undertreatment of PID in female partners and possible missed opportunities to diagnose other STDs are of concern and have not been evaluated in comparison with patient-delivered therapy and partner referral. This approach should not be considered a routine partner management strategy in MSM because of the high risk for coexisting undiagnosed STDs or HIV infection.

Section 17.3

Antibiotic-Resistant Gonorrhea Infections

Excerpted from "Antibiotic-Resistant Gonorrhea (ARG)
Basic Information," by the Centers for Disease Control and
Prevention (CDC, www.cdc.gov), April 5, 2011.

The development of antibiotic resistance in *Neisseria gonorrhoeae* is a growing public health concern, in particular because the United States gonorrhea control strategy relies on effective antibiotic therapy. Since antibiotics were first used for treatment of gonorrhea, *N. gonorrhoeae* has progressively developed resistance to the antibiotic drugs prescribed to treat it: Sulfanilamide, penicillin, tetracycline, and ciprofloxacin. Currently, CDC STD treatment guidelines recommend dual therapy with the injectable cephalosporin ceftriaxone and either azithromycin or doxycycline to treat all uncomplicated gonococcal infections among adults and adolescents in the United States. Dual therapy is recommended to address the potential emergence of gonococcal cephalosporin resistance. Given the ability of *N. gonorrhoeae* to develop antibiotic resistance, it is critical to continuously monitor gonococcal antibiotic resistance and encourage research and development of new treatment regimens for gonorrhea.

Trends

In 1993, ciprofloxacin (a fluoroquinolone) and cephalosporins (ceftriaxone and cefixime) were the recommended treatments for gonorrhea. However, in the late 1990s and early 2000s, ciprofloxacin resistance was detected in Hawaii and the West Coast, and by 2004, ciprofloxacin resistance was detected among men who have sex with men (MSM) with gonorrhea. By 2006, 13.8% of isolates exhibited resistance to ciprofloxacin, and ciprofloxacin resistance was present in all regions of the country, including the heterosexual population. On April 13, 2007, CDC stopped recommending fluoroquinolones as treatment for gonococcal infections for all persons in the United States.

Susceptibility testing for the cephalosporin antibiotics is being conducted on ceftriaxone, cefixime, and cefpodoxime. CDC has observed recent worrisome trends in decreasing cephalosporin susceptibility, especially to oral cephalosporins such as cefixime. So far, none of the *N. gonorrhoeae* isolates tested have exhibited resistance, and CDC has not received any reports of clinical treatment failures to any cephalosporin in the United States.

In 2010, 27.2% of isolates collected were resistant to penicillin, tetracycline, ciprofloxacin, or a combination of these antimicrobials.

Challenges

A major challenge to monitoring emerging antimicrobial resistance of *N. gonorrhoeae* is the substantial decline in capability of laboratories to perform essential gonorrhea culture techniques required for antibiotic susceptibility testing. This decline results from an increased use of newer non-culture-based laboratory technology, such as a diagnostic test called the Nucleic Acid Amplification Test (NAAT). Currently, there is no reliable technology that allows for antibiotic susceptibility testing from non-culture specimens. Increased laboratory culture capacity is needed.

Chapter 18

Herpes

Chapter Contents

Section 18.1—Genital Herpes 148

Section 18.2—Oral Herpes 151

Section 18.3—Treating and Managing Herpes 155

Section 18.1

Genital Herpes

Excerpted from "Genital Herpes—CDC Fact Sheet," by the Centers for Disease Control and Prevention (CDC, www.cdc.gov), January 31, 2012.

What is genital herpes?

Genital herpes is a sexually transmitted disease (STD) caused by the herpes simplex viruses type 1 (HSV-1) or type 2 (HSV-2). Most genital herpes is caused by HSV-2. Most individuals have no or only minimal signs or symptoms from HSV-1 or HSV-2 infection. When signs do occur, they typically appear as one or more blisters on or around the genitals or rectum. The blisters break, leaving tender ulcers (sores) that may take two to four weeks to heal the first time they occur. Typically, another outbreak can appear weeks or months after the first, but it almost always is less severe and shorter than the first outbreak. Although the infection can stay in the body indefinitely, the number of outbreaks tends to decrease over a period of years.

How common is genital herpes?

Results of a nationally representative study show that genital herpes infection is common in the United States. Nationwide, 16.2%, or about one out of six, people 14 to 49 years of age have genital HSV-2 infection. Over the past decade, the percentage of Americans with genital herpes infection in the United States has remained stable.

Genital HSV-2 infection is more common in women (approximately one out of five women 14 to 49 years of age) than in men (about one out of nine men 14 to 49 years of age). Transmission from an infected male to his female partner is more likely than from an infected female to her male partner.

How do people get genital herpes?

HSV-1 and HSV-2 can be found in and released from the sores that the viruses cause, but they also are released between outbreaks from skin that does not appear to have a sore. Generally, a person can only get HSV-2 infection during sexual contact with someone who has a genital HSV-2 infection. Transmission can occur from an infected partner who does not have a visible sore and may not know that he or she is infected.

HSV-1 can cause genital herpes, but it more commonly causes infections of the mouth and lips, so-called fever blisters. HSV-1 infection of the genitals can be caused by oral-genital or genital-genital contact with a person who has HSV-1 infection. Genital HSV-1 outbreaks recur less regularly than genital HSV-2 outbreaks.

What are the signs and symptoms of genital herpes?

Most people infected with HSV-2 are not aware of their infection. However, if signs and symptoms occur during the first outbreak, they can be quite pronounced. The first outbreak usually occurs within two weeks after the virus is transmitted, and the sores typically heal within two to four weeks. Other signs and symptoms during the primary episode may include a second crop of sores, and flu-like symptoms, including fever and swollen glands. However, most individuals with HSV-2 infection never have sores, or they have very mild signs that they do not even notice or that they mistake for insect bites or another skin condition.

People diagnosed with a first episode of genital herpes can expect to have several (typically four or five) outbreaks (symptomatic recurrences) within a year. Over time these recurrences usually decrease in frequency. It is possible that a person becomes aware of the first episode years after the infection is acquired.

What are the complications of genital herpes?

Genital herpes can cause recurrent painful genital sores in many adults, and herpes infection can be severe in people with suppressed immune systems. Regardless of severity of symptoms, genital herpes frequently causes psychological distress in people who know they are infected.

In addition, genital HSV can lead to potentially fatal infections in babies. It is important that women avoid contracting herpes during pregnancy because a newly acquired infection during late pregnancy poses a greater risk of transmission to the baby. If a woman has active genital herpes at delivery, a cesarean delivery is usually performed. Fortunately, infection of a baby from a woman with herpes infection is rare.

149

Herpes may play a role in the spread of HIV [human immunodeficiency virus], the virus that causes AIDS [acquired immunodeficiency syndrome]. Herpes can make people more susceptible to HIV infection, and it can make HIV-infected individuals more infectious.

How is genital herpes diagnosed?

The signs and symptoms associated with HSV-2 can vary greatly. Health care providers can diagnose genital herpes by visual inspection if the outbreak is typical, and by taking a sample from the sore(s) and testing it in a laboratory. HSV infections can be diagnosed between outbreaks by the use of a blood test. Blood tests, which detect antibodies to HSV-1 or HSV-2 infection, can be helpful, although the results are not always clear-cut.

How can herpes be prevented?

The surest way to avoid transmission of sexually transmitted diseases, including genital herpes, is to abstain from sexual contact, or to be in a long-term mutually monogamous relationship with a partner who has been tested and is known to be uninfected.

Genital ulcer diseases can occur in both male and female genital areas that are covered or protected by a latex condom, as well as in areas that are not covered. Correct and consistent use of latex condoms can reduce the risk of genital herpes.

Persons with herpes should abstain from sexual activity with uninfected partners when lesions or other symptoms of herpes are present. It is important to know that even if a person does not have any symptoms he or she can still infect sex partners. Sex partners of infected persons should be advised that they may become infected and they should use condoms to reduce the risk. Sex partners can seek testing to determine if they are infected with HSV. A positive HSV-2 blood test most likely indicates a genital herpes infection.

Section 18.2

Oral Herpes

Oral herpes is an infection of the lips, mouth, or gums due to the herpes simplex virus. It causes small, painful blisters commonly called cold sores or fever blisters. Oral herpes is also called herpes labialis.

Causes

Oral herpes is a common infection of the mouth area. It is caused by the herpes simplex virus type 1 (HSV-1). Most people in the United States are infected with this virus by age 20.

After the first infection, the virus goes to sleep (becomes dormant) in the nerve tissues in the face. Sometimes, the virus later wakes up (reactivates), causing cold sores.

Herpes virus type 2 (HSV-2) usually causes genital herpes. However, sometimes HSV-2 is spread to the mouth during oral sex, causing oral herpes.

Herpes viruses spread easily. You can catch this virus if you have intimate or personal contact with someone who is infected. You can also catch it if you touch items infected with the herpes virus, such as infected razors, towels, dishes, and other shared items. Parents may spread the virus to their children during regular daily activities.

Symptoms

Some people get mouth ulcers when they first come into contact with HSV-1 virus. Others have no symptoms. Symptoms usually occur in kids between one and five years old.

Symptoms may be mild or severe.

They usually appear within one to three weeks after you come into contact with the virus. They may last up to three weeks.

Warning symptoms include:

• itching of the lips or skin around mouth;

- burning near the lips or mouth area;
- tingling near the lips or mouth area.

Before blisters appear, you may have:

- sore throat;
- fever;
- swollen glands;
- painful swallowing.

Blisters or a rash may form on your:

- gums;
- lips;
- mouth;
- throat.

Many blisters are called an outbreak. You may have:

- red blisters that break open and leak;
- small blisters filled with clear yellowish fluid;
- several smaller blisters may grow together into a large blister.

As the blister heals, it gets yellow and crusty, eventually turning into pink skin.

Symptoms may be triggered by:

- menstruation or hormone changes;
- being out in the sun;
- fever;
- stress.

If the symptoms return later, they are usually more mild.

Exams and Tests

Your doctor or nurse can diagnose oral herpes by looking at your mouth area. Sometimes, a sample of the sore is taken and sent to a laboratory for closer examination. Tests may include:

- viral culture;

- viral DNA [deoxyribonucleic acid] test;

- Tzanck test to check for HSV.

Treatment

Symptoms may go away on their own without treatment in one to two weeks.

Your health care provider can prescribe medicines to fight the virus. This is called antiviral medicine. It can help reduce pain and make your symptoms go away sooner. Medicines used to treat mouth sores include:

- acyclovir;

- famciclovir;

- valacyclovir.

These medicines work best if you take them when you have warning signs of a mouth sore, before any blisters develop. If you get mouth sores frequently, your doctor may tell you to take these medicines all the time.

Antiviral skin creams may also be used. However, they are expensive and often only shorten the outbreak by a few hours to a day.

The following steps can also help make you feel better:

- Apply ice or a warm washcloth to the sores to help ease pain.

- Wash the blister gently with germ-fighting (antiseptic) soap and water. This helps prevent spreading the virus to other body areas.

- Avoid hot beverages, spicy and salty foods, and citrus.

- Gargle with cool water or eat popsicles.

- Rinse with salt water.

- Take a pain reliever such as acetaminophen (Tylenol).

Outlook (Prognosis)

Oral herpes usually goes away by itself in one to two weeks. However, it may come back.

Herpes infection may be severe and dangerous if:

- it occurs in or near the eye;
- you have a weakened immune system due to certain diseases and medications.

Possible Complications

Herpes infection of the eye is a leading cause of blindness in the United States. It causes scarring of the cornea.

Other complications of oral herpes may include:

- return of mouth sores and blisters;
- spread of the virus to other skin areas;
- bacterial skin infection;
- widespread body infection, which may be life threatening in people who have a weakened immune system due to atopic dermatitis, cancer, or HIV [human immunodeficiency virus] infection.

When to Contact a Medical Professional

Call for an appointment with your health care provider if you have:

- symptoms that are severe or that don't go away after two weeks;
- sores or blisters near your eyes;
- herpes symptoms and a weakened immune system due to certain diseases or medicines.

Prevention

Here are some tips to prevent mouth sores:

- Apply sunblock or lip balm containing zinc oxide to your lips before you go outside.
- A moisturizing balm to prevent the lips from becoming too dry may also help.
- Avoid direct contact with herpes sores.
- Wash items such as towels and linens in boiling hot water after each use.
- Do not share utensils, straws, glasses, or other items if someone has oral herpes.

154

Do not have oral sex if you have oral herpes, especially if you have blisters. You can spread the virus to the genitals, causing herpes simplex virus 2, or genital herpes. Both oral and genital herpes viruses can sometimes be spread even when you do not have mouth sores or blisters.

Section 18.3

Treating and Managing Herpes

Excerpted from "Genital Herpes Fact Sheet," by the
Office on Women's Health, part of the U.S. Department of Health
and Human Services, August 10, 2009.

Herpes symptoms can come and go, but the virus stays inside your body even after all signs of the infection have gone away. In most people, the virus becomes active from time to time, creating an outbreak. Some people have herpes virus outbreaks only once or twice. People who have a first outbreak can expect to have four or five outbreaks within a year. Over time, the outbreaks tend to occur less often and be less severe. Experts don't know what causes the virus to become active. Some women say the virus comes back when they are sick, under stress, out in the sun, or during their period.

Doctors can diagnose genital herpes by looking at visible sores if the outbreak is typical and by taking a sample from the sore for testing in a lab. Some cases of herpes are harder to diagnose, especially between outbreaks. Blood tests that look for antibodies to HSV-1 or HSV-2 can help to detect herpes infection in people without symptoms or between outbreaks.

What is the treatment for genital herpes?

Genital herpes cannot be cured; the virus will always be in your body. But the antiviral drugs acyclovir, valacyclovir, and famciclovir can shorten outbreaks and make them less severe, or stop them from happening. Valacyclovir (brand name Valtrex) also can lower your risk of passing the infection to someone else.

Depending on your needs, your doctor can give you drugs to take right after getting outbreak symptoms or drugs to take on a regular basis to try to stop outbreaks from happening. Talk to your doctor about treatment options.

During outbreaks, these steps can speed healing and help keep the infection from spreading to other sites of the body or to other people:

- Keep the infected area clean and dry.

- Try not to touch the sores.

- Wash hands after contact.

- Avoid sexual contact from the time you first notice symptoms until the sores have healed.

Is there a cure for genital herpes?

No. Once you have the virus, it stays in your body and there is a chance that you will have outbreaks. Medicine can shorten and stop outbreaks from happening.

Research is underway to develop new ways to protect women from the herpes virus and prevent its spread. One large study is testing a herpes vaccine for women. Researchers are also working to make gels or creams that would kill the virus before it could infect someone.

Can genital herpes cause problems during pregnancy?

Yes. If the mother is having her first outbreak near the time of delivery, she is much more likely to pass the virus to her baby. If the outbreak is not the first one, the baby's risk of getting the virus is very low. Babies born with herpes may be premature or may die, or they may have brain damage, severe rashes, or eye problems. Doctors may do a cesarean delivery if the mother has herpes sores near the birth canal to lower the risk of passing the virus. Fortunately, most women with genital herpes have healthy babies. Also, medicines can help babies born with herpes if they are treated right away.

It is not yet known if all genital herpes drugs are safe for pregnant women to take. Some doctors may recommend acyclovir be taken either as a pill or intravenously (IV, or a needle into a vein) during pregnancy. Let your doctor know if you have genital herpes, even if you are not having an outbreak. He or she will help you manage it safely during pregnancy.

Can I breastfeed if I have genital herpes?

If you have genital herpes, you can keep breastfeeding as long as the sores are covered. Herpes is spread through contact with sores and can be dangerous to a newborn. If you have sores on your nipple or areola, the darker skin around the nipple, you should stop breastfeeding on that breast. Pump or hand express your milk from that breast until the sore clears. Pumping will help keep up your milk supply and prevent your breast from getting overly full. You can store your milk to give to your baby in a bottle at another feeding. If the parts of your breast pump that contact the milk also touch the sore(s) while pumping, you should throw the milk away.

Can genital herpes cause other problems?

Genital herpes infection usually does not cause serious health problems in healthy adults. People whose immune systems don't work properly, such as people with HIV [human immunodeficiency virus], can have severe outbreaks that are long-lasting. Sometimes, people with normal immune systems can get herpes infection in the eye. But this is less common with HSV-2 infection.

Herpes may play a role in the spread of HIV, the virus that causes AIDS [acquired immunodeficiency syndrome]. Herpes sores can make it easier for HIV to get into your body. Also, herpes can make people who are HIV-positive more infectious.

Living with herpes can be hard to cope with even if you have no symptoms. At first, you might feel embarrassed or ashamed. You might worry whether having herpes will affect your relationship with your sexual partner or keep you from having meaningful relationships in the future. Keep in mind that millions of people have herpes. And not unlike many other health issues, treatment can help you manage the infection. After a little time, most people with herpes are able to adjust to the diagnosis and move on. Let your doctor know if you're having a hard time adjusting. Talking to someone about your feelings may help.

What can I do to keep from getting genital herpes?

There are things you can do to lower your risk of getting genital herpes:

- Don't have sex. The surest way to prevent any STI, including genital herpes, is to practice abstinence, or not having vaginal, oral, or anal sex. Keep in mind, you can get genital herpes from close contact other than sexual intercourse.

157

- Be faithful. Having a sexual relationship with one partner who has been tested for herpes and is not infected is another way to lower your risk of getting infected. Be faithful to each other, meaning that you only have sex with each other and no one else.

- Use condoms. Use condoms correctly and every time you have any type of sex. For vaginal sex, use a latex male condom or a female polyurethane condom. For anal sex, use a latex male condom. For oral sex, use a dental dam. Keep in mind that condoms may not cover all infected areas, so you can still get herpes even if you use a condom.

- Know that some methods of birth control, like birth control pills, shots, implants, or diaphragms, will not protect you from STIs. If you use one of these methods, be sure to also use a latex condom or dental dam correctly and every time you have sex.

- Talk with your sex partner(s) about STIs and using condoms. It's up to you to make sure you are protected. If your partner is infected, take steps to lower your risk of getting herpes from your partner.

- Talk frankly with your doctor and your sex partner(s) about any STIs you or your partner has or has had. If you feel embarrassed, try to put this aside. Your doctor is there to help you with any and all health problems. Also, being open with your partners can help you protect your health and the health of others.

- Know the symptoms. Learn the common symptoms of genital herpes and other STIs. Do not have oral-genital contact if you or your partner has any signs of oral herpes, such as a fever blister. Seek medical help right away if you think you may have genital herpes or another STI. Don't have sexual contact until you have seen your doctor.

What should I do if I have genital herpes?

- See your doctor for testing and treatment right away.

- Follow your doctor's orders and finish all the medicine that you are given. Even if the symptoms go away, you still need to finish all of the medicine.

- Avoid having any sexual activity while you are being treated for genital herpes and while you have any symptoms of an outbreak.

- Be sure to tell your sexual partners, so they can be tested.

- Remember that genital herpes is a lifelong disease. Even though you may have long periods with no symptoms, you can still pass the virus to another person. Talk with your doctor about what you can do to have fewer future outbreaks, and how to prevent passing the virus to another person.

What should I do if my partner has genital herpes?

- Get tested to find out if you also are infected with the herpes virus.

- Avoid having any sexual activity while your partner is being treated for a genital herpes outbreak or if your partner has symptoms of an outbreak, such as open sores.

- Use condoms correctly and every time you have sex to lower your risk of becoming infected. Keep in mind that you can become infected with the herpes virus since condoms do not always cover all infected areas. Also, the virus can spread even if no symptoms are present.

- Talk to your partner about using daily suppressive therapy to reduce the number of outbreaks and lower the risk of infecting you with the virus.

Chapter 19

Hepatitis

Chapter Contents

Section 19.1—What Is Hepatitis? 162

Section 19.2—Hepatitis and HIV Coinfection 174

Section 19.3—Treating Hepatitis 178

Section 19.1

What Is Hepatitis?

Excerpted from "Hepatitis B FAQs for the Public,"
by the Centers for Disease Control and Prevention
(CDC, www.cdc.gov), June 9, 2009.

What is hepatitis?

Hepatitis means inflammation of the liver. Toxins, certain drugs, some diseases, heavy alcohol use, and bacterial and viral infections can all cause hepatitis. Hepatitis is also the name of a family of viral infections that affect the liver; the most common types are hepatitis A, hepatitis B, and hepatitis C.

What is the difference between hepatitis A, hepatitis B, and hepatitis C?

Hepatitis A, hepatitis B, and hepatitis C are diseases caused by three different viruses. Although each can cause similar symptoms, they have different modes of transmission and can affect the liver differently. Hepatitis A appears only as an acute or newly occurring infection and does not become chronic. People with hepatitis A usually improve without treatment. Hepatitis B and hepatitis C can also begin as acute infections, but in some people, the virus remains in the body, resulting in chronic disease and long-term liver problems. There are vaccines to prevent hepatitis A and B; however, there is not one for hepatitis C. If a person has had one type of viral hepatitis in the past, it is still possible to get the other types.

What is hepatitis B?

Hepatitis B is a contagious liver disease that ranges in severity from a mild illness lasting a few weeks to a serious, lifelong illness. It results from infection with the hepatitis B virus. Hepatitis B can be either acute or chronic.

Acute hepatitis B virus infection is a short-term illness that occurs within the first six months after someone is exposed to the hepatitis

B virus. Acute infection can—but does not always—lead to chronic infection.

Chronic hepatitis B virus infection is a long-term illness that occurs when the hepatitis B virus remains in a person's body.

How common is acute hepatitis B in the United States?

In 2007, there were an estimated 43,000 new hepatitis B virus infections in the United States. However, the official number of reported hepatitis B cases is much lower. Many people don't know they are infected or may not have symptoms and therefore never seek the attention of medical or public health officials.

Has the number of people in the United States with acute hepatitis B been decreasing?

Yes, rates of acute hepatitis B in the United States have declined by approximately 82% since 1990. At that time, routine hepatitis B vaccination of children was implemented and has dramatically decreased the rates of the disease in the United States, particularly among children.

How common is chronic hepatitis B in the United States?

In the United States, an estimated 800,000 to 1.4 million persons have chronic hepatitis B virus infection.

How common is chronic hepatitis B outside the United States?

Globally, chronic hepatitis B affects approximately 350 million people and contributes to an estimated 620,000 deaths worldwide each year.

How likely is it that acute hepatitis B will become chronic?

The likelihood depends upon the age at which someone becomes infected. The younger a person is when infected with hepatitis B virus, the greater his or her chance of developing chronic hepatitis B. Approximately 90% of infected infants will develop chronic infection. The risk goes down as a child gets older. Approximately 25%–50% of children infected between the ages of 1 and 5 years will develop chronic hepatitis. The risk drops to 6%–10% when a person is infected over

163

5 years of age. Worldwide, most people with chronic hepatitis B were infected at birth or during early childhood.

How is hepatitis B spread?

Hepatitis B is spread when blood, semen, or other body fluid infected with the hepatitis B virus enters the body of a person who is not infected. People can become infected with the virus during activities such as the following:

- Birth (spread from an infected mother to her baby during birth)
- Sex with an infected partner
- Sharing needles, syringes, or other drug-injection equipment
- Sharing items such as razors or toothbrushes with an infected person
- Direct contact with the blood or open sores of an infected person
- Exposure to blood from needle sticks or other sharp instruments

Can a person spread hepatitis B and not know it?

Yes. Many people with chronic hepatitis B virus infection do not know they are infected since they do not feel or look sick. However, they still can spread the virus to others and are at risk of serious health problems themselves.

Can hepatitis B be spread through sex?

Yes. Among adults in the United States, hepatitis B is most commonly spread through sexual contact and accounts for nearly two-thirds of acute hepatitis B cases. In fact, hepatitis B is 50–100 times more infectious than HIV [human immunodeficiency virus] and can be passed through the exchange of body fluids, such as semen, vaginal fluids, and blood.

Can hepatitis B be spread through food?

Unlike hepatitis A, it is not spread routinely through food or water. However, there have been instances in which hepatitis B has been spread to babies when they have received food pre-chewed by an infected person.

What are ways hepatitis B is not spread?

Hepatitis B virus is not spread by sharing eating utensils, breastfeeding, hugging, kissing, holding hands, coughing, or sneezing.

Who is at risk for hepatitis B?

Although anyone can get hepatitis B, some people are at greater risk, such as those who do or are the following:

- Have sex with an infected person
- Have multiple sex partners
- Have a sexually transmitted disease
- Are men who have sexual contact with other men
- Inject drugs or share needles, syringes, or other drug equipment
- Live with a person who has chronic hepatitis B
- Are infants born to infected mothers
- Are exposed to blood on the job
- Are hemodialysis patients
- Travel to countries with moderate to high rates of hepatitis B

If I think I have been exposed to the hepatitis B virus, what should I do?

If you are concerned that you might have been exposed to the hepatitis B virus, call your health professional or your health department. If a person who has been exposed to hepatitis B virus gets the hepatitis B vaccine and/or a shot called HBIG (hepatitis B immune globulin) within 24 hours, hepatitis B infection may be prevented.

How long does the hepatitis B virus survive outside the body?

Hepatitis B virus can survive outside the body at least seven days. During that time, the virus can still cause infection if it enters the body of a person who is not infected.

How should blood spills be cleaned from surfaces to make sure that hepatitis B virus is gone?

All blood spills—including those that have already dried—should be cleaned and disinfected with a mixture of bleach and water (one part household bleach to 10 parts water). Gloves should always be used when cleaning up any blood spills. Even dried blood can present a risk to others.

If I had hepatitis B in the past, can I get it again?

No, once you recover from hepatitis B, you develop antibodies that protect you from the virus for life. An antibody is a substance found in the blood that the body produces in response to a virus. Antibodies protect the body from disease by attaching to the virus and destroying it. However, some people, especially those infected during early childhood, remain infected for life because they never clear the virus from their bodies.

Can I donate blood, organs, or semen if I have hepatitis B?

No, if you have ever tested positive for the hepatitis B virus, experts recommend that you not donate blood, organs, or semen because this can put the recipient at great risk.

Does acute hepatitis B cause symptoms?

Sometimes. Although a majority of adults develop symptoms from acute hepatitis B virus infection, many young children do not. Adults and children over the age of five years are more likely to have symptoms. Seventy percent of adults will develop symptoms from the infection.

What are the symptoms of acute hepatitis B?

Symptoms of acute hepatitis B, if they appear, can include the following:
- Fever
- Fatigue
- Loss of appetite
- Nausea
- Vomiting
- Abdominal pain
- Dark urine
- Clay-colored bowel movements
- Joint pain
- Jaundice (yellow color in the skin or the eyes)

How soon after exposure to hepatitis B will symptoms appear?

On average, symptoms appear 90 days (or three months) after exposure, but they can appear any time between six weeks and six months after exposure.

How long do acute hepatitis B symptoms last?

Symptoms usually last a few weeks, but some people can be ill for as long as six months.

Can a person spread hepatitis B without having symptoms?

Yes. Many people with hepatitis B have no symptoms, but these people can still spread the virus.

What are the symptoms of chronic hepatitis B?

Some people have ongoing symptoms similar to acute hepatitis B, but most individuals with chronic hepatitis B remain symptom free for as long as 20 or 30 years. About 15%–25% of people with chronic hepatitis B develop serious liver conditions, such as cirrhosis (scarring of the liver) or liver cancer. Even as the liver becomes diseased, some people still do not have symptoms, although certain blood tests for liver function might begin to show some abnormalities.

How will I know if I have hepatitis B?

Talk to your health professional. Since many people with hepatitis B do not have symptoms, doctors diagnose the disease by one or more blood tests. These tests look for the presence of antibodies or antigens and can help determine whether you:

- have acute or chronic infection;
- have recovered from infection;
- are immune to hepatitis B;
- could benefit from vaccination.

How serious is chronic hepatitis B?

Chronic hepatitis B is a serious disease that can result in long-term health problems, including liver damage, liver failure, liver cancer, or even death. Approximately 2,000–4,000 people die every year from hepatitis B-related liver disease.

What are antigens and antibodies?

An antigen is a substance on the surface of a virus that causes a person's immune system to recognize and respond to it. When the body is exposed to an antigen, the body views it as foreign material and takes steps to neutralize the antigen by producing antibodies. An antibody is a substance found in the blood that the body produces in response to a virus. Antibodies protect the body from disease by attaching to the virus and destroying it.

What are the common blood tests available to diagnose hepatitis B?

There are many different blood tests available to diagnose hepatitis B. They can be ordered as an individual test or as a series of tests. Ask your health professional to explain what he or she hopes to learn from the tests and when you will get the results.

What can people with chronic hepatitis B do to take care of their liver?

People with chronic hepatitis B should be monitored regularly by a doctor experienced in caring for people with hepatitis B. They should avoid alcohol because it can cause additional liver damage. They also should check with a health professional before taking any prescription pills, supplements, or over-the-counter medications, as these can potentially damage the liver.

Can hepatitis B be prevented?

Yes. The best way to prevent hepatitis B is by getting the hepatitis B vaccine. The hepatitis B vaccine is safe and effective and is usually given as three to four shots over a six-month period.

What is the hepatitis B vaccine series?

The hepatitis B vaccine series is a sequence of shots that stimulate a person's natural immune system to protect against HBV. After the vaccine is given, the body makes antibodies that protect a person against the virus. An antibody is a substance found in the blood that is produced in response to a virus invading the body. These antibodies are then stored in the body and will fight off the infection if a person is exposed to the hepatitis B virus in the future.

Who should get vaccinated against hepatitis B?

Hepatitis B vaccination is recommended for the following people:

- All infants, starting with the first dose of hepatitis B vaccine at birth

- All children and adolescents younger than 19 years of age who have not been vaccinated

- People whose sex partners have hepatitis B

- Sexually active persons who are not in a long-term, mutually monogamous relationship.

- Persons seeking evaluation or treatment for a sexually transmitted disease

- Men who have sexual contact with other men

- People who share needles, syringes, or other drug-injection equipment

- People who have close household contact with someone infected with the hepatitis B virus

- Health care and public safety workers at risk for exposure to blood or blood-contaminated body fluids on the job

- People with end-stage renal disease, including predialysis, hemo-dialysis, peritoneal dialysis, and home dialysis patients

- Residents and staff of facilities for developmentally disabled persons

- Travelers to regions with moderate or high rates of hepatitis B

- People with chronic liver disease

- People with HIV infection

- Anyone who wishes to be protected from hepatitis B virus infection

In order to reach individuals at risk for hepatitis B, vaccination is also recommended for anyone in or seeking treatment from the following:

- Sexually transmitted disease treatment facilities
- HIV testing and treatment facilities
- Facilities providing drug-abuse treatment and prevention services
- Health care settings targeting services to injection drug users
- Health care settings targeting services to men who have sex with men
- Chronic hemodialysis facilities and end-stage renal disease programs
- Correctional facilities
- Institutions and nonresidential day care facilities for developmentally disabled persons

When should a person get the hepatitis B vaccine series?

Children and Adolescents

- All children should get their first dose of hepatitis B vaccine at birth and complete the vaccine series by 6–18 months of age.
- All children and adolescents younger than 19 years of age who have not yet gotten the vaccine should also be vaccinated. "Catch-up" vaccination is recommended for children and adolescents who were never vaccinated or who did not get the entire vaccine series.

Adults

- Any adult who is at risk for hepatitis B virus infection or who wants to be vaccinated should talk to a health professional about getting the vaccine series.

Is the hepatitis B vaccine recommended before international travel?

The risk for hepatitis B virus infection in international travelers is generally low, although people traveling to certain countries are at risk. Travelers to regions with moderate or high rates of hepatitis B should get the hepatitis B vaccine.

How is the hepatitis B vaccine series given?

The hepatitis B vaccine is usually given as a series of three or four shots over a six-month period.

Is the hepatitis B vaccine series effective?

Yes, the hepatitis B vaccine is very effective at preventing hepatitis B virus infection. After receiving all three doses, hepatitis B vaccine provides greater than 90% protection to infants, children, and adults immunized before being exposed to the virus.

Is the hepatitis B vaccine safe?

Yes, the hepatitis B vaccine is safe. Soreness at the injection site is the most common side effect reported. As with any medicine, there are very small risks that a serious problem could occur after getting the vaccine. However, the potential risks associated with hepatitis B are much greater than the risks the vaccine poses. Since the vaccine became available in 1982, more than 100 million people have received hepatitis B vaccine in the United States and no serious side effects have been reported.

Is it harmful to have an extra dose of hepatitis B vaccine or to repeat the entire hepatitis B vaccine series?

No, getting extra doses of hepatitis B vaccine is not harmful.

What should be done if hepatitis B vaccine series was not completed?

Talk to your health professional to resume the vaccine series as soon as possible. The series does not need to be restarted.

Who should not receive the hepatitis B vaccine?

The hepatitis B vaccine is not recommended for people who have had serious allergic reactions to a prior dose of hepatitis B vaccine or to any part of the vaccine. Also, it not recommended for anyone who is allergic to yeast because yeast is used when making the vaccine. Tell your doctor if you have any severe allergies.

Are booster doses of hepatitis B vaccine necessary?

It depends. A "booster" dose of hepatitis B vaccine is a dose that increases or extends the effectiveness of the vaccine. Booster doses are recommended only for hemodialysis patients and can be considered for other people with a weakened immune system. Booster doses are not recommended for persons with normal immune status who have been fully vaccinated.

Is there a vaccine that will protect me from both hepatitis A and hepatitis B?

Yes, there is a combination vaccine that protects people from both hepatitis A and hepatitis B. The combined hepatitis A and B vaccine is usually given as three separate doses over a six-month period.

Can I get the hepatitis B vaccine at the same time as other vaccines?

Yes. Getting two different vaccines at the same time has not been shown to be harmful.

Where can I get the hepatitis B vaccine?

Talk to your doctor or health professional or call your health department. Some clinics offer free or low-cost vaccines.

What is hepatitis B immune globulin (HBIG)?

Hepatitis B immune globulin is a substance made from human blood samples that contains antibodies against the hepatitis B virus. It is given as a shot and can provide short-term protection (approximately three months) against hepatitis B.

Are pregnant women tested for hepatitis B?

Yes. When a pregnant woman comes in for prenatal care, she will be given a series of routine blood tests, including one that checks for the presence of hepatitis B virus infection. This test is important because women infected with this virus can pass hepatitis B to their babies during birth. But this can be prevented by giving the infant HBIG and the first hepatitis B vaccine at birth, and then completing the series.

What if a pregnant woman has hepatitis B?

If a pregnant woman has hepatitis B, she can pass the infection to her baby during birth. But this can be prevented through a series of vaccinations and HBIG for her baby beginning at birth. Without vaccination, babies born to women with hepatitis B virus infection can develop chronic infection, which can lead to serious health problems.

How does a baby get hepatitis B?

A baby can get hepatitis B from an infected mother during childbirth.

Can a baby be protected from getting hepatitis B from his or her mother during birth?

Yes, almost all cases of hepatitis B can be prevented if a baby born to an infected woman receives the necessary shots at the recommended times The infant should receive a shot called hepatitis B immune globulin (HBIG) and the first dose of hepatitis B vaccine within 12 hours of birth. Two or three additional shots of vaccine are needed over the next 1–15 months to help prevent hepatitis B. The timing and total number of shots will be influenced by several factors, including the type of vaccine and the baby's age and weight. In addition, experts recommend that the baby be tested after completion of the vaccine series to make sure he or she is protected from the disease. To best protect your baby, follow the advice of his or her doctor.

What happens if a baby gets hepatitis B?

Most newborns who become infected with hepatitis B virus do not have symptoms, but they have a 90% chance of developing chronic hepatitis B. This can eventually lead to serious health problems, including liver damage, liver cancer, and even death.

Do babies need the hepatitis B vaccine even if a pregnant woman does not have hepatitis B?

Yes. The hepatitis B vaccine is recommended for all infants. CDC recommends that the infant get the first shot before leaving the hospital.

Why is the hepatitis B vaccine recommended for all babies?

Hepatitis B vaccine is recommended for all babies so that they will be protected from a serious but preventable disease. Babies and young children are at much greater risk for developing a chronic infection if infected, but the vaccine can prevent this.

Section 19.2

Hepatitis and HIV Coinfection

Excerpted from "Hepatitis C Virus and HIV Coinfection," by the Centers for Disease Control and Prevention (CDC, www.cdc.gov), September 2002. Reviewed and revised by David A. Cooke, MD, FACP, July 10, 2012.

Coinfection with HIV and hepatitis C virus (HCV) is a significant problem, especially among injection drug users (IDUs). Care for individuals living with both diseases is complex. Coinfected IDUs can be treated successfully, although the caregiving team should have expertise in liver disease, HIV [human immunodeficiency syndrome], and addiction.

Many IDUs Are Coinfected with HIV and HCV

HIV has been an important and familiar health and social crisis for two decades. Less familiar, but also important, is HCV infection. These two viruses are similar in a number of ways, and infection with both is a serious problem.

Both HCV and HIV are transmitted by exposure to infected blood. About one-quarter of the people infected with HIV also have HCV.

The majority of coinfected people are IDUs. HCV is acquired relatively soon after individuals begin injecting drugs.

Within five years of beginning to inject, 50% to 80% of IDUs are infected with HCV. As a result, many IDUs who become infected with HIV are already infected with HCV. It is estimated that 50% to 90% of IDUs with HIV also have HCV infection.

Why Is HIV-HCV Coinfection Important?

The introduction in the mid-1990s of highly active antiretroviral therapy (HAART) for HIV has caused a sharp drop in the number of deaths from AIDS [acquired immunodeficiency syndrome]. This means that people with HIV are living longer. Therefore, if they are coinfected, the complications from HCV have more time to develop. These complications (cirrhosis, liver cancer, end-stage liver disease) generally develop over 20–30 years. Liver disease from HCV is now the leading non-AIDS cause of death in the United States in coinfected individuals with HIV.

Treatment for each disease is complicated, expensive, and has side effects. This poses difficult issues for patients who are living with both HIV and HCV.

Finally, coinfection is important because it has a disproportionate impact on certain communities, including those in prison and jail and communities of color.

Effects of Coinfection on HIV and HCV

HIV's Effect on HCV

Studies have shown that HIV infection in a person who is also infected with HCV results in higher levels of HCV in the blood, more rapid progression to HCV-related liver disease, and increased risk for cirrhosis and liver cancer. As a result, HCV is now regarded as an opportunistic infection in people with HIV infection, although it is not considered an AIDS-defining illness.

HCV's Effect on HIV

These effects are less well understood. Some research suggests that infection with genotype 1 HCV is associated with more rapid progression to AIDS or death, although this is still controversial. (HCV has several genetic variations, called genotypes. Most people with HCV infection in the United States have genotype 1. Genotypes 2 and 3 are more common in Europe.) Some evidence also indicates that HCV is associated with impaired CD4+ [cluster of differentiation 4] T cell recovery during antiretroviral therapy.

Care and Treatment of Coinfected IDUs

Coinfected IDUs should do the following:

- Stop injecting drugs, get into substance abuse treatment, and stay in treatment; if they are not able to stop, they should use sterile syringes and equipment and not share drug solution, syringes, or preparation equipment (needles, drug solution containers, water, cotton filters).

- Stop drinking alcoholic beverages; if they are not able to stop, they should limit drinking because alcohol contributes to liver damage; when appropriate, they should be referred to alcohol treatment and relapse-prevention programs.

• Practice safer personal care and sexual behaviors (not sharing toothbrushes and razors, using condoms consistently, limiting the number of sex partners, getting treatment for sexually transmitted diseases).

• Be immunized against hepatitis A and hepatitis B, unless they are already immune from past exposure.

• Get regular checkups to monitor overall health and status of liver disease; coinfected individuals on HAART may be at increased risk of liver toxicity and should be closely monitored.

Treatment for Chronic Hepatitis C

The Food and Drug Administration (FDA) has approved four antiviral drugs for the treatment of chronic hepatitis C: Alpha interferon or an improved form of interferon, called pegylated interferon; ribavirin; boceprevir; and telaprevir.

Most patients are treated with a triple combination: Interferon and ribavirin, plus either boceprevir or telaprevir. Ribavirin, boceprevir, and telaprevir can only be used as part of combination therapy and never as single medications. Triple therapy has significantly better rates of cure than two drug regimens.

Treatment Issues for Coinfected Individuals

Treatment for each of these diseases involves long-term therapy with multiple powerful drugs. Adherence to either treatment regimen is critically important to their success, and for HIV, to prevent resistance from developing. These issues are compounded for individuals who are living with both treatment regimens.

Treatment for either disease also has side effects, which should be closely monitored. Therapy with interferon alone appears to be reasonably well tolerated in coinfected patients.

However, combination therapy can have serious toxicities, and there are a number of important interactions among drugs used to treat hepatitis C and HIV. It is very important that your physician is aware of all of the medications you are taking and is notified immediately of any changes.

Another factor to consider is that effectiveness of treatment may be influenced by factors such as the person's age, how healthy he or she is at the beginning of therapy, the degree of existing liver disease, the person's CD4 count, and the extent of any other HIV-related illnesses.

Additional Issues for IDUs

Coping with coinfection and the demands of antiviral therapy pose particular challenges for coinfected IDUs:

- Many IDUs also drink alcohol and abstaining from drinking may be difficult.

- For those IDUs who have stopped injecting, using interferon can trigger a desire to inject again because its effects can resemble drug withdrawal (feeling "drug sick"); in addition, interferon is given by injection. If the person continues to inject or begins again, there may be a high risk of HCV reinfection.

Although treatment of coinfection is complicated for IDUs, they can be successfully treated, and those who have stopped injecting have response rates similar to non-IDUs. A key aspect of their care is close monitoring by a caregiving team that has expertise in liver disease, HIV, and addiction medicine.

Section 19.3

Treating Hepatitis

Hepatitis B Treatment Information

The future looks bright for those who are chronically infected with the hepatitis B virus (HBV).

Only 10 years ago, there were no options. Now, there are promising drugs that can slow down liver damage caused by the virus. This means that there will be less damage done to the liver, and less chance of developing serious liver disease later on. With all of the exciting new research, there is great hope that a complete cure is on the horizon for people living with chronic hepatitis B.

What Treatments Are Currently Approved for HBV?

The good news is that there are several promising treatment options. Currently, there are seven FDA [U.S. Food and Drug Administration] approved drugs in the United States to treat chronic HBV: Intron A (Interferon Alpha), Pegasys (Pegylated Interferon), Epivir HBV (Lamivudine), Hepsera (Adefovir), Baraclude (Entecavir), Tyzeka (Telbivudine), and Viread (Tenofovir).

You and your doctor will need to discuss the treatment options before deciding which one is best for you.

For many patients, these medications will decrease or stop hepatitis B virus reproduction. This results in patients feeling better within a month or two because liver damage from the virus is slowed down, or even reversed in some cases. Although the FDA has approved these drugs for chronic hepatitis B, they do not provide a complete cure at this time. They do, however, significantly decrease the risk of progressive liver damage from the hepatitis B virus. To learn more about these approved drugs as well as the experimental drugs still being tested, visit the Hepatitis B Foundation's HBV Drug Watch at www.hepb.org.

Does Every Patient Need to Be Treated?

It is important to know that not every patient with chronic HBV needs to be on medication. Patients with active signs of liver disease may benefit the most from treatment.

However, all chronically infected patients should be seen by their doctor at least once a year (or more frequently) for regular medical follow-up care, whether they start treatment or not. Talk to your doctor about approved treatments or whether there are any clinical trials of new HBV drugs that you might be eligible for and could benefit from.

What about Clinical Trials?

Clinical trials are carefully controlled studies that are used to determine whether new drugs, treatments, or medical products are safe and effective. People volunteer to participate in these trials as they can provide patients the opportunity to potentially benefit from the latest advances in medical science. There are many HBV treatments that are currently in clinical trial, and many new and promising treatments on the horizon. To help you learn more, the Hepatitis B Foundation maintains a list of hepatitis B clinical trials on its website at www.hepb.org.

How Can I Learn More about Treatment for HBV?

First, talk to your doctor. If he or she is unfamiliar with the latest treatment advances, contact a liver specialist (hepatologist). Be sure to visit the Hepatitis B Foundation website at www.hepb.org for a national directory of liver specialists, an updated Drug Watch, and HBV clinical trial sites. Call 215-489-4900 or email info@hepb.org for more personalized information and referrals. You can also visit the National Institutes of Health (NIH) clinical trials site at www.clinicaltrials.gov or Center Watch at www.centerwatch.com.

Approved Drugs for Adults

The future looks bright for individuals living with chronic hepatitis B. Only a decade ago there were no treatment options. Although there is still no complete cure for hepatitis B, there are seven approved drugs for adults (two for children) and many promising new drugs in development. Current treatments seem to be most effective in those who show signs of active liver disease.

Not every person with chronic hepatitis B needs to be on medication. You should talk to your doctor about whether you are a good candidate for drug therapy or a clinical trial. Be sure that you understand the pros and cons of each treatment option.

Whether you decide to start treatment or not, it is very important to be seen by a liver specialist or doctor knowledgeable about hepatitis B on a regular basis.

Approved Hepatitis B Drugs in the United States

- Interferon Alpha (Intron A) is given by injection several times a week for six months to a year, or sometimes longer. The drug can cause side effects such as flu-like symptoms, depression, and headaches. Approved 1991 and available for both children and adults.

- Pegylated Interferon (Pegasys) is given by injection once a week usually for six months to a year. The drug can cause side effects such as flu-like symptoms and depression. Approved May 2005 and available only for adults.

- Lamivudine (Epivir-HBV, Zeffix, or Heptodin) is a pill that is taken once a day, with few side effects, for at least one year or longer. Approved 1998 and available for both children and adults.

- Adefovir Dipivoxil (Hepsera) is a pill taken once a day, with few side effects, for at least one year or longer. Approved September 2002 for adults. Pediatric clinical trials are in progress.

- Entecavir (Baraclude) is a pill taken once a day, with few side effects, for at least one year or longer. Approved April 2005 for adults. Pediatric clinical trials are in progress.

- Telbivudine (Tyzeka, Sebivo) is a pill taken once a day, with few side effects, for at least one year or longer. Approved October 2006 for adults.

- Tenofovir (Viread) is a pill taken once a day, with few side effects, for at least one year or longer. Approved August 2008 for adults.

Although the FDA has approved these seven drugs for chronic hepatitis B, they do not provide a complete cure, except in rare cases (a "cure" generally means that a person loses the hepatitis B virus and develops protective surface antibodies).

The drugs, however, significantly decrease the risk of liver damage from the hepatitis B virus by slowing down or stopping the virus from reproducing. As with HIV, it appears that combination therapy will probably be the most effective method of combating chronic hepatitis B infections.

Cost Comparison of Hepatitis B Drug Therapy

What does it cost for the different approved HBV drug therapies? See the cost comparison of the approved therapies at http://www.hepb .org/pdf/2011_Drug_Comparison.pdf.

HBF Drug Watch

With promising new compounds in development for hepatitis B, there is great hope that a cure will be found in the near future.

Visit the HBF Drug Watch [http://www.hepb.org/professionals/ hbf_drug_watch.htm] for a complete list of approved hepatitis B drugs and compounds in development, as well as a list of Hepatitis B Clinical Trials.

Chapter 20

HIV/AIDS

Chapter Contents

Section 20.1—How HIV Causes AIDS 184

Section 20.2—How the Immune System Reacts to HIV 198

Section 20.3—Questions and Answers about HIV
                        Transmission 200

Section 20.4—HIV Signs and Symptoms.................................. 212

Section 20.5—Testing for HIV... 214

Section 20.6—HIV and Its Treatment 219

Section 20.7—Living with HIV 232

Section 20.8—How Can I Pay for HIV Care? 241

Section 20.9—The Affordable Care Act and People
                        Living with HIV/AIDS 245

Section 20.1

How HIV Causes AIDS

Excerpted from "More on How HIV Causes AIDS," by the National
Institute of Allergy and Infectious Diseases (NIAID, www.niaid.nih.gov),
part of the National Institutes of Health, January 5, 2009.

Overview

Untreated HIV [human immunodeficiency virus] disease is characterized by a gradual deterioration of immune function. Most notably, crucial immune cells called CD4 positive (CD4+) T cells are disabled and killed during the typical course of infection. These cells, sometimes called "T-helper cells," play a central role in the immune response, signaling other cells in the immune system to perform their special functions.

A healthy, uninfected person usually has 800 to 1,200 CD4+ T cells per cubic millimeter (mm^3) of blood. During untreated HIV infection, the number of these cells in a person's blood progressively declines. When the CD4+ T cell count falls below 200/mm^3, a person becomes particularly vulnerable to the opportunistic infections and cancers that typify AIDS [acquired immunodeficiency syndrome], the end stage of HIV disease. People with AIDS often suffer infections of the lungs, intestinal tract, brain, eyes, and other organs, as well as debilitating weight loss, diarrhea, neurologic conditions, and cancers such as Kaposi sarcoma and certain types of lymphomas.

Most scientists think that HIV causes AIDS by directly inducing the death of CD4+ T cells or interfering with their normal function, and by triggering other events that weaken a person's immune function. For example, the network of signaling molecules that normally regulates a person's immune response is disrupted during HIV disease, impairing a person's ability to fight other infections. The HIV-mediated destruction of the lymph nodes and related immunologic organs also plays a major role in causing the immunosuppression seen in people with AIDS. Immunosuppression by HIV is confirmed by the fact that medicines, which interfere with the HIV lifecycle, preserve CD4+ T cells and immune function as well as delay clinical illness.

Scope of the HIV Epidemic

Although HIV was first identified in 1983, studies of previously stored blood samples indicate that the virus entered the U.S. population sometime in the late 1970s. In the United States, 1,106,391 cases of AIDS, and 597,499 deaths among people with AIDS had been reported to the Centers for Disease Control and Prevention (CDC) by the end of 2008 and 2007, respectively. Approximately 40,000 new HIV infections occur each year in the United States, 70 percent of them among men and 30 percent among women. Of the new infections, approximately 40 percent are from male-to-male contact, 30 percent from heterosexual contact, and 25 percent from injection drug use. Minority groups in the United States have also been disproportionately affected by the epidemic.

Worldwide, an estimated 33 million people were living with HIV as of December 2008, according to the Joint United Nations Programme on HIV/AIDS (UNAIDS). Through 2008, cumulative AIDS-associated deaths worldwide numbered more than 33 million. Globally, approximately 2.7 million new HIV infections and approximately 1.7 million AIDS-related deaths, including an estimated 280,000 children under 15 years old, occurred in the year 2008 alone.

HIV belongs to a class of viruses called retroviruses. Retroviruses are RNA (ribonucleic acid) viruses, and to replicate (duplicate) they must make a DNA (deoxyribonucleic acid) copy of their RNA. It is the DNA genes that allow the virus to replicate.

Like all viruses, HIV can replicate only inside cells, commandeering the cell's machinery to reproduce. Only HIV and other retroviruses, however, once inside a cell, use an enzyme called reverse transcriptase to convert their RNA into DNA, which can be incorporated into the host cell's genes.

HIV belongs to a subgroup of retroviruses known as lentiviruses, or "slow" viruses. The course of infection with these viruses is characterized by a long interval between initial infection and the onset of serious symptoms.

Other lentiviruses infect nonhuman species. For example, the feline immunodeficiency virus (FIV) infects cats and the simian immunodeficiency virus (SIV) infects monkeys and other nonhuman primates. Like HIV in humans, these animal viruses primarily infect immune system cells, often causing immune deficiency and AIDS-like symptoms. These viruses and their hosts have provided researchers with useful, albeit imperfect, models of the HIV disease process in people.

185

without being killed, thus acting as reservoirs of HIV. CD4+ T cells also serve as important reservoirs of HIV; a small proportion of these cells harbor HIV in a stable, inactive form. Normal immune processes may activate these cells, resulting in the production of new HIV virions.

Cell-to-cell spread of HIV also can occur through the CD4-mediated fusion of an infected cell with an uninfected cell.

Reverse Transcription

In the cytoplasm of the cell, HIV reverse transcriptase converts viral RNA into DNA, the nucleic acid form in which the cell carries its genes. Fifteen of the 26 antiviral drugs approved in the United States for treating people with HIV infection work by interfering with this stage of the viral life cycle.

Integration

The newly made HIV DNA moves to the cell's nucleus, where it is spliced into the host's DNA with the help of HIV integrase. HIV DNA that enters the DNA of the cell is called a provirus. Several drugs that target the integrase enzyme are in the early stages of development and are being investigated for their potential as antiretroviral agents.

Transcription

For a provirus to produce new viruses, RNA copies must be made that can be read by the host cell's protein-making machinery. These copies are called messenger RNA (mRNA), and production of mRNA is called transcription, a process that involves the host cell's own enzymes. Viral genes in concert with the cellular machinery control this process; the tat gene, for example, encodes a protein that accelerates transcription. Genomic RNA is also transcribed for later incorporation in the budding virion.

Cytokines, proteins involved in the normal regulation of the immune response, also may regulate transcription. Molecules such as tumor necrosis factor (TNF)-alpha and interleukin (IL)-6, secreted in elevated levels by the cells of HIV-infected people, may help to activate HIV proviruses. Other infections, by organisms such as Mycobacterium tuberculosis, also may enhance transcription by inducing the secretion of cytokines.

Translation

After HIV mRNA is processed in the cell's nucleus, it is transported to the cytoplasm. HIV proteins are critical to this process; for example, a protein encoded by the rev gene allows mRNA encoding HIV structural proteins to be transferred from the nucleus to the cytoplasm. Without the rev protein, structural proteins are not made. In the cytoplasm, the virus co-opts the cell's protein-making machinery—including structures called ribosomes—to make long chains of viral proteins and enzymes, using HIV mRNA as a template. This process is called translation.

Assembly and Budding

Newly made HIV core proteins, enzymes, and genomic RNA gather inside the cell and an immature viral particle forms and buds off from the cell, acquiring an envelope that includes both cellular and HIV proteins from the cell membrane. During this part of the viral life cycle, the core of the virus is immature and the virus is not yet infectious. The long chains of proteins and enzymes that make up the immature viral core are now cut into smaller pieces by a viral enzyme called protease.

This step results in infectious viral particles. Drugs called protease inhibitors interfere with this step of the viral life cycle. FDA has approved eight such drugs—saquinavir, ritonavir, indinavir, amprenavir, nelfinavir, fosamprenavir, atazanavir, and lopinavir—for marketing in the United States. An HIV inhibitor that targets a unique step in the viral life cycle, very late in the process of viral maturation, has been identified and is currently undergoing further development.

Recently, researchers have discovered that virus budding from the host cell is much more complex than previously thought. Binding between the HIV Gag protein and molecules in the cell directs the accumulation of HIV components in special intracellular sacks, called multivesicular bodies (MVB), that normally function to carry proteins out of the cell. In this way, HIV actively hitchhikes out of the cell in the MVB by hijacking normal cell machinery and mechanisms. Discovery of this budding pathway has revealed several potential points for intervening in the viral replication cycle.

Transmission of HIV

Among adults, HIV is spread most commonly during sexual intercourse with an infected partner. During intercourse, the virus can enter the body through the mucosal linings of the vagina, vulva, penis, or rectum or, rarely, via the mouth and possibly the upper gastrointestinal tract after oral sex. The likelihood of transmission is increased by factors that may damage these linings, especially other sexually transmitted infections that cause ulcers or inflammation.

Research suggests that immune system cells of the dendritic cell type, which live in the mucosa, may begin the infection process after sexual exposure by binding to and carrying the virus from the site of infection to the lymph nodes where other immune system cells become infected. A molecule on the surface of dendritic cells, DC-SIGN, may be critical for this transmission process.

HIV also can be transmitted by contact with infected blood, most often by the sharing of needles or syringes contaminated with minute quantities of blood containing the virus. The risk of acquiring HIV from blood transfusions is extremely small in the United States, as all blood products in this country are screened routinely for evidence of the virus.

Almost all HIV-infected children in the United States get the virus from their mothers before or during birth. In the United States, approximately 25 percent of pregnant HIV-infected women not receiving antiretroviral therapy have passed on the virus to their babies. In 1994, researchers showed that a specific regimen of the drug AZT (zidovudine) can reduce the risk of transmission of HIV from mother to baby by two-thirds. The use of combinations of antiretroviral drugs and simpler drug regimens has further reduced the rate of mother-to-child HIV transmission in the United States.

In developing countries, cheap and simple antiviral drug regimens have been proven to significantly reduce mother-to-child transmission at birth in resource-poor settings. Unfortunately, the virus also may be transmitted from an HIV-infected mother to her infant via breastfeeding. Moreover, due to the use of medicines to prevent transmission at delivery, breastfeeding may become the most common mode of HIV infection in infants. Thus, development of affordable alternatives to breastfeeding is greatly needed.

Early Events in HIV Infection

Once it enters the body, HIV infects a large number of CD4+ cells and replicates rapidly. During this acute or primary phase of infection, the blood contains many viral particles that spread throughout the body, seeding various organs, particularly the lymphoid organs.

Two to four weeks after exposure to the virus, up to 70 percent of HIV-infected people suffer flu-like symptoms related to the acute infection. Their immune systems fight back with killer T cells (CD8+ T cells) and B-cell-produced antibodies, which dramatically reduce HIV levels. A person's CD4+ T cell count may rebound somewhat and even approach its original level. A person may then remain free of

HIV-related symptoms for years despite continuous replication of HIV in the lymphoid organs that had been seeded during the acute phase of infection.

One reason that HIV is unique is the fact that despite the body's aggressive immune responses, which are sufficient to clear most viral infections, some HIV invariably escapes. This is due in large part to the high rate of mutations that occur during the process of HIV replication. Even when the virus does not avoid the immune system by mutating, the body's best soldiers in the fight against HIV—certain subsets of killer T cells that recognize HIV—may be depleted or become dysfunctional.

In addition, early in the course of HIV infection, people may lose HIV-specific CD4+ T cell responses that normally slow the replication of viruses. Such responses include the secretion of interferons and other antiviral factors, and the orchestration of CD8+ T cells.

Finally, the virus may hide within the chromosomes of an infected cell and be shielded from surveillance by the immune system. Such cells can be considered as a latent reservoir of the virus. Because the antiviral agents currently in our therapeutic arsenal attack actively replicating virus, they are not effective against hidden, inactive viral DNA (so-called provirus). New strategies to purge this latent reservoir of HIV have become one of the major goals for current research efforts.

Course of HIV Infection

Among people enrolled in large epidemiologic studies in Western countries, the median time from infection with HIV to the development of AIDS-related symptoms has been approximately 10 to 12 years in the absence of antiretroviral therapy. Researchers, however, have observed a wide variation in disease progression. Approximately 10 percent of HIV-infected people in these studies have progressed to AIDS within the first two to three years following infection, while up to 5 percent of people in the studies have stable CD4+ T cell counts and no symptoms even after 12 or more years.

Factors such as age or genetic differences among individuals, the level of virulence of an individual strain of virus, and coinfection with other microbes may influence the rate and severity of disease progression. Drugs that fight the infections associated with AIDS have improved and prolonged the lives of HIV-infected people by preventing or treating conditions such as *Pneumocystis carinii* pneumonia, cytomegalovirus disease, and diseases caused by a number of fungi.

HIV Coreceptors and Disease Progression

Recent research has shown that most infecting strains of HIV use a coreceptor molecule called CCR5, in addition to the CD4 molecule, to enter certain of its target cells. HIV-infected people with a specific mutation in one of their two copies of the gene for this receptor may have a slower disease course than people with two normal copies of the gene. Rare individuals with two mutant copies of the CCR5 gene appear, in most cases, to be completely protected from HIV infection. Mutations in the gene for other HIV coreceptors also may influence the rate of disease progression.

Viral Burden and Disease Progression

Numerous studies show that people with high levels of HIV in their bloodstreams are more likely to develop new AIDS-related symptoms or die than those with lower levels of virus. For instance, in the Multicenter AIDS Cohort Study (MACS), investigators showed that the level of HIV in an untreated person's plasma six months to a year after infection—the so-called viral set point—is highly predictive of the rate of disease progression; that is, patients with high levels of virus are much more likely to get sicker faster than those with low levels of virus. The MACS and other studies have provided the rationale for providing aggressive antiretroviral therapy to HIV-infected people, as well as for routinely using newly available blood tests to measure viral load when initiating, monitoring, and modifying anti-HIV therapy.

Potent combinations of three or more anti-HIV drugs known as highly active antiretroviral therapy, or HAART, can reduce a person's viral burden (amount of virus in the circulating blood) to very low levels and in many cases delay the progression of HIV disease for prolonged periods. Before the introduction of HAART therapy, 85 percent of patients survived an average of three years following AIDS diagnosis. Today, 95 percent of patients who start therapy before they get AIDS survive on average three years following their first AIDS diagnosis. For those who start HAART after their first AIDS event, survival is still very high at 85 percent, averaging three years after AIDS diagnosis.

Antiretroviral regimens, however, have yet to completely and permanently suppress the virus in HIV-infected people. Recent studies have shown that, in addition to the latent HIV reservoir discussed in the preceding text, HIV persists in a replication-competent form in resting CD4+ T cells even in people receiving aggressive antiretroviral therapy who have no readily detectable HIV in their blood. Investigators around the world are working to develop the next generation of anti-HIV drugs that can stop HIV, even in these biologic scenarios.

A treatment goal, along with reduction of viral burden, is the reconstitution of the person's immune system, which may have become sufficiently damaged that it cannot replenish itself. Various strategies for assisting the immune system in this regard are being tested in clinical trials in tandem with HAART, such as the Evaluation of Subcutaneous Proleukin in a Randomized International Trial (ESPRIT) trial exploring the effects of the T cell growth factor, IL-2.

HIV Is Active in the Lymph Nodes

Although HIV-infected people often show an extended period of clinical latency with little evidence of disease, the virus is never truly completely latent although individual cells may be latently infected. Researchers have shown that even early in disease, HIV actively replicates within the lymph nodes and related organs, where large amounts of virus become trapped in networks of specialized cells with long, tentacle-like extensions. These cells are called follicular dendritic cells (FDCs). FDCs are located in hot spots of immune activity in lymphoid tissue called germinal centers. They act like flypaper, trapping invading pathogens (including HIV) and holding them until B cells come along to start an immune response.

Over a period of years, even when little virus is readily detectable in the blood, significant amounts of virus accumulate in the lymphoid tissue, both within infected cells and bound to FDCs. In and around the germinal centers, numerous CD4+ T cells are probably activated by the increased production of cytokines such as TNF-alpha and IL-6 by immune system cells within the lymphoid tissue. Activation allows uninfected cells to be more easily infected and increases replication of HIV in already infected cells.

While greater quantities of certain cytokines such as TNF-alpha and IL-6 are secreted during HIV infection, other cytokines with key roles in the regulation of normal immune function may be secreted in decreased amounts. For example, CD4+ T cells may lose their capacity to produce IL-2, a cytokine that enhances the growth of other T cells and helps to stimulate other cells' response to invaders. Infected cells also have low levels of receptors for IL-2, which may reduce their ability to respond to signals from other cells.

Breakdown of Lymph Node Architecture

Ultimately, with chronic cell activation and secretion of inflammatory cytokines, the fine and complex inner structure of the lymph node breaks down and is replaced by scar tissue. Without this structure, cells in the lymph node cannot communicate and the immune system cannot function properly. Investigators also have reported recently that this scarring reduces the ability of the immune system to replenish itself following antiretroviral therapy that reduces the viral burden.

Role of CD8+ T Cells

CD8+ T cells are critically important in the immune response to HIV. These cells attack and kill infected cells that are producing virus. Thus, vaccine efforts are directed toward eliciting or enhancing these killer T cells, as well as eliciting antibodies that will neutralize the infectivity of HIV.

CD8+ T cells also appear to secrete soluble factors that suppress HIV replication. Several molecules, including RANTES [Regulated upon activation, normal T-cell expressed, and secreted], MIP [macrophage inflammatory protein]-1alpha, MIP-1beta, and MDC [macrophage-derived chemokine] appear to block HIV replication by occupying the coreceptors necessary for many strains of HIV to enter their target cells. There may be other immune system molecules—including the so-called CD8 antiviral factor (CAF), the defensins (type of antimicrobials), and others yet undiscovered—that can suppress HIV replication to some degree.

Rapid Replication and Mutation of HIV

HIV replicates rapidly; several billion new virus particles may be produced every day. In addition, the HIV reverse transcriptase enzyme makes many mistakes while making DNA copies from HIV RNA. As a consequence, many variants or strains of HIV develop in a person, some of which may escape destruction by antibodies or killer T cells. Additionally, different strains of HIV can recombine to produce a wide range of variants.

During the course of HIV disease, viral strains emerge in an infected person that differ widely in their ability to infect and kill different cell types, as well as in their rate of replication. Scientists are investigating why strains of HIV from people with advanced disease appear to be more virulent and infect more cell types than strains obtained earlier from the same person. Part of the explanation may be the expanded ability of the virus to use other coreceptors, such as CXCR4 [chemokine (C-X-C motif) receptor 4].

Theories of Immune System Cell Loss in HIV Infection

Researchers around the world are studying how HIV destroys or disables CD4+ T cells, and many think that a number of mechanisms may occur simultaneously in an HIV-infected person. Data suggest that billions of CD4+ T cells may be destroyed every day, eventually overwhelming the immune system's capacity to regenerate.

Direct Cell Killing

Infected CD4+ T cells may be killed directly when large amounts of virus are produced and bud out from the cell surface, disrupting the cell membrane, or when viral proteins and nucleic acids collect inside the cell, interfering with cellular machinery.

Apoptosis

Infected CD4+ T cells may be killed when the regulation of cell function is distorted by HIV proteins, probably leading to cell suicide by a process known as programmed cell death or apoptosis. Recent reports indicate that apoptosis occurs to a greater extent in HIV-infected people, both in their bloodstreams and lymph nodes. Apoptosis is closely associated with the aberrant cellular activation seen in HIV disease.

Uninfected cells also may undergo apoptosis. Investigators have shown in cell cultures that the HIV envelope alone or bound to antibodies sends an inappropriate signal to CD4+ T cells causing them to undergo apoptosis, even if not infected by HIV.

Innocent Bystanders

Uninfected cells may die in an innocent bystander scenario: HIV particles may bind to the cell surface, giving them the appearance of an infected cell and marking them for destruction by killer T cells after antibody attaches to the viral particle on the cell. This process is called antibody-dependent cellular cytotoxicity.

Killer T cells also may mistakenly destroy uninfected cells that have consumed HIV particles and that display HIV fragments on their surfaces. Alternatively, because HIV envelope proteins bear some resemblance to certain molecules that may appear on CD4+ T cells, the body's immune responses may mistakenly damage such cells as well.

Anergy

Researchers have shown in cell cultures that CD4+ T cells can be turned off by activation signals from HIV that leaves them unable to respond to further immune stimulation. This inactivated state is known as anergy.

Damage to Precursor Cells

Studies suggest that HIV also destroys precursor cells that mature to have special immune functions, as well as the microenvironment of the bone marrow and the thymus needed for developing such cells. These organs probably lose the ability to regenerate, further compounding the suppression of the immune system.

Central Nervous System Damage

Although monocytes and macrophages can be infected by HIV, they appear to be relatively resistant to being killed by the virus. These cells, however, travel throughout the body and carry HIV to various organs, including the brain, which may serve as a hiding place or "reservoir" for the virus that may be relatively resistant to most anti-HIV drugs.

Neurologic manifestations of HIV disease are seen in up to 50 percent of HIV-infected people, to varying degrees of severity. People infected with HIV often experience the following:

- Cognitive symptoms, including impaired short-term memory, reduced concentration, and mental slowing

- Motor symptoms such as fine motor clumsiness or slowness, tremor, and leg weakness

- Behavioral symptoms including apathy, social withdrawal, irritability, depression, and personality change

More serious neurologic manifestations in HIV disease typically occur in patients with high viral loads, generally when a person has advanced HIV disease or AIDS.

Neurologic manifestations of HIV disease are the subject of many research projects. Current evidence suggests that although nerve cells do not become infected with HIV, supportive cells within the brain, such as astrocytes and microglia (as well as monocyte/macrophages that have migrated to the brain) can be infected with the virus. Researchers postulate that infection of these cells can cause a disruption of normal neurologic functions by altering cytokine levels, by delivering aberrant signals, and by causing the release of toxic products in the brain. The use of anti-HIV drugs frequently reduces the severity of neurologic symptoms, but in many cases does not, for reasons that are unclear. The impact of long-term therapy and long-term HIV disease on neurologic function is also unknown and under intensive study.

Role of Immune Activation in HIV Disease

During a normal immune response, many parts of the immune system are mobilized to fight an invader. CD4+ T cells, for instance, may quickly multiply and increase their cytokine secretion, thereby signaling other cells to perform their special functions. Scavenger cells called macrophages may double in size and develop numerous organelles, including lysosomes that contain digestive enzymes used to process ingested pathogens. Once the immune system clears the foreign antigen, it returns to a relative state of quiescence.

Paradoxically, although it ultimately causes immune deficiency, HIV infection for most of its course is characterized by immune system hyperactivation, which has negative consequences. As noted above, HIV replication and spread are much more efficient in activated CD4+ cells. Chronic immune system activation during HIV disease also may result in a massive stimulation of B cells, impairing the ability of these cells to make antibodies against other pathogens.

Chronic immune activation also can result in apoptosis, and an increased production of cytokines that not only may increase HIV replication but also have other deleterious effects. Increased levels of TNF-alpha, for example, may be at least partly responsible for the severe weight loss or wasting syndrome seen in many HIV-infected people.

The persistence of HIV and HIV replication plays an important role in the chronic state of immune activation seen in HIV-infected people. In addition, researchers have shown that infections with other organisms activate immune system cells and increase production of the virus in HIV-infected people. Chronic immune activation due to persistent infections, or the cumulative effects of multiple episodes of immune activation and bursts of virus production, likely contribute to the progression of HIV disease.

Section 20.2

How the Immune System Reacts to HIV

"Immune System 101," from AIDS.gov, part of the U.S.
Department of Health and Human Services, August 22, 2011.

Your immune system works because your body is able to recognize "self" and "non-self." This means that your body is able to tell if an invader (virus, bacteria, parasite, or other another person's tissues) has entered it—even if you aren't consciously aware that anything has happened. Your body recognizes this invader and uses a number of different tactics to destroy it.

Major Players of the Immune System

Lymph nodes (also called lymph glands): These small, bean-shaped structures are part of your lymphatic system. That system is made up of tissues and organs (bone marrow, spleen, thymus, and lymph nodes) that produce and store cells that fight infection and disease, along with the clear fluid, lymph, that carries those cells to different parts of the body. Lymph nodes filter the lymphatic fluid and store special cells that can trap cancer cells or bacteria that are traveling through your body in the lymph fluid. Lymph nodes are critical for your body's immune response and many of your immune reactions begin there. When you have an infection, your lymph nodes can get larger and feel tender or sore.

Thymus: A small organ located just behind your breastbone. This is where your T-cells mature (That's why they are called T-cells. The T is for thymus.)

Spleen: The largest lymphatic organ in the body—it's about the size of your fist. Your spleen is located in the upper-left part of your abdomen. It contains white blood cells that fight infection or disease. Your spleen also helps control the amount of blood in your body and destroys old and damaged blood cells.

Bone marrow: The yellow tissue in the center of your bones that is responsible for making white blood cells that are destined to become lymphocytes.

Lymphocytes: A small white blood cell that plays a large role in defending the body against disease. There are two main types of lymphocytes: B-cells and T-cells. B-cells make antibodies that attack bacteria and toxins. T-cells help destroy infected or cancerous cells and attack body cells themselves when they have been taken over by viruses or have become cancerous.

The Immune System in Action

Your immune system has many different ways of fighting off foreign invaders. When confronted with a virus, your body responds by activating specific processes of the immune system. First your body recognizes a foreign antigen and delivers it to the lymph system, where it is ingested by a macrophage.

Then the macrophage processes the virus and displays the antigens for that particular virus on its own exterior. This antigen then signals a helper T- cell.

Next the T-cell reads this signal and sounds the alarm for other parts of your immune system to respond.

The B-cell responds to this call and comes to read the antigen from the surface of the macrophage.

The B-cell then becomes activated and produces millions of antibodies that are specific to the antigen. These antibodies are released into your body to attach to the virus particles.

These antibodies are important because the invading virus may outnumber your own immune system cells. The antibodies attach to the antigens and hold on tight.

These antibodies then send a signal to other macrophages and other immune cells to come and engulf and destroy the antibody and whatever it has captured.

The final stage of your immune response involves the suppressor T-cell. Once the number of invaders has dropped significantly and the infection has resolved, the suppressor T-cell will signal the other cells of the immune system to rest. This is important as prolonged activation of your immune response could eventually lead to damage to your healthy cells.

How HIV Affects This Complex Process

HIV disrupts this process by directly infecting the helper T-cells. Your initial immune response does get rid of a great deal of HIV, but some of it manages to survive and infect these important cells. Once the infected helper T-cells are activated, they work to create new viruses instead of doing the job they are supposed to do in your immune system. In addition, many helper T-cells are destroyed in the HIV replication process.

Section 20.3

Questions and Answers about HIV Transmission

"HIV Transmission," by the Centers for Disease Control and Prevention (CDC, www.cdc.gov), March 25, 2010.

How is HIV passed from one person to another?

HIV [human immunodeficiency virus] can be detected in several fluids and tissue of a person living with HIV. It is important to understand however, that finding a small amount of HIV in a body fluid or tissue does not mean that HIV is transmitted by that body fluid or tissue. Only specific fluids (blood, semen, vaginal secretions, and breast milk) from an HIV-infected person can transmit HIV. These specific fluids must come in contact with a mucous membrane or damaged tissue or be directly injected into the bloodstream (from a needle or syringe) for transmission to possibly occur.

In the United States, HIV is most commonly transmitted through specific sexual behaviors (anal or vaginal sex) or sharing needles with an infected person. It is less common for HIV to be transmitted through oral sex or for an HIV-infected woman to pass the virus to her baby before or during childbirth or after birth through breastfeeding or by prechewing food for her infant. In the United States, it is also possible to acquire HIV through exposure to infected blood, transfusions of infected blood, blood products, or organ transplantation, though this risk is extremely remote due to rigorous testing of the U.S. blood supply and donated organs.

Some healthcare workers have become infected after being stuck with needles containing HIV-infected blood or, less frequently, when infected blood comes in contact with a worker's open cut or is splashed into a worker's eyes or inside their nose. There has been only one instance of patients being infected by an HIV-infected dentist.

Which body fluids transmit HIV?

These body fluids have been shown to contain high concentrations of HIV:

- Blood
- Semen
- Vaginal fluid
- Breast milk
- Other body fluids containing blood

The following are additional body fluids that may transmit the virus that health care workers may come into contact with:

- Fluid surrounding the brain and the spinal cord
- Fluid surrounding bone joints
- Fluid surrounding an unborn baby

How well does HIV survive outside the body?

Scientists and medical authorities agree that HIV does not survive well outside the body, making the possibility of environmental transmission remote. HIV is found in varying concentrations or amounts in blood, semen, vaginal fluid, breast milk, saliva, and tears. To obtain data on the survival of HIV, laboratory studies have required the use of artificially high concentrations of laboratory-grown virus. Although these unnatural concentrations of HIV can be kept alive for days or even weeks under precisely controlled and limited laboratory conditions, CDC studies have shown that drying of even these high concentrations of HIV reduces the amount of infectious virus by 90 to 99 percent within several hours. Since the HIV concentrations used in laboratory studies are much higher than those actually found in blood or other specimens, drying of HIV-infected human blood or other body fluids reduces the theoretical risk of environmental transmission to that which has been observed—essentially zero. Incorrect interpretations of conclusions drawn from laboratory studies have in some instances caused unnecessary alarm.

Results from laboratory studies should not be used to assess specific personal risk of infection because (1) the amount of virus studied is not found in human specimens or elsewhere in nature, and (2) no one has been identified as infected with HIV due to contact with an environmental surface. Additionally, HIV is unable to reproduce outside its living host (unlike many bacteria or fungi, which may do so under suitable conditions), except under laboratory conditions; therefore, it does not spread or maintain infectiousness outside its host.

Can I get HIV from anal sex?

Yes. In fact, unprotected (without a condom) anal sex (intercourse) is considered to be very risky behavior. It is possible for either sex partner to become infected with HIV during anal sex. HIV can be found in the blood, semen, preseminal fluid, or vaginal fluid of a person infected with the virus. In general, the person receiving the semen is at greater risk of getting HIV because the lining of the rectum is thin and may allow the virus to enter the body during anal sex. However, a person who inserts his penis into an infected partner also is at risk because HIV can enter through the urethra (the opening at the tip of the penis) or through small cuts, abrasions, or open sores on the penis.

Not having (abstaining from) sex is the most effective way to avoid HIV. If people choose to have anal sex, they should use a latex condom. Most of the time, condoms work well. However, condoms are more likely to break during anal sex than during vaginal sex. Thus, even with a condom, anal sex can be risky. A person should use generous amounts of water-based lubricant in addition to the condom to reduce the chances of the condom breaking.

Can I get HIV from vaginal sex?

Yes, it is possible for either partner to become infected with HIV through vaginal sex (intercourse). In fact, it is the most common way the virus is transmitted in much of the world. HIV can be found in the blood, semen (cum), preseminal fluid (precum), or vaginal fluid of a person infected with the virus.

In women, the lining of the vagina can sometimes tear and possibly allow HIV to enter the body. HIV can also be directly absorbed through the mucous membranes that line the vagina and cervix.

In men, HIV can enter the body through the urethra (the opening at the tip of the penis) or through small cuts or open sores on the penis.

Risk for HIV infection increases if you or a partner has a sexually transmitted disease (STD).

Not having (abstaining from) sex is the most effective way to avoid HIV. If you choose to have vaginal sex, use a latex condom to help protect both you and your partner from HIV and other STDs. Studies have shown that latex condoms are very effective, though not perfect, in preventing HIV transmission when used correctly and consistently. If either partner is allergic to latex, plastic (polyurethane) condoms for either the male or female can be used.

Can I get HIV from oral sex?

Yes, it is possible for either partner to become infected with HIV through performing or receiving oral sex, though it is a less common mode of transmission than other sexual behaviors (anal and vaginal sex). There have been a few cases of HIV transmission from performing oral sex on a person infected with HIV. While no one knows exactly what the degree of risk is, evidence suggests that the risk is less than that of unprotected anal or vaginal sex.

If the person performing oral sex has HIV, blood from his or her mouth may enter the body of the person receiving oral sex through:

- the lining of the urethra (the opening at the tip of the penis);
- the lining of the vagina or cervix;
- the lining of the anus; or
- directly into the body through small cuts or open sores.

If the person receiving oral sex has HIV, their blood, semen (cum), preseminal fluid (precum), or vaginal fluid may contain the virus. Cells lining the mouth of the person performing oral sex may allow HIV to enter their body.

The risk of HIV transmission increases:

- if the person performing oral sex has cuts or sores around or in their mouth or throat;
- if the person receiving oral sex ejaculates in the mouth of the person performing oral sex; or
- if the person receiving oral sex has another sexually transmitted disease (STD).

Not having (abstaining from) sex is the most effective way to avoid HIV.

If you choose to perform oral sex, and your partner is male, use the following guidelines:

- Use a latex condom on the penis.

- If you or your partner is allergic to latex, plastic (polyurethane) condoms can be used.

Studies have shown that latex condoms are very effective, though not perfect, in preventing HIV transmission when used correctly and consistently. If either partner is allergic to latex, plastic (polyurethane) condoms for either the male or female can be used.

If you choose to have oral sex, and your partner is female, use a latex barrier (such as a natural rubber latex sheet, a dental dam, or a cut-open condom that makes a square) between your mouth and the vagina. A latex barrier such as a dental dam reduces the risk of blood or vaginal fluids entering your mouth. Plastic food wrap also can be used as a barrier.

If you choose to perform oral sex with a male or female partner and this sex includes oral contact with your partner's anus (anilingus or rimming), use a latex barrier (such as a natural rubber latex sheet, a dental dam, or a cut-open condom that makes a square) between your mouth and the anus. Plastic food wrap also can be used as a barrier.

How can I prevent HIV transmission when using sex toys?

If you choose to share sex toys with your partner, such as dildos or vibrators, each partner should use a new condom on the sex toy; and be sure to clean sex toys between each use.

Can I get HIV from injecting drugs?

Yes. At the start of every intravenous injection, blood is introduced into the needle and syringe. HIV can be found in the blood of a person infected with the virus. The reuse of a blood-contaminated needle or syringe by another drug injector (sometimes called direct syringe sharing) carries a high risk of HIV transmission because infected blood can be injected directly into the bloodstream.

Sharing drug equipment (or works) can be a risk for spreading HIV. Infected blood can be introduced into drug solutions by the following:

- Using blood-contaminated syringes to prepare drugs

- Reusing water

- Reusing bottle caps, spoons, or other containers (spoons and cookers) used to dissolve drugs in water and to heat drug solutions

- Reusing small pieces of cotton or cigarette filters (cottons) used to filter out particles that could block the needle

Street sellers of syringes may repackage used syringes and sell them as sterile syringes. For this reason, people who continue to inject drugs should obtain syringes from reliable sources of sterile syringes, such as pharmacies.

It is important to know that sharing a needle or syringe for any use, including skin popping and injecting steroids, can put one at risk for HIV and other blood-borne infections.

Is there a connection between HIV and other sexually transmitted diseases?

Yes. Having a sexually transmitted disease (STD) can increase a person's risk of becoming infected with HIV, whether the STD causes open sores or breaks in the skin (e.g., syphilis, herpes, chancroid) or does not cause breaks in the skin (e.g., chlamydia, gonorrhea).

If the STD infection causes irritation of the skin, breaks or sores may make it easier for HIV to enter the body during sexual contact. Even when the STD causes no breaks or open sores, the infection can stimulate an immune response in the genital area that can make HIV transmission more likely.

In addition, if an HIV-infected person is also infected with another STD, that person is three to five times more likely than other HIV-infected persons to transmit HIV through sexual contact.

Not having (abstaining from) sexual intercourse is the most effective way to avoid all STDs, including HIV. For those who choose to be sexually active, the following HIV prevention activities are highly effective:

- Engaging in behaviors that do not involve vaginal or anal intercourse or oral sex

- Having sex with only one uninfected partner

- Using latex condoms every time you have sex

Are health care workers at risk of getting HIV on the job?

The risk of health care workers being exposed to HIV on the job is very low, especially if they carefully follow universal precautions (i.e., using protective practices and personal protective equipment to prevent HIV and other blood-borne infections). It is important to remember that casual, everyday contact with an HIV-infected person does not expose health care workers or anyone else to HIV. For health care workers on the job, the main risk of HIV transmission is through accidental injuries from needles and other sharp instruments that may be contaminated with the virus; however, even this risk is small. Scientists estimate that the risk of infection from a needle stick is less than 1 percent, a figure based on the findings of several studies of health care workers who received punctures from HIV-contaminated needles or were otherwise exposed to HIV-contaminated blood.

Are patients in a health care setting at risk of getting HIV?

Although HIV transmission is possible in health care settings, it is extremely rare. Medical experts emphasize that the careful practice of infection control procedures, including universal precautions (i.e., using protective practices and personal protective equipment to prevent HIV and other blood-borne infections), protects patients as well as health care providers from possible HIV transmission in medical and dental offices and hospitals.

In 1990, the CDC reported on an HIV-infected dentist in Florida who apparently infected some of his patients while doing dental work. Studies of viral DNA [deoxyribonucleic acid] sequences linked the dentist to six of his patients who were also HIV-infected. The CDC has not yet been able to establish how the transmission took place. No additional studies have found any evidence of transmission from provider to patient in health care settings.

CDC has documented rare cases of patients contracting HIV in health care settings from infected donor tissue. Most of these cases occurred due to failures in following universal precautions and infection control guidelines. Most also occurred early in the HIV epidemic, before established screening procedures were in place.

Have people been infected with HIV from being stuck by needles in non-health care settings?

No. While it is possible to get infected with HIV if you are stuck with a needle that is contaminated with HIV, there are no documented cases of transmission outside of a health-care setting.

CDC has received inquiries about used needles left by HIV-infected injection drug users in coin return slots of pay phones, the underside of gas pump handles, and on movie theater seats. Some reports have falsely indicated that CDC "confirmed" the presence of HIV in the needles. CDC has not tested such needles nor has CDC confirmed the presence or absence of HIV in any sample related to these rumors. The majority of these reports and warnings appear to be rumors/myths.

CDC was informed of one incident in Virginia of a needle stick from a small-gauge needle (believed to be an insulin needle) in a coin return slot of a pay phone and a needle found in a vending machine that did not cause a needle-stick injury. There was an investigation by the local police and health department and there was no report of anyone contracting an infectious disease from these needles.

Discarded needles are sometimes found in the community. These needles are believed to have been discarded by persons who use insulin or inject illicit drugs. Occasionally the public and certain workers (e.g., sanitation workers or housekeeping staff) may sustain needle-stick injuries involving inappropriately discarded needles. Needle-stick injuries can transfer blood and blood-borne pathogens (e.g., hepatitis B, hepatitis C, and HIV), but the risk of transmission is extremely low and there are no documented cases of transmission outside of a health care setting.

CDC does not recommend routinely testing discarded needles to assess the presence or absence of infectious agents in the needles. Management of exposed persons should be done on a case-by-case basis to determine (1) the risk of a blood-borne pathogen infection in the source and (2) the nature of the injury. Anyone who is injured from a needle-stick in a community setting should contact their health-care provider or go to an emergency room as soon as possible. Antiretroviral medications given shortly after being stuck by a needle infected with HIV can reduce the risk of HIV infection. The health-care provider should then report the injury to the local or state health department.

Are lesbians or other women who have sex with women at risk for HIV?

Female-to-female transmission of HIV appears to be a rare occurrence. However, there are case reports of female-to-female transmission of HIV. The well-documented risk of female-to-male transmission of HIV shows that vaginal secretions and menstrual blood may contain the virus and that mucous membrane (e.g., oral, vaginal) exposure to these secretions has the potential to lead to HIV infection.

In order to reduce the risk of HIV transmission, women who have sex with women should do the following:

- Avoid exposure of a mucous membrane, such as the mouth (especially non-intact tissue), to vaginal secretions and menstrual blood.

- Use condoms consistently and correctly each and every time for sexual contact with men or when using sex toys. Sex toys should not be shared. No barrier methods for use during oral sex have been evaluated as effective by the Food and Drug Administration (FDA). However, natural rubber latex sheets, dental dams, cut open condoms, or plastic wrap may offer some protection from contact with body fluids during oral sex and possibly reduce the risk of HIV transmission.

- Know your own and your partner's HIV status. This knowledge can help uninfected women begin and maintain behavioral changes that reduce the risk of becoming infected. For women who are found to be infected, it can assist in getting early treatment and avoiding infecting others.

Can I get HIV from getting a tattoo or through body piercing?

A risk of HIV transmission does exist if instruments contaminated with blood are either not sterilized or disinfected or are used inappropriately between clients. CDC recommends that single-use instruments intended to penetrate the skin be used once, then disposed of. Reusable instruments or devices that penetrate the skin and/or contact a client's blood should be thoroughly cleaned and sterilized between clients.

Personal service workers who do tattooing or body piercing should be educated about how HIV is transmitted and take precautions to prevent transmission of HIV and other blood-borne infections in their settings.

If you are considering getting a tattoo or having your body pierced, ask staff at the establishment what procedures they use to prevent the spread of HIV and other blood-borne infections, such as the hepatitis B virus. You also may call the local health department to find out what sterilization procedures are in place in the local area for these types of establishments.

Can HIV be transmitted by kissing?

It depends on the type of kissing. There is no risk from closed-mouth kissing.

There are extremely rare cases of HIV being transmitted via deep French kissing but in each case, infected blood was exchanged due to bleeding gums or sores in the mouth. Because of this remote risk, it is recommended that individuals who are HIV-infected avoid deep, open-mouth French kissing with a non-infected partner, as there is a potential risk of transferring infected blood.

Can HIV be transmitted by human bite?

It is very rare, but in specific circumstances HIV can be transmitted by a human bite. In 1997, CDC published findings from a state health department investigation of an incident that suggested blood-to-blood transmission of HIV by a human bite. There have been other rare reports in the medical literature in which HIV appeared to have been transmitted by a human bite. Biting is not a common way of transmitting HIV, in fact, there are numerous reports of bites that did not result in HIV infection. Severe trauma with extensive tissue damage and the presence of blood were reported in each of the instances where transmission was documented or suspected. Bites that do not involve broken skin have no risk for HIV transmission, as intact skin acts as a barrier to HIV transmission.

Can HIV be transmitted by being scratched?

No. There is no risk of transmission from scratching because there is no transfer of body fluids between individuals. Any person with open wounds should have them treated as soon as possible.

Can HIV be transmitted by being spit on by an HIV-infected person?

No. In some persons living with HIV, the virus has been detected in saliva, but in extremely low quantities. Contact with saliva alone has never been shown to result in transmission of HIV, and there is no documented case of transmission from an HIV-infected person spitting on another person.

Can I get HIV from casual contact (shaking hands, hugging, using a toilet, drinking from the same glass, or the sneezing and coughing of an infected person)?

No. HIV is not transmitted by day-to-day contact in the workplace, schools, or social settings. HIV is not transmitted through shaking hands, hugging, or a casual kiss. You cannot become infected from a toilet seat, a drinking fountain, a doorknob, dishes, drinking glasses, food, or pets.

HIV is not an airborne or food-borne virus, and it does not live long outside the body.

Although contact with blood and other body substances can occur in households, transmission of HIV is rare in this setting. A small number of transmission cases have been reported in which a person became infected with HIV as a result of contact with blood or other body secretions from an HIV-infected person in the household.

Persons living with HIV and persons providing home care for those living with HIV should be fully educated and trained regarding appropriate infection-control procedures.

Can I get HIV from mosquitoes?

No. From the start of the HIV epidemic there has been concern about HIV transmission from biting and bloodsucking insects, such as mosquitoes. However, studies conducted by the CDC and elsewhere have shown no evidence of HIV transmission from mosquitoes or any other insects—even in areas where there are many cases of AIDS [acquired immunodeficiency syndrome] and large populations of mosquitoes. Lack of such outbreaks, despite intense efforts to detect them, supports the conclusion that HIV is not transmitted by insects.

The results of experiments and observations of insect-biting behavior indicate that when an insect bites a person, it does not inject its own or a previously bitten person's or animal's blood into the next person bitten. Rather, it injects saliva, which acts as a lubricant so the insect can feed efficiently. Diseases such as yellow fever and malaria are transmitted through the saliva of specific species of mosquitoes. However, HIV lives for only a short time inside an insect and, unlike organisms that are transmitted via insect bites, HIV does not reproduce (and does not survive) in insects. Thus, even if the virus enters a mosquito or another insect, the insect does not become infected and cannot transmit HIV to the next human it bites.

There also is no reason to fear that a mosquito or other insect could transmit HIV from one person to another through HIV-infected blood left on its mouth parts. Several reasons help explain why this is so. First, infected people do not have constantly high levels of HIV in their blood streams. Second, insect mouth parts retain only very small amounts of blood on their surfaces. Finally, scientists who study insects have determined that biting insects normally do not travel from one person to the next immediately after ingesting blood. Rather, they fly to a resting place to digest the blood meal.

Can I get HIV while playing sports?

There are no documented cases of HIV being transmitted during participation in sports. The very low risk of transmission during sports participation would involve sports with direct body contact in which bleeding might be expected to occur.

If someone is bleeding, their participation in the sport should be interrupted until the wound stops bleeding and is both antiseptically cleaned and securely bandaged. There is no risk of HIV transmission through sports activities where bleeding does not occur.

Has HIV been transmitted from body fluids placed in restaurant food?

No incident of food being contaminated with HIV-infected blood or semen has been reported to CDC. Furthermore, CDC has received no reports of HIV infection resulting from eating food, including condiments.

HIV does not live long outside the body. Even if small amounts of HIV-infected blood or semen was consumed, exposure to the air, heat from cooking, and stomach acid would destroy the virus. Therefore, there is no risk of contracting HIV from eating food.

Has CDC discovered a mutated version of HIV that is transmitted through the air?

No, this story is not true. Many scientific studies have been conducted to examine all the possible ways that HIV is transmitted. These studies have not shown HIV to be transmitted through air, water, insects, or casual contact.

Section 20.4

HIV Signs and Symptoms

"HIV/AIDS 101: Signs and Symptoms," by the Centers for Disease
Control and Prevention (CDC, www.cdc.gov), June 2012.

HIV-Positive without Symptoms

Many people who are HIV [human immunodeficiency virus]-positive
do not have symptoms of HIV infection. Often people only begin to feel
sick when they progress toward AIDS (acquired immunodeficiency
syndrome). Sometimes people living with HIV go through periods of
being sick and then feel fine.

While the virus itself can sometimes cause people to feel sick, most
of the severe symptoms and illnesses of HIV disease come from the
opportunistic infections that attack a damaged immune system. It
is important to remember that some symptoms of HIV infection are
similar to symptoms of many other common illnesses, such as the flu,
or respiratory or gastrointestinal infections.

Early Stages of HIV: Signs and Symptoms

As early as two to four weeks after exposure to HIV (but up to three
months later), people can experience an acute illness, often described
as "the worst flu ever." This is called acute retroviral syndrome (ARS),
or primary HIV infection, and it's the body's natural response to HIV
infection. During primary HIV infection, there are higher levels of virus circulating in the blood, which means that people can more easily
transmit the virus to others.

Symptoms can include the following:

- Fever

- Chills

- Rash

- Night sweats

- Muscle aches

- Sore throat
- Fatigue
- Swollen lymph nodes
- Ulcers in the mouth

It is important to remember, however, that not everyone gets ARS when they become infected with HIV.

Chronic Phase or Latency: Signs and Symptoms

After the initial infection and seroconversion, the virus becomes less active in the body, although it is still present. During this period, many people do not have any symptoms of HIV infection. This period is called the chronic or latency phase. This period can last up to 10 years—sometimes longer.

AIDS: Signs and Symptoms

When HIV infection progresses to AIDS, many people begin to suffer from fatigue, diarrhea, nausea, vomiting, fever, chills, night sweats, and even wasting syndrome at late stages. Many of the signs and symptoms of AIDS come from opportunistic infections which occur in patients with a damaged immune system.

Section 20.5

Testing for HIV

This section contains text excerpted from "The Role of STD Detection and Treatment in HIV Prevention," by the Centers for Disease Control and Prevention (CDC, www.cdc.gov), September 1, 2010; from "Pre-Post-Test Counseling," from AIDS.gov, part of the U.S. Department of Health and Human Services, October 11, 2010; and from "Testing for HIV," by AIDSinfo (www.aidsinfo.nih.gov), part of the U.S. Department of Health and Human Services, November 2011.

The Role of STD Detection and Treatment in HIV Prevention

Testing and treatment of sexually transmitted diseases (STDs) can be an effective tool in preventing the spread of HIV [human immunodeficiency virus], the virus that causes AIDS [acquired immunodeficiency syndrome].

What is the link between STDs and HIV infection?

Individuals who are infected with STDs are at least two to five times more likely than uninfected individuals to acquire HIV infection if they are exposed to the virus through sexual contact. In addition, if an HIV-infected individual is also infected with another STD, that person is more likely to transmit HIV through sexual contact than other HIV-infected persons.

There is substantial biological evidence demonstrating that the presence of other STDs increases the likelihood of both transmitting and acquiring HIV.

- **Increased susceptibility:** STDs appear to increase susceptibility to HIV infection by two mechanisms. Genital ulcers (e.g., syphilis, herpes, or chancroid) result in breaks in the genital tract lining or skin. These breaks create a portal of entry for HIV. Additionally, inflammation resulting from genital ulcers or non-ulcerative STDs (e.g., chlamydia, gonorrhea, and trichomoniasis) increase the concentration of cells in genital secretions that can serve as targets for HIV (e.g., CD4+ cells).

- **Increased infectiousness:** STDs also appear to increase the risk of an HIV-infected person transmitting the virus to his or her sex partners. Studies have shown that HIV-infected individuals who are also infected with other STDs are particularly likely to shed HIV in their genital secretions. For example, men who are infected with both gonorrhea and HIV are more than twice as likely to have HIV in their genital secretions than are those who are infected only with HIV. Moreover, the median concentration of HIV in semen is as much as 10 times higher in men who are infected with both gonorrhea and HIV than in men infected only with HIV. The higher the concentration of HIV in semen or genital fluids, the more likely it is that HIV will be transmitted to a sex partner.

How can STD treatment slow the spread of HIV infection?

Evidence from intervention studies indicates that detecting and treating STDs may reduce HIV transmission.

- STD treatment reduces an individual's ability to transmit HIV. Studies have shown that treating STDs in HIV-infected individuals decreases both the amount of HIV in genital secretions and how frequently HIV is found in those secretions.

- Herpes can make people more susceptible to HIV infection, and it can make HIV-infected individuals more infectious. It is critical that all individuals, especially those with herpes, know whether they are infected with HIV and, if uninfected with HIV, take measures to protect themselves from infection with HIV.

- Among individuals with both herpes and HIV, trials are underway studying if treatment of the genital herpes helps prevent HIV transmission to partners.

Pre- and Post-Test Counseling

General Pre-Test and Post-Test Information

Counseling before and after an HIV [human immunodeficiency virus] test is important because it provides critical information about HIV itself and about the testing process. While counseling services may not be available in all health care settings, many testing sites do offer these services. If you would like access to pre-test and post-test counseling, be sure to inquire about the availability of these services at your chosen test site. If they do not have them readily available, the staff may be able to direct you to alternate service providers who do.

Pre-test counseling sessions generally include the following:

- Information about the HIV test—what it tests for, what it might not tell you, and how long it will take you to get your results

- Information about how HIV is transmitted and how you can protect yourself from infection

- Information about the confidentiality of your test results

- A clear, easy-to-understand explanation of what your test results mean

Once the results are available, you will usually be given the results in private and in person. Post-test counseling generally includes the following:

- Clear communication about what your test result means

- HIV prevention counseling, if your results are negative

- A confirmatory test, called a Western blot test, if your results are positive. The results of that test should be available within two weeks.

If Your HIV Test Is Positive

- Your counselor will discuss what it means to live a healthy life with HIV and how you can keep from infecting others.

- Your counselor will also talk about treatments for HIV and can link you to a physician for immediate care. Getting into treatment quickly is important—it can help you keep your immune system healthy and keep you from progressing to AIDS [acquired immunodeficiency syndrome].

- All HIV-positive test results must be reported to your state health department for data tracking. Many states then report data to the CDC [Centers for Disease Control and Prevention], but no personal information (name, address, etc.) is ever shared when those data are reported.

HIV Pre-Test and Post-Test Counseling for Pregnant Women

CDC has outlined these recommendations for HIV counseling and testing of pregnant women:

- All pregnant women should be tested for HIV as early as possible during pregnancy, and HIV screening should be included in the routine panel of prenatal screening tests.

- Patients should be informed that HIV screening is recommended for all pregnant women and that it will be performed unless they decline (opt-out screening).

- If a pregnant woman declines to be tested for HIV, her healthcare providers should explore and address her reasons for declining HIV testing.

- Pregnant women should receive appropriate health education, including information about HIV and its transmission, as a routine part of prenatal care.

- Access to clinical care, prevention counseling, and support services is essential for women with positive HIV test results.

- HIV screening should be repeated in the third trimester of pregnancy for women known to be at high risk for HIV.

- Repeat HIV testing in the third trimester is also recommended for all women in areas with higher rates of HIV or AIDS and for women receiving healthcare in facilities with at least one diagnosed HIV case per 1,000 pregnant women per year.

Testing for HIV

I may have been exposed to HIV (human immunodeficiency virus). What should I do?

Get tested. The only way to know if you're infected with the virus is to get an HIV test.

Although some people newly infected with HIV may have flu-like symptoms, such as fever, sore throat, and rash, HIV can't be diagnosed by symptoms. Getting tested is the only way to know if you're infected with HIV.

What is the most common HIV test?

The most common HIV test is the HIV antibody test. The HIV antibody test checks for HIV antibodies in a person's blood, urine, or fluids from the mouth.

When a person becomes infected with HIV, the body begins to produce antibodies to HIV. Generally it takes about three months to produce enough antibodies to be detected by an HIV antibody test. (For some people, it can take up to six months.) The time period between infection and the appearance of detectable HIV antibodies is called the window period. Because HIV antibodies are not yet detectable, the HIV antibody test is not useful during the window period.

What HIV test is used during the window period?

The plasma HIV RNA (ribonucleic) test (also called a viral load test) can detect HIV in a person's blood within nine days of infection, before the body develops detectable HIV antibodies. The plasma HIV RNA test is recommended when recent infection is very likely—for example, immediately after a person has had unprotected sex with a partner infected with HIV, and especially if the person also has flu-like symptoms.

Detecting HIV at the earliest stage of infection lets people take steps right away to prevent HIV transmission. This is important because immediately after infection the amount of HIV in the body is very high, increasing the risk of HIV transmission. Starting treatment at this earliest stage of infection may also be considered.

What does it mean to test HIV positive?

To be diagnosed with HIV, a person must have positive results from two HIV tests. The first test may be either an HIV antibody test (using blood, urine, or fluids from the mouth) or a plasma HIV RNA test (using blood). The second test (always using blood) must be a Western blot test. The Western blot test confirms that a person has HIV.

How long does it take to get HIV test results?

Results of the first antibody test are generally available within a few days. (Rapid HIV antibody tests can produce results within an hour.) Results of the plasma HIV RNA test and Western blot are available in a few days to a few weeks.

If I test HIV positive now, will I always test HIV positive?

Yes. There's no cure for HIV. Because you will always be infected with the virus, you will always test HIV positive. However, treatment with anti-HIV medications can keep you healthy and protect you from AIDS (acquired immunodeficiency syndrome)-related illnesses.

If a pregnant woman tests positive for HIV, will her baby be born with HIV?

In the United States and Europe, fewer than two babies in 100 born to mothers infected with HIV are infected with the virus. This is because most mothers infected with HIV and their babies receive anti-HIV medications to prevent mother-to-child transmission of HIV.

Where can I find information on HIV testing locations?

Many hospitals, medical clinics, and community organizations offer HIV testing. To find an HIV testing site near you, visit www.hivtest.org.

Section 20.6

HIV and Its Treatment

Excerpted from "HIV and Its Treatment," by AIDSinfo
(www.aidsinfo.nih.gov), part of the U.S. Department of Health
and Human Services, November 11, 2011.

What is HIV/AIDS?

HIV stands for human immunodeficiency virus. HIV attacks and destroys the infection-fighting CD4 cells of the immune system. Loss of CD4 cells makes it difficult for the immune system to fight infections.

AIDS stands for acquired immunodeficiency syndrome. AIDS is the most advanced stage of HIV infection.

How is HIV transmitted?

HIV is transmitted (spread) from one person to another through specific body fluids—blood, semen, genital fluids, and breast milk. Having unprotected sex and sharing drug needles with a person infected by HIV are the most common ways HIV is transmitted.

You can't get HIV by shaking hands, hugging, or closed-mouth kissing with a person who has HIV. And HIV isn't spread through objects such as toilet seats, doorknobs, dishes, or drinking glasses used by a person with HIV.

Although it takes many years for symptoms of HIV to develop, a person infected with HIV can spread the disease at any stage of HIV infection. Detecting HIV during the earliest stages of infection and starting treatment well before symptoms of HIV develop can help people with HIV stay healthy. Treatment can also reduce the risk of HIV transmission.

What is the treatment for HIV?

Antiretroviral therapy (ART) is the recommended treatment for HIV infection. ART involves taking a combination (regimen) of three or more anti-HIV medications daily. ART prevents HIV from multiplying and destroying infection-fighting CD4 cells. This helps the body fight off life-threatening infections and cancer.

Although anti-HIV medications can't cure HIV, people with HIV are enjoying healthy lives and living longer thanks to ART.

Can treatment prevent HIV from advancing to AIDS?

Yes. Treatment with anti-HIV medications prevents HIV from multiplying and destroying the immune system. This helps the body fight off life-threatening infections and cancers and prevents HIV from advancing to AIDS.

Although it takes many years, without treatment HIV can advance to AIDS. To be diagnosed with AIDS, a person infected with HIV must either have a CD4 count less than 200 cells/mm^3 or have an AIDS-defining condition. The CD4 count of a healthy person ranges from 500 to 1,200 cells/mm^3. People infected with HIV with CD4 counts less than 500 cells/mm^3 should begin ART. AIDS-defining conditions are serious and life-threatening illnesses. Having an AIDS-defining condition indicates that a person's HIV infection has advanced to AIDS.

What illnesses are considered AIDS-defining conditions?

The Centers for Disease Control and Prevention (CDC) considers several illnesses AIDS-defining conditions.

Pneumocystis jiroveci pneumonia, tuberculosis, and toxoplasmosis are examples of AIDS-defining conditions.

I may have been exposed to HIV. What should I do?

Get tested. The only way to know if you're infected with the virus is to get an HIV test.

Although some people newly infected with HIV may have flu-like symptoms, such as fever, sore throat, and rash, HIV can't be diagnosed by symptoms. Getting tested is the only way to know if you're infected with HIV.

What is the most common HIV test?

The most common HIV test is the HIV antibody test. The HIV antibody test checks for HIV antibodies in a person's blood, urine, or fluids from the mouth.

When a person becomes infected with HIV, the body begins to produce antibodies to HIV. Generally it takes about three months to produce enough antibodies to be detected by an HIV antibody test. (For some people, it can take up to six months.) The time period between infection and the appearance of detectable HIV antibodies is called the window period. Because HIV antibodies are not yet detectable, the HIV antibody test is not useful during the window period.

What HIV test is used during the window period?

The plasma HIV RNA [ribonucleic acid] test (also called a viral load test) can detect HIV in a person's blood within nine days of infection, before the body develops detectable HIV antibodies. The plasma HIV RNA test is recommended when recent infection is very likely—for example, immediately after a person has had unprotected sex with a partner infected with HIV, and especially if the person also has flu-like symptoms.

Detecting HIV at the earliest stage of infection lets people take steps right away to prevent HIV transmission. This is important because immediately after infection the amount of HIV in the body is very high, increasing the risk of HIV transmission. Starting treatment at this earliest stage of infection may also be considered.

What does it mean to test HIV positive?

To be diagnosed with HIV, a person must have positive results from two HIV tests. The first test may be either an HIV antibody test (using blood, urine, or fluids from the mouth) or a plasma HIV RNA test (using blood). The second test (always using blood) must be a Western blot test. The Western blot test confirms that a person has HIV.

How long does it take to get HIV test results?

Results of the first antibody test are generally available within a few days. (Rapid HIV antibody tests can produce results within an hour.) Results of the plasma HIV RNA test and Western blot are available in a few days to a few weeks.

If I test HIV positive now, will I always test HIV positive?

Yes. There's no cure for HIV. Because you will always be infected with the virus, you will always test HIV positive. However, treatment with anti-HIV medications can keep you healthy and protect you from AIDS-related illnesses.

If a pregnant woman tests positive for HIV, will her baby be born with HIV?

In the United States and Europe, fewer than two babies in 100 born to mothers infected with HIV are infected with the virus. This is because most mothers infected with HIV and their babies receive anti-HIV medications to prevent mother-to-child transmission of HIV.

Seeing an HIV Health Care Provider

I just tested HIV positive. What should I look for in a health care provider?

Look for a health care provider who has experience treating HIV and AIDS. You may want to see a specialist in HIV.

You need a health care provider with whom you feel comfortable. You will be working closely together to make many decisions regarding your treatment.

What can I expect at my first health care provider visit?

Your health care provider will ask you questions about your health and lifestyle, do a physical exam, and order blood tests. Your health care provider will also discuss what it means to have HIV and how it might affect your life. Your first visit is a good time to ask your health care provider questions.

What questions should I ask my health care provider?

Ask your health care provider about the following:

- The benefits and risks of HIV treatment
- How HIV treatment may affect your lifestyle
- Lab tests used to monitor HIV infection

- How to avoid getting other infections

- How to avoid transmitting HIV

Write down your questions so you remember them when you visit your health care provider.

What tests will my health care provider order?

You will have three very important blood tests at your first medical appointment, including a CD4 count, a viral load test, and drug-resistance testing.

- The CD4 count measures the number of CD4 cells in a sample of blood. CD4 cells are infection-fighting cells of the body's immune system. HIV destroys CD4 cells, making it hard for the body to fight off infections. Because the CD4 count indicates the level of HIV damage to the immune system, the test is key to deciding when to start HIV treatment. A goal of treatment is to prevent HIV from destroying CD4 cells.

- A viral load test measures the amount of HIV in a sample of blood. A goal of HIV treatment is to keep a person's viral load so low that the virus can't be detected by a viral load test.

- Drug-resistance testing identifies which anti-HIV medications will or will not be effective against a person's strain of HIV.

Your CD4 count, viral load test, and drug-resistance testing results will provide an initial measure of your HIV infection before you start treatment. Once you start treatment, your health care provider will compare future test results with your initial results to monitor your HIV infection.

Your health care provider may also order other tests, such as a blood cell count, kidney and liver function tests, and tests for sexually transmitted infections (STIs) and other diseases.

When will I begin HIV treatment?

Starting HIV treatment is a big step. When to begin treatment depends on your health and your readiness to take a combination of anti-HIV medications (a regimen) every day. Once you begin taking anti-HIV medications, you will probably need to take them for the rest of your life.

Your health care provider will help you decide if you are ready to start treatment. Once you start treatment, your health care provider will help you find ways to stick to your treatment regimen.

223

What happens if I don't start treatment right away?

If you don't start treatment right away, you should have a CD4 count and viral load test once every three to six months. Your health care provider will use the test results to monitor your infection and help you decide when to start treatment.

When to Start Anti-HIV Medications

I just tested HIV positive. Do I need to start treatment?

Even though you have HIV, you may not need to start treatment right away. When to start anti-HIV medications (also called antiretrovirals) depends on several factors, including the following:

- Your overall health

- How well your immune system is working (CD4 count)

- The amount of HIV in your blood (viral load)

- Whether you're pregnant

- Your ability and willingness to commit to lifelong treatment

You and your health care provider will work together to decide on the best time to start treatment.

Can anti-HIV medications really help?

Yes. Although anti-HIV medications can't cure HIV, treatment can keep you healthy and improve your quality of life.

HIV attacks the immune system, destroying the system's CD4 cells. This makes it hard for the body to fight infection. But anti-HIV medications can prevent HIV from multiplying. Reducing the amount of HIV in your body gives the immune system a chance to recover and produce more infection-fighting CD4 cells. An increase in CD4 count indicates that treatment is working.

Once you start treatment—and take your anti-HIV medications exactly as directed—it's possible to have an undetectable viral load within three to six months. An undetectable viral load means that the level of HIV in your blood is too low to be detected by a viral load test. You aren't cured. There is still some HIV in your body. However, an undetectable viral load indicates that your anti-HIV medications are working effectively to keep you healthy and reduce your risk of transmitting HIV.

How will I know when to start anti-HIV medications?

It's time to start treatment if the following are true:

- Your CD4 count is less than 500 cells/mm^3.
- You have AIDS.
- You're pregnant.
- You have HIV-related kidney disease.
- You need treatment for hepatitis B virus (HBV).

Some research suggests that it may be helpful to start treatment early, when the CD4 count is greater than 500 cells/mm^3. You and your health care provider may want to discuss the benefits and risks of starting treatment early.

If anti-HIV medications can help me stay healthy, why wait to start treatment?

Successful HIV treatment depends on a lifelong commitment to take anti-HIV medications exactly as directed (treatment adherence). If you and your health care provider feel you're not ready to closely follow an HIV regimen for the rest of your life, you may decide to delay treatment. Delaying treatment will give you and your health care provider time to address any issues that may make adherence difficult.

Recommended HIV Treatment Regimens

What is the treatment for HIV?

Antiretroviral therapy (ART) is the recommended treatment for HIV. ART involves taking a combination of anti-HIV medications (a regimen) every day. Anti-HIV medications (also called antiretrovirals) are grouped into six drug classes according to how they fight HIV. The six classes are non-nucleoside reverse transcriptase inhibitors (NNRTIs), nucleoside reverse transcriptase inhibitors (NRTIs), protease inhibitors (PIs), fusion inhibitors, CCR5 antagonists, and integrase inhibitors.

Recommended HIV treatment regimens include three or more anti-HIV medications from at least two different drug classes. Taking a combination of anti-HIV medications from different classes is the most effective way to control the virus. Some anti-HIV medications are available in combination (two or more medications in one pill).

Anti-HIV medications are approved by the U.S. Food and Drug Administration (FDA).

How will I know which anti-HIV medications to take?

The best combination of anti-HIV medications for you depends on your individual needs. Factors that you and your health care provider will consider when selecting your HIV regimen include the following:

- Other diseases or conditions you may have

- Possible side effects of anti-HIV medications

- How anti-HIV medications may interact with other medications you take

- Your drug-resistance testing results

- Complexity of the regimen—how many pills to take every day and how often, and if pills must be taken with or without food

- Any personal issues that may make following a regimen difficult (such as depression or alcohol or drug abuse)

What are the recommended regimens for people taking anti-HIV medications for the first time?

After considering your individual needs, you and your health care provider may select one of the following regimens recommended for people taking anti-HIV medications for the first time:

- Atripla (a combination of three anti-HIV medications in one pill)

- Reyataz + Norvir + Truvada (Truvada is a combination of two anti-HIV medications in one pill.)

- Prezista + Norvir + Truvada

- Isentress + Truvada

Women who are planning on becoming pregnant or are in the first trimester of pregnancy should not use Atripla or Sustiva. (Sustiva, which is one of the medications in Atripla, can harm an unborn baby.) If you are pregnant or expect to become pregnant soon, talk to your health care provider about the benefits and risks of taking anti-HIV medications.

Because individual needs vary, these recommended HIV treatment regimens may not be right for everyone. If none of the preferred regimens is right for you, your health care provider will help you select an alternative regimen based on your needs.

Will I have side effects from the anti-HIV medications in my regimen?

Anti-HIV medications can cause side effects. Side effects vary depending on the anti-HIV medication. And people taking the same medication may not have the same side effects. Before starting treatment, discuss possible side effects with your health care provider or pharmacist.

Most side effects from anti-HIV medications are manageable. However, side effects that become unbearable or life threatening call for a change in medications. Side effects that may seem minor, such as fever, nausea, fatigue, or rash, can indicate serious problems. Once you start treatment, always discuss any side effects from your anti-HIV medications with your health care provider.

What is treatment adherence?

Treatment adherence means adhering to (following) your treatment regimen—taking the correct dose of each anti-HIV medication at the correct time and exactly as prescribed. Adherence is very important for successful HIV treatment.

Why is adherence important?

Adherence affects the success of HIV treatment in two ways:

- Good adherence to an HIV treatment regimen helps anti-HIV medications work effectively to reduce the amount of HIV in the body (viral load). Skipping medications, even occasionally, gives HIV the chance to multiply rapidly. Preventing the virus from multiplying is the best way to stay healthy.

- Good adherence to an HIV treatment regimen also helps prevent drug resistance. Drug resistance develops when the virus mutates (changes form), becoming resistant to certain anti-HIV medications. One or more anti-HIV medications in a treatment regimen can become ineffective as a result of drug resistance.

Skipping medications makes it easier for drug resistance to develop. HIV can develop resistance to the anti-HIV medications in a person's current regimen or to other, similar anti-HIV medications not yet taken, limiting options for successful HIV treatment. And drug-resistant strains of HIV can be transmitted to others, too.

Although there are many different anti-HIV medications and treatment regimens, studies show that a person's first regimen offers the best chance for long-term treatment success. Adhering to your regimen from the start will help ensure your HIV treatment is successful.

Why is treatment adherence sometimes difficult?

There are several reasons why adhering to an HIV treatment regimen can be difficult. Most treatment regimens involve taking several pills every day—with or without food, or before or after other medications. Other factors that can make treatment adherence difficult include the following:

- Difficulty taking medications (such as trouble swallowing pills)
- Side effects from medications (for example, fatigue or diarrhea)
- Daily schedule issues (including a busy schedule, shift work, or travel away from home)
- Being sick or depressed
- Alcohol or drug abuse

What can I do to adhere to my HIV treatment regimen?

Before you start treatment, be certain you're committed to taking anti-HIV medications every day as directed. Talk to your health care provider about any issues that may make adherence difficult, such as the following:

- Possible side effects from the anti-HIV medications in your regimen
- How other medications you take may interact with your anti-HIV medications
- Your schedule at home and at work
- Any personal issues such as depression or alcohol or drug abuse
- Lack of health insurance to pay for anti-HIV medications

Understanding issues that can make adherence difficult will help you and your health care provider select the best regimen for you. Some people may find that adhering to an HIV treatment regimen becomes more difficult over time. So, talk to your health care provider about adherence at every visit.

Following an HIV Treatment Regimen

How can I prepare for adherence before I start HIV treatment?

Being prepared to take anti-HIV medications every day is a first step to treatment success. Planning ahead will help you adhere to your treatment regimen when you start treatment.

Begin by talking to your health care provider. Make sure you understand why you're starting HIV treatment and why treatment adherence is important. Discuss these important details about your treatment regimen:

- Each anti-HIV medication in your regimen

- The dose of each medication

- How many pills in each dose

- When to take each medication

- How to take each medication—with or without food

- Possible side effects from each medication, including serious side effects

- Possible interactions between the anti-HIV medications in your regimen and other medications you take

- How to store your medications

Tell your health care provider if you have any personal issues, such as depression or alcohol or drug abuse, that can make adherence difficult. If needed, your health care provider may recommend resources to help you address these issues before you start treatment.

How can I maintain adherence after I start treatment?

You may consider one or more of the following strategies to help you adhere to your regimen:

- Use a seven-day pill box. Once a week, fill the pill box with your medications for the entire week.

- Take your medications at the same time every day.

- Use a timer, an alarm clock, or your cell phone alarm to remind you to take your medications.

229

- Enlist your family members, friends, or coworkers to remind you to take your medications.

- Keep your medications nearby. Keep a backup supply of medications in your briefcase or purse or at work.

- Plan ahead for changes in your daily routine, including weekends and holidays. If you're going away, pack enough medications to last the entire trip.

- Use a medication diary to stay on track. Write down the name of each medication; include the dose, number of pills to take, and when to take them. Check off each medication as you take it. Reviewing your diary will help you identify the times you're most likely to skip medications.

- Keep all your medical appointments. Write down the date and time of health care provider visits on your calendar or daily schedule. If you run low on medications before your next visit, call your health care provider to renew your prescriptions.

- Get additional tips on adherence by joining a support group for people living with HIV.

What should I do if I forget to take my medications?

Unless your health care provider tells you otherwise, take a medication you missed as soon as you remember that you skipped it. However, if it's almost time for the next dose of the medication, don't take the missed dose and just continue on your regular medication schedule. Don't take a double dose of a medication to make up for a missed dose.

What should I do if I have problems adhering to my treatment regimen?

Tell your health care provider that you're having difficulty following your regimen. Together you can identify the reasons why you're skipping medications.

Tell your health care provider about any side effects from the medications in your regimen. Side effects are a major reason treatment adherence can be difficult. A regimen that involves taking many pills at many times during the day can also make adherence difficult. Based on why you're having problems with adherence, your health care provider may adjust or change your regimen.

Preventing HIV Transmission

How is HIV transmitted?

HIV is transmitted (spread) through the blood, semen, genital fluids, or breast milk of an infected person. The spread of the virus is called HIV transmission. The most common ways people become infected with HIV are by having unprotected sex with a person infected with HIV or sharing drug needles or syringes with a person infected with HIV.

Women infected with HIV can transmit the virus to their babies during pregnancy or childbirth or by breastfeeding. If you are a woman who has HIV, talk to your health care provider about ways to prevent pregnancy. And if you are pregnant or plan to become pregnant, ask your health care provider how you can protect your baby from HIV.

I am taking anti-HIV medications and my viral load is undetectable. Can I still infect another person with HIV?

Your anti-HIV medications are doing a good job of controlling your infection. The amount of HIV in your blood is so low that a viral load test can't detect the virus. However, having an undetectable viral load doesn't mean you're cured. You still have HIV. And although having an undetectable viral load reduces the risk of HIV transmission, you can still infect another person with the virus.

How can I prevent transmitting HIV?

To prevent infecting another person with HIV, do the following:

- Use a condom every time you have sex.
- If you inject drugs, don't share your needles or syringes.
- Don't share your razor, toothbrush, or other items that may have your blood on them.
- Take your anti-HIV medications according to your health care provider's directions.
- If you are a mother infected with HIV, don't breastfeed your baby.

Talk to your health care provider about how HIV is transmitted and ways to prevent spreading the virus. At each visit, discuss any high-risk behaviors (such as having unprotected sex or sharing drug needles) with your health care provider.

Talking about high-risk behaviors can be difficult. And making changes, even when we want to, isn't always easy. However, it's important to be honest with your health care provider about any high-risk activities. Discussing ways to prevent HIV transmission can reduce your chances of infecting another person with the virus.

Can I put my partner who is also infected with HIV at risk?

It's important to use condoms and not share drug needles even if your partner is also infected with HIV. You and your partner may have different strains of the virus. Your partner's HIV could act differently in your body or cause the anti-HIV medications you take to be less effective. And your strain of HIV could have the same effects on your partner.

Section 20.7

Living with HIV

Excerpted from "Living with HIV/AIDS," by the Division of HIV/AIDS Prevention, Centers for Disease Control and Prevention (CDC, www.cdc.gov), June 21, 2007. Reviewed by David A. Cooke, MD, FACP, July 10, 2012.

HIV (human immunodeficiency virus) is the virus that causes acquired immunodeficiency syndrome (AIDS).

Although infection with HIV is serious, people with HIV and AIDS are living longer, healthier lives today, thanks to new and effective treatments. This text will help you understand how you can live with HIV and keep yourself healthy.

What is HIV and how did I get it?

HIV is the virus that causes AIDS. The first cases of AIDS were identified in the United States in 1981, but the virus probably existed here and in other parts of the world for many years before that. In 1984, scientists proved that HIV causes AIDS.

Ways you might have gotten HIV:

- Having unprotected sex (sex without a condom) with someone who has HIV

- Sharing a needle to inject drugs or sharing drug works with someone who has HIV

- Having a mother who was infected with HIV when you were born

- From a blood transfusion (However, it is unlikely you got infected that way because all blood in the United States has been tested for HIV since 1985.)

Ways you did not get (and no one else can get) HIV:

- Just working with or being around someone who has HIV

- Being stung or bitten by an insect

- Sitting on toilet seats

- Doing everyday things like sharing a meal

What is the difference between HIV and AIDS?

HIV is the virus that causes the disease AIDS. Although HIV causes AIDS, a person can be infected with HIV for many years before AIDS develops.

When HIV enters your body, it infects specific cells in your immune system. These cells are called CD4 [cluster of differentiation] cells or helper T cells. They are important parts of your immune system and help your body fight infection and disease. When your CD4 cells are not working well, you are more likely to get sick.

Usually, CD4 cell counts in someone with a healthy immune system range from 500 to 1,800 per cubic millimeter of blood. AIDS is diagnosed when your CD4 cell count goes below 200. Even if your CD4 cell count is over 200, AIDS can be diagnosed if you have HIV and certain diseases such as tuberculosis or *Pneumocystis carinii* pneumonia (PCP).

There are general stages of HIV infection that you may go through before AIDS develops.

- **Infection:** The earliest stage is right after you are infected. HIV can infect cells and copy itself before your immune system has started to respond. You may have felt flu-like symptoms during this time.

233

- **Response:** The next stage is when your body responds to the virus. Even if you don't feel any different, your body is trying to fight the virus by making antibodies against it. This is called seroconversion, when you go from being HIV negative to HIV positive.

- **No symptoms:** You may enter a stage in which you have no symptoms. This is called asymptomatic infection. You still have HIV and it may be causing damage that you can't feel.

- **Symptoms:** Symptomatic HIV infection is when you develop symptoms, such as certain infections, including PCP.

- **AIDS:** AIDS is diagnosed when you have a variety of symptoms, infections, and specific test results. There is no single test to diagnose AIDS.

How long does it take to go from HIV infection to a diagnosis of AIDS?

There is no one answer to this question because everyone is different. Estimates of the average length of time for progression from HIV to AIDS are being developed. Before antiretroviral therapy became available in 1996, scientists estimated that AIDS would develop within 10 years in about half the people with HIV. Since 1996, new medical treatments have been developed that can prevent or cure some of the illnesses associated with AIDS, though they cannot cure AIDS itself.

Various factors, including your genetic makeup, can influence the time between HIV infection and the development of AIDS.

There is a shorter time between HIV infection and AIDS when a person has the following characteristics:

- Older age

- Infection with more than one type of HIV

- Poor nutrition

- Severe stress

There is a longer time between HIV infection and AIDS when a person has the following characteristics:

- Closely adhering to your doctor's recommendations

- Eating healthy foods

- Taking care of yourself

What is clear is that you have some control over the progression of HIV infection.

How can I stay healthy longer?

There are many things you can do for yourself to stay healthy. Here are a few.

Make sure you have a health care provider who knows how to treat HIV. Begin treatment promptly once your doctor tells you to. Keep your appointments. Follow your doctor's instructions. If your doctor prescribes medicine for you, take the medicine just the way he or she tells you to because taking only some of your medicine gives your HIV infection more chance to fight back. If you get sick from your medicine, call your doctor for advice; don't make changes to your medicine on your own or because of advice from friends. Get immunizations (shots) to prevent infections such as pneumonia and flu. Your doctor will tell you when to get these shots. Practice safe sex to reduce your risk of getting a sexually transmitted disease (STD) or another strain of HIV. If you smoke or use drugs not prescribed by your doctor, quit. Eat healthy foods. This will help keep you strong, keep your energy and weight up, and help your body protect itself. Exercise regularly. Get enough sleep and rest. Take time to relax. Many people find that meditation or prayer, along with exercise and rest, help them cope with the stress of having HIV or AIDS.

There are also many things you can do to protect your health when you prepare food or eat, when you travel, and when you're around pets and other animals.

What can I expect when I go to the doctor?

During your first appointment your doctor will ask you questions, examine you, take a blood sample, and do some other tests. Your doctor also may do a skin test for tuberculosis and give you some immunizations (shots).

Tell your doctor about any health problems you are having so that you can get treatment. You also should ask your doctor any questions you have about HIV or AIDS, such as the following:

- What to do if your medicine makes you sick

- Where to get help for quitting smoking or using drugs

- How to create a healthier diet how to minimize the chance that you will spread HIV to your partners

Your blood sample is used for many tests, including the CD4 cell count and viral load. Your CD4 cell count tells you how many CD4 cells you have in your blood. If you are getting treatment, your CD4 cell counts indicate how well it is working. If your CD4 cell count rises, your body is better able to fight infection. Viral load testing measures the amount of HIV in your blood. Your viral load helps predict what will happen next with your HIV infection if you don't get treatment.

Keep your follow-up appointments with your doctor. At these appointments you and your doctor will talk about your test results, and he or she may prescribe medicine for you.

What are some of the other diseases I could get?

Because HIV damages your immune system, you may have a higher chance of getting certain diseases, called opportunistic infections. They are so named because an HIV-infected person's weakened immune system gives these diseases the opportunity to develop. Fortunately, people with HIV who are taking medicine can go a long time before their immune system is damaged enough to allow an opportunistic infection to occur. That's why it is so important to get tested and start treatment early. Many people may not know they have HIV until AIDS and an opportunistic infection develop. Many germs can cause opportunistic infections.

Examples of common opportunistic infections include the following:

- *Pneumocystis carinii* pneumonia
- Mycobacterium avium complex
- Cytomegalovirus
- Tuberculosis
- Toxoplasmosis
- Cryptosporidiosis
- Hepatitis C
- Human papillomavirus

Certain symptoms can occur with opportunistic infections, such as the following:

- Breathing problems
- Mouth problems, such as thrush (white spots), sores, change in taste, dryness, trouble swallowing, or loose teeth

- Fever for more than two days
- Weight loss
- Change in vision or floaters (moving lines or spots in your vision)
- Diarrhea
- Skin rashes or itching

Tell your doctor right away if you have any of these problems. Your doctor can treat most of your HIV-related problems, but sometimes you may need to go to a specialist. Visit a dentist at least twice a year and more often if you have mouth problems.

How do I protect other people from my HIV?

Things you should do:

- Abstain from sex. The surest way to avoid transmission of STDs, including a different strain of HIV, is to not have sexual intercourse.

- Use condoms correctly and consistently. Correct and consistent use of the male latex condom can reduce the risk for STD transmission. However, no protective method is 100% effective. Condom use cannot guarantee absolute protection against any STD. If you are allergic to latex, you can use polyurethane condoms. Condoms lubricated with spermicides are no more effective than other lubricated condoms in protecting against the transmission of HIV and other STDs. If you use condoms incorrectly, they can slip off or break, which reduces their protective effects. Inconsistent use, such as not using condoms with every act of intercourse, can lead to STD transmission because transmission can occur with just one act of intercourse.

- Use protection during oral sex. A condom or dental dam (a square piece of latex used by dentists) can be used. Do not reuse these items.

- Tell others that you have HIV. Tell people you've had sex with. This can be difficult, but they need to know so they can get the help they need. Your local public health department may help you find these people and tell them they have been exposed to HIV. If they have HIV, this may help them get care and avoid spreading HIV to others. Tell people you are planning on having sex with. Practicing safe sex will help protect your health and that of your partners.

- If you are a man and had sex with a woman who became pregnant, you need to tell the woman that you have HIV, even if you are not the father of the baby. If she has HIV, she needs to get early medical care for her own health and her baby's health.

Things you should not do:

- Don't share sex toys. Keep sex toys for your own use only.
- Don't share drug needles or drug works. Use a needle exchange program if one is available. Seek help if you inject drugs. You can fight HIV much better if you don't have a drug habit.
- Don't donate blood, plasma, or organs.
- Don't share razors or toothbrushes. HIV can be spread through fresh blood on such items.

Is there special advice for women with HIV?

Yes. If you are a woman with HIV, your doctor should check you for STDs and perform a Pap test at least once a year.

As a woman with HIV, you are more likely to have abnormal Pap test results. Infection with HIV means your body is less effective in controlling all types of viruses. The human papillomavirus (HPV) is a specific virus that can infect cervical cells (the cells that the Pap test looks at). Your doctor may recommend a special test that can look for HPV as part of your exam. If your Pap test result is abnormal, your doctor may need to repeat it or do other tests. If you have had an abnormal Pap test result in the past, tell your doctor.

If you are thinking about avoiding pregnancy or becoming pregnant, talk with your doctor. You might ask some of the following questions:

- What birth control methods are best for me?
- Will HIV cause problems for me during pregnancy or delivery?
- Will my baby have HIV?
- Will treatment for my HIV infection cause problems for my baby?

If I choose to get pregnant, what medical and community programs and support groups can help me and my baby?

If you become pregnant, talk to your doctor right away about medical care for you and your baby. You also need to plan for your child's future in case you get sick.

Your HIV treatment will not change very much from what it was before you became pregnant. You should have a Pap test and tests for STDs during your pregnancy. Your doctor will order tests and suggest medicines for you to take. Talk with him or her about all the pros and cons of taking medicine while you are pregnant.

Talk with your doctor about how you can prevent giving HIV to your baby. It is very important that you get good care early in your pregnancy. The chances of passing HIV to your baby before or during birth are about one in four, or 25%, but treatment with antiretroviral medicines has been shown to greatly lower this risk. Your doctor will want you to take these medicines to increase your baby's chance of not getting HIV.

Although you are pregnant, to avoid catching other diseases and to avoid spreading HIV, you should still use condoms each time you have sex. Even if your partner already has HIV, he should still use condoms.

After birth, your baby will need to be tested for HIV, even if you took antiretroviral medicines while you were pregnant. Your baby will need to take medicine to prevent HIV infection and PCP. Talk with your doctor about your baby's special medical needs. Because HIV infection can be passed through breast milk, you should not breastfeed your baby.

Where can I find help in dealing with HIV?

If you are living with HIV or AIDS, you may need many kinds of support: Medical, emotional, psychological, and financial. Your doctor, your local health and social services departments, local AIDS service organizations, and libraries can help you in finding all kinds of help, such as the following:

- Answers to your questions about HIV and AIDS

- Doctors, insurance, and help in making health care decisions

- Food, housing, and transportation

- Planning to meet financial and daily needs

- Support groups for you and your loved ones

- Home nursing care

- Help in legal matters, including Americans with Disabilities Act (ADA) claims

- Confidential help in applying for Social Security disability benefits

Many people living with HIV feel better if they can talk with other people who also have HIV. Here are some ways to find support.

- Contact your local AIDS service organization. Look under "AIDS" or "Social Service Organizations" in the yellow pages of your telephone book.

- Contact a local hospital, church, or American Red Cross chapter for referrals.

- Read HIV newsletters or magazines.

- Join support groups or Internet forums.

- Volunteer to help others with HIV.

- Be an HIV educator or public speaker, or work on a newsletter.

- Attend social events to meet other people who have HIV.

Today, thousands of people are living with HIV or AIDS. Many are leading full, happy, and productive lives. You can too if you work with your doctor and others and take the steps outlined in this text to stay healthy.

Section 20.8

How Can I Pay for HIV Care?

"Paying for HIV Care," by the Office on Women's Health
(www.womenshealth.gov), July 1, 2011.

Paying for everyday needs and health care is hard for many people, including those living with HIV/AIDS [human immunodeficiency virus/ acquired immunodeficiency syndrome]. HIV/AIDS drugs are expensive, and many people find it hard to buy the medicines they need. Some people with HIV/AIDS are not able to work. Other people may have problems getting the housing they need. Studies show that people with HIV/AIDS are better able to take care of their health when all their basic needs, like housing, are met. Services are available to help people with HIV/AIDS pay for health care, medicine, housing, and other basic needs.

Getting and Keeping Health Insurance

Many people who are infected with HIV are able to live full lives with no signs of their infection for a long time. The main way these people will be paying for HIV care is with health insurance. Even when you seem to be doing fine with HIV, you will have expenses. At first you may need screenings and doctor visits, but eventually you will need expensive medicine and other care.

Today, most Americans living with HIV get their insurance from Medicaid [www.medicaid.gov] or Medicare [www.medicare.gov]. These are government-run insurance programs. Medicare is for people over 65 and people with disabilities. Medicaid is for people with low incomes and people with disabilities. Some people get health insurance through their employer. There are also people who have to buy plans on their own. This might include people working for small businesses that don't offer insurance. Getting coverage has been difficult for people living with HIV/AIDS. Nearly 30 percent of people with HIV don't have any insurance at all. People with HIV can also get assistance from the AIDS Drug Assistance Program [ftp://ftp.hrsa.gov/hab/B.ADAP.final.pdf].

This program helps people who cannot afford to pay for their HIV medications.

In addition to Medicare and Medicaid, other health insurance is changing because of health care reform. Learn more about how to get the health insurance you need at HealthCare.gov.

The Health Insurance Portability and Accountability Act of 1996 (HIPAA) helps people with HIV/AIDS keep their health insurance. Part of the law protects people when they lose or change jobs by offering insurance "portability" to qualifying people. The law also sets guidelines to keep people's medical information private.

Disability Benefits for People Who Cannot Work

If you have HIV/AIDS and cannot work, you may qualify for help from the Social Security Administration. The money you get can help you pay for basic needs, such as food, clothing, and shelter. Benefits are paid under two programs:

- The Social Security Disability Insurance Program [www.social security.gov/disability] is for people who have worked and paid Social Security taxes. The amount of money you get each month depends on how much you earned while you were working. You also will qualify for Medicare after you have been getting disability benefits for 24 months. Medicare is a federal health insurance program. It helps pay for medical care, HIV drugs, and other services.

- The Supplemental Security Income (SSI) program [www.social security.gov/ssi] is for people who have little income and few resources. If you get SSI, you most likely will be able to get food stamps and Medicaid, too.

If your Social Security benefits are very low and you have limited other income and resources, you may qualify for both programs.

Medicare and Medicaid for Working People with Disabilities

Special rules make it possible for people with disabilities receiving Social Security benefits or Supplemental Security Income (SSI) to work and still receive monthly payments and Medicare or Medicaid. Social Security calls these rules work incentives. Contact your state Social Security office to find out if you can make use of these programs.

Medicaid

Medicaid is a federally sponsored health program for people with low income. Each state runs its own Medicaid program. Medicaid does not pay money to you; instead, it sends payments directly to your doctors. You must qualify to get Medicaid. Most adults with HIV who qualify for Medicaid:

- are disabled;

- have low income;

- have limited assets;

- have families with dependent children and meet certain income and resource standards.

Medicaid was expanded under health care reform. So if you haven't qualified before, you might now. You apply to Medicaid in the state where you live. Each state has different rules as to whether you qualify. You can get an application at your local Medicaid office. You can also call your local Social Security office. Learn more from the Centers for Medicare and Medicaid Services [www.cms.gov).

- Financial support during pregnancy—If you are pregnant, Medicaid may pay for your prenatal care. If you are pregnant and HIV-positive, Medicaid might pay for counseling, medicine to lower the risk of passing HIV to your baby, and treatment for HIV. You can stay on Medicaid for about 90 days after you deliver your baby. It may continue for one year after you deliver your baby. This depends on the rules in your state. Each state makes its own Medicaid rules. If you don't think you qualify for Medicaid, check again. You may be able to get it while pregnant because the income limits are raised for pregnant women to provide prenatal care and HIV treatment.

- Early and Periodic Screening, Diagnostic, and Treatment (EPSDT)—The Early and Periodic Screening, Diagnostic, and Treatment (EPSDT) service is Medicaid's preventive child health program for children under 21. EPSDT offers access to Medicaid services and screenings that may be important for a child with HIV but are not covered for the rest of the Medicaid population.

Ryan White HIV/AIDS Program

This federal program helps people with HIV/AIDS who have nowhere else to turn for the care they need. It pays for doctor visits,

HIV/AIDS drugs, and supportive services for people with HIV/AIDS. In some cases, family members can receive services through a Ryan White program for women, infants, children, and youth, even though they are not diagnosed with HIV. Call your state's HIV/AIDS hotline [hab.hrsa.gov/gethelp/statehotlines.html] to ask about care or medicines through Ryan White or other programs.

Programs That Help Pay for HIV/AIDS Medicines

You can get help paying for HIV/AIDS drug treatment:

- Ryan White AIDS Drug Assistance Program (ADAP) gives HIV drugs to people with HIV/AIDS who don't have health insurance that pays for HIV drugs. For example, it covers people with low incomes who may not be disabled and can't get public health insurance, like Medicaid. This drug program is run by your state and may have different rules than other states. Call your state's HIV/AIDS hotline to ask about the ADAP program in your state.

- Patient assistance programs [www.pparx.org] are offered by some drug companies to give medicines at a lower cost or for free to people who can't afford them. Ask your doctor to contact the program for you.

- Clinical trials [www.womenshealth.gov/hiv-aids/research -clinical-trials-hiv-aids] offer people with HIV a way to try new HIV medicines that aren't yet available to the public. AIDS clinical trials are research studies in which new treatments for AIDS and HIV infection are tested in humans. These studies help determine if the drugs are useful and safe in treating HIV/AIDS. These HIV drugs are free for the person in the trial.

Medicare Part D Prescription Drug Coverage

If you get your medications through Medicare Part D coverage, health care reform may make drugs more affordable for you. People whose HIV drugs are paid for with Medicare Part D may fall into the "donut hole" in drug coverage. This means that the costs are high enough that Medicare stops paying for them, and you pay the rest. When your drug costs increase much more in the same year, a type of emergency coverage kicks in, and Medicare pays for your drugs again. For people paying for all of their drugs while in this "donut hole," health care reform now gives them a 50 percent discount on brand-name drugs. More discounts will go into effect in coming years.

Housing Opportunities for Persons with AIDS (HOPWA)

You can get help with health services, legal assistance, and housing at HousingWorks.org .The U.S. Department of Housing and Urban Development (HUD), Office of HIV/AIDS Housing runs the Housing Opportunities for Persons With AIDS (HOPWA) program [portal.hud.gov/hudportal/HUD?src=/program_offices/comm_planning/aidshousing/programs]. Their programs provide HIV/AIDS housing that includes short- and long-term rental assistance, live-in medical facilities, and housing sites developed just for people living with AIDS.

Section 20.9

The Affordable Care Act and People Living with HIV/AIDS

Excerpted from "The Affordable Care Act and People Living with
HIV or AIDS," HealthCare.gov, part of the U.S. Department of
Health and Human Services, September 13, 2010.

If you or a loved one is living with HIV [human immunodeficiency virus] or AIDS [acquired immunodeficiency syndrome], you know how far our nation has come in treating and reducing the spread of the disease—and how much more we need to do.

People living with HIV and AIDS have always had a difficult time obtaining access to health coverage. Medicaid, Medicare, and the Ryan White HIV/AIDS Program have provided a critical safety net. But today, nearly 30% of people living with HIV do not have any health insurance coverage, and many others have limited coverage. In addition, people living with HIV and AIDS have faced hurdles to getting quality care from qualified providers.

The Affordable Care Act passed by Congress and signed by President Obama in March 2010 helps make it easier and fairer for people living with HIV or AIDS to get the coverage and care they need. It will do the following:

- Stop insurance discrimination: As early as September 23, 2010, insurers will no longer be able to deny coverage to children because they have HIV or AIDS. And insurers won't be able to rescind coverage for adults or children unless they can show evidence of fraud or intentional misrepresentation of a material fact in an application.

• Increase access to coverage: Starting in 2014, adults also may not be denied coverage based on their HIV status, and no one may be charged higher premiums because of their HIV status or any other disability. The Affordable Care Act will also broaden Medicaid eligibility so that low-income people living with HIV won't have to wait for an AIDS diagnosis to become eligible. Tax credits will help middle class Americans better afford coverage also starting in 2014.

• Improve quality of coverage: Annual and lifetime limits on coverage can keep people living with HIV/AIDS from getting the care they need. Ending lifetime limits and phasing out annual limits will ensure that coverage is there when people need it, which is what the Affordable Care Act will do starting as early as September 23, 2010. In addition, under the Affordable Care Act, many private insurance plans will soon be required to cover recommended preventive services like regular check-ups and HIV screening tests at no additional cost—helping people stay healthy and access life-saving treatments more quickly. In January, as a result of the Affordable Care Act, Medicare will adopt a similar policy.

• Provide better care: The Affordable Care Act also makes key investments in our health care system, including expanding the health care workforce and increasing funding for community health centers.

Chapter 21

Human Papillomavirus (HPV)

Chapter Contents

Section 21.1—What Is Genital HPV Infection and
How Does It Affect Women?................................. 248

Section 21.2—HPV and Men 254

Section 21.3—Recurrent Respiratory Papillomatosis 259

Section 21.4—Pap Tests and Cervical Cancer
Screening to Check for HPV 262

Section 21.5—Making Sense of Your HPV Test Results 264

Section 21.6—What You Should Know When You Are
Diagnosed with Genital Warts 271

Section 21.7—Treating HPV and Related Problems 273

Section 21.8—HPV Infection and Cancer 276

Section 21.1

What Is Genital HPV Infection and How Does It Affect Women?

This section includes text from "Genital HPV Infection—Fact Sheet," by the Centers for Disease Control and Prevention (CDC, www.cdc.gov), November 7, 2011, and text excerpted from "Human Papillomavirus (HPV) and Genital Warts Fact Sheet," by the Office on Women's Health (www .womenshealth.gov), part of the U.S. Department of Health and Human Services, January 1, 2009.

Genital HPV Infection

Genital human papillomavirus (also called HPV) is the most common sexually transmitted disease (STD). There are more than 40 HPV types that can infect the genital areas of males and females. These HPV types can also infect the mouth and throat. Most people who become infected with HPV do not even know they have it.

HPV is not the same as herpes or HIV (human immunodeficiency virus, the virus that causes AIDS [acquired immunodeficiency syndrome]). These are all viruses that can be passed on during sex, but they cause different symptoms and health problems.

What are the signs, symptoms, and potential health problems of HPV?

Most people with HPV do not develop symptoms or health problems from it. In 90% of cases, the body's immune system clears HPV naturally within two years. But, sometimes, HPV infections are not cleared and can cause the following:

- Genital warts

- Rarely, warts in the throat (a condition called recurrent respiratory papillomatosis, or RRP (When this occurs in children it is called juvenile-onset RRP [JORRP].)

- Cervical cancer and other, less common but serious cancers, including cancers of the vulva, vagina, penis, anus, and oropharynx (back of throat including base of tongue and tonsils)

The types of HPV that can cause genital warts are not the same as the types that can cause cancers. There is no way to know which people who get HPV will go on to develop cancer or other health problems.

Genital warts usually appear as a small bump or group of bumps in the genital area. They can be small or large, raised or flat, or shaped like a cauliflower. Health care providers can diagnose warts by looking at the genital area during an office visit. Warts can appear within weeks or months after sexual contact with an infected partner—even if the infected partner has no signs of genital warts. If left untreated, genital warts might go away, remain unchanged, or increase in size or number. They will not turn into cancer.

Cervical cancer usually does not have symptoms until it is quite advanced. For this reason, it is important for women to get regular screening for cervical cancer. Screening tests can find early signs of disease so that problems can be treated early, before they ever turn into cancer.

Other HPV-related cancers might not have signs or symptoms until they are advanced and hard to treat. These include cancers of the vulva, vagina, penis, anus, and oropharynx (back of throat including base of tongue and tonsils).

RRP is a condition in which warts grow in the throat. These growths can sometimes block the airway, causing a hoarse voice or troubled breathing.

HPV and Genital Warts Facts

Genital HPV is the most common sexually transmitted infection (STI) in the United States. About 20 million Americans ages 15 to 49 currently have HPV. And at least half of all sexually active men and women get genital HPV at some time in their lives.

What is the difference between the high-risk and low-risk types of HPV?

Some types of HPV can cause cervical cancer. These types of HPV are called high risk. Having high-risk HPV is not the same as having cervical cancer. But high-risk HPV can lead to cancer. Most often, high-risk HPV causes no health problems and goes away on its own. High-risk HPV cases that don't go away are the biggest risk factor for cervical cancer. If you have high-risk HPV, your doctor can look for changes on your cervix during Pap tests. Changes can be treated to try to prevent cervical cancer. Be sure to have regular Pap tests so changes can be found early.

Low-risk HPV can cause genital warts. Warts can form weeks, months, or years after sexual contact with an infected person. In women genital warts can grow in the following areas:

- Inside and around the outside of the vagina

- On the vulva (lips or opening to the vagina), cervix, or groin

- In or around the anus

In men, genital warts can grow in the following areas:

- On the penis

- On the scrotum, thigh, or groin

- In or around the anus

Rarely, genital warts grow in the mouth or throat of a person who had oral sex with an infected person.

The size of genital warts varies. Some are so small you can't see them. They can be flat and flesh-colored or look bumpy like cauliflower. They often form in clusters or groups. They may itch, burn, or cause discomfort.

Low-risk HPV doesn't always cause warts. In fact, most people with low-risk HPV never know they are infected. This is because they don't get warts or any other symptoms.

How do women get HPV?

Genital HPV is passed by skin-to-skin and genital contact. It is most often passed during vaginal and anal sex. Although much less common, it is possible to pass HPV during oral sex or hand-to-genital contact.

Should I get the HPV vaccine?

It depends on your age and whether you already have had sex.

Two vaccines (Cervarix and Gardasil) can protect girls and young women against the types of HPV that cause most cervical cancers. The vaccines work best when given before a person's first sexual contact, when she could be exposed to HPV. Both vaccines are recommended for 11- and 12-year-old girls. But the vaccines also can be used in girls as young as 9 and in women through age 26 who did not get any or all of the shots when they were younger. These vaccines are given in a series of three shots. It is best to use the same vaccine brand for all three doses. Ask your doctor which brand vaccine is best for you. The vaccine does not replace the need to wear condoms to lower your risk of getting other types of HPV and other sexually transmitted infections. Women who have had the HPV vaccine still need to have regular Pap tests.

Studies are also being done on HPV vaccines for males.

How do I know if I have an HPV infection?

Most women who have HPV infections never know it. This is one reason why you need regular Pap tests. A Pap test is when a cell sample is taken from your cervix and looked at with a microscope.

A Pap test can find changes on the cervix caused by HPV. To do a Pap test, your doctor will use a small brush to take cells from your cervix. It's simple, fast, and the best way to find out if your cervix is healthy.

If you are age 30 or older, your doctor may also do an HPV test with your Pap test. This is a DNA [deoxyribonucleic acid] test that detects most of the high-risk types of HPV. It helps with cervical cancer screening. If you're younger than 30 years old and have had an abnormal Pap test result, your doctor may give you an HPV test. This test will show if HPV caused the abnormal cells on your cervix.

One other way to tell if you have an HPV infection is if you have genital warts.

Do I still need a Pap test if I got the HPV vaccine?

Yes. There are three reasons why:

1. The vaccine does not protect against all HPV types that cause cancer.

2. Women who don't get all the vaccine doses (or at the right time) might not be fully protected.

3. Women may not fully benefit from the vaccine if they got it after getting one or more of the four HPV types.

How often should I get a Pap test?

Follow these guidelines:

- Have a Pap test every two years starting at age 21. Women 30 and older who have had three normal Pap tests in a row can now have one every three years.

- If you are older than 65, you may be able to stop having Pap tests. Discuss your needs with your doctor.

- If you had your cervix taken out as part of a hysterectomy, you do not need further Pap tests if the surgery was not due to cancer.

- Talk with your doctor or nurse about when to begin testing, how often you should be tested, and when you can stop.

What happens if I have an abnormal Pap test?

An abnormal result does not mean you have HPV or cervical cancer. Other reasons for an abnormal Pap test result include the following:

- Yeast infections

- Irritation

- Hormone changes

If your Pap test is abnormal, your doctor may do the test again. You may also have an HPV test or these tests:

- **Colposcopy:** A device is used to look closely at your cervix. It lets the doctor look at any abnormal areas.

- **Schiller test:** The test involves coating the cervix with an iodine solution. Healthy cells turn brown and abnormal cells turn white or yellow.

- **Biopsy:** A small amount of cervical tissue is taken out and looked at under a microscope. This way the doctor can tell if the abnormal cells are cancer.

Could I have HPV even if my Pap test was normal?

Yes. You can have HPV but still have a normal Pap test. Changes on your cervix may not show up right away; or they may never appear. For women older than 30 who get an HPV test and a Pap test, a negative result on both the Pap and HPV tests means no cervical changes or HPV were found on the cervix. This means you have a very low chance of getting cervical cancer in the next few years.

How do I protect myself from HPV?

Using condoms may reduce the risk of getting genital warts and cervical cancer. But condoms don't always protect you from HPV. The best ways to protect yourself from HPV are to do the following:

- Not have sex
- Be faithful, meaning you and your partner only have sex with each other and no one else

If I had HPV that went away on its own, can I get it again?

Yes. There are many types of HPV, so you can get HPV again.

How do I protect my partner from HPV after my warts have gone away?

Even if you think the warts have gone away, there may be some you can't see. And even after the warts are treated, the HPV virus may remain. Using condoms may reduce your risk of passing on genital warts.

How does HPV affect a pregnancy?

Most women who had genital warts, but no longer have them, do not have problems during pregnancy or birth. For women who have genital warts during pregnancy, the warts may grow or become larger and bleed. In rare cases, a pregnant woman can pass HPV to her baby during vaginal delivery. Rarely, a baby who is exposed to HPV gets warts in the throat or voice box.

If the warts block the birth canal, a woman may need to have a cesarean section (C-section) delivery. But HPV infection or genital warts are not sole reasons for a C-section.

How can I be sure I don't get cervical cancer?

While there are no sure ways to prevent cervical cancer, you can lower your risk by doing the following:

- Getting regular Pap tests: The best time to get a Pap test is 10 to 20 days after the first day of your last period. Don't have the test done during your period. Also, for two days before your Pap test don't have sex or use douches, vaginal medicines (unless your doctor tells you to), or spermicides. Talk to your doctor about how often to get Pap tests.
- Not smoking: Smoking can raise your risk of cervical cancer.
- Being faithful: This means you and your partner only have sex with each other and no one else.
- Using a condom every time you have vaginal, anal, or oral sex: Condoms don't always protect you from HPV. But they may reduce your risk of getting genital warts and cervical cancer.

Section 21.2

HPV and Men

"HPV and Men Fact Sheet," by the Centers for Disease
Control and Prevention (CDC, www.cdc.gov), December 19, 2011.

What is genital human papillomavirus (HPV)?

Genital human papillomavirus (HPV) is a common virus. Most sexually active people in the United States will have HPV at some time in their lives. There are more than 40 types of HPV that are passed on through sexual contact. These types can infect the genital areas of men, including the skin on and around the penis or anus. They can also infect the mouth and throat.

How do men get HPV?

HPV is passed on through genital contact—most often during vaginal and anal sex. HPV may also be passed on during oral sex. Since HPV usually causes no symptoms, most men and women can get HPV—and pass it on—without realizing it. People can have HPV even if years have passed since they had sex. Even men with only one lifetime sex partner can get HPV.

What are the health problems caused by HPV in men?

Most men who get HPV (of any type) never develop any symptoms or health problems. But some types of HPV can cause genital warts. Other types can cause cancers of the penis, anus, or oropharynx (back of the throat, including base of the tongue and tonsils.) The types of HPV that can cause genital warts are not the same as the types that can cause cancer.

Note: Anal cancer is not the same as colorectal cancer. Colorectal cancer is more common than anal cancer, and is not caused by HPV.

How common are HPV-related health problems in men?

- About 1% of sexually active men in the United States have genital warts at any one time.

- Cancers of the penis, anus, and oropharynx are uncommon, and only a subset of these cancers are actually related to HPV. Each year in the United States there are about 400 men who get HPV-related cancer of the penis; 1,500 men who get HPV-related cancer of the anus; and 5,600 men who get cancers of the oropharynx (back of throat), but many of these cancers are related to tobacco and alcohol use, not HPV.

Some men are more likely to develop HPV-related diseases than others:

- Gay and bisexual men (who have sex with other men) are about 17 times more likely to develop anal cancer than men who only have sex with women.
- Men with weakened immune systems, including those who have HIV (human immunodeficiency virus), are more likely than other men to develop anal cancer. Men with HIV are also more likely to get severe cases of genital warts that are harder to treat.

What are the signs and symptoms?

Most men who get HPV never develop any symptoms or health problems. But for those who do develop health problems, these are some of the signs and symptoms:

Symptoms of genital warts include the following:

- One or more growths on the penis, testicles, groin, thighs, or in/around the anus may be a symptom of genital warts.
- Warts may be single, grouped, raised, flat, or cauliflower-shaped. They usually do not hurt.
- Warts may appear within weeks or months after sexual contact with an infected person.

Anal cancer symptoms include the following:

- Anal bleeding, pain, itching, or discharge
- Swollen lymph nodes in the anal or groin area
- Changes in bowel habits or the shape of your stool

Sometimes there are no signs or symptoms.
Penile cancer symptoms include the following:

- The first signs may be changes in color, skin thickening, or a build-up of tissue on the penis.

- Later signs may include a growth or sore on the penis. It is usually painless, but in some cases, the sore may be painful and bleed.

Cancers of the oropharynx include the following:

- Sore throat or ear pain that doesn't go away
- Constant coughing
- Pain or trouble swallowing or breathing
- Weight loss
- Hoarseness or voice changes that last more than two weeks
- Lump or mass in the neck

Is there a test for HPV in men?

Currently, there is no HPV test recommended for men. The only approved HPV tests on the market are for screening women for cervical cancer. They are not useful for screening for HPV-related cancers or genital warts in men.

Screening for anal cancer is not routinely recommended for men. This is because more research is needed to find out if it can actually prevent anal cancer. However, some experts do recommend yearly anal cancer screening (anal Pap tests) for gay, bisexual, and HIV-positive men—since anal cancer is more common in these men.

There is no approved test to find genital warts for men or women. However, most of the time, you can see genital warts. If you think you may have genital warts, you should see a health care provider.

There is no test for men to check one's overall HPV status. But HPV usually goes away on its own, without causing health problems. So an HPV infection that is found today will most likely not be there a year or two from now.

Screening tests are not available for penile cancer.

You can check for any abnormalities on your penis, scrotum, or around the anus. See your doctor if you find warts, blisters, sores, ulcers, white patches, or other abnormal areas on your penis—even if they do not hurt.

Is there a treatment or cure for HPV?

There is no treatment or cure for HPV. But there are ways to treat the health problems caused by HPV in men.

Genital warts can be treated with medicine, removed (surgery), or frozen off. Some of these treatments involve a visit to the doctor. Others can be done at home by the patient himself. No one treatment is better than another. But warts often come back within a few months after treatment—so several treatments may be needed. Treating genital warts may not necessarily lower a man's chances of passing HPV on to his sex partner. If warts are not treated, they may go away on their own, stay the same, or grow (in size or number). They will not turn into cancer.

Cancers of the penis, anus, and oropharynx can be treated with surgery, radiation therapy, and chemotherapy. Often, two or more of these treatments are used together. Patients should decide with their doctors which treatments are best for them.

Are there ways to lower my chances of getting HPV?

A safe and effective HPV vaccine (Gardasil) can protect boys and men against the HPV types that cause most genital warts and anal cancers. It is given in three shots over six months.

Condoms (if used with every sex act, from start to finish) may lower your chances of passing HPV to a partner or developing HPV-related diseases. But HPV can infect areas that are not covered by a condom—so condoms may not fully protect against HPV.

Because HPV is so common and usually invisible, the only sure way to prevent it is not to have sexual contact. Even people with only one lifetime sex partner can get HPV, if their partner was infected with HPV.

I heard about a new HPV vaccine. Can it help me?

If you are 26 or younger, there is an HPV vaccine that can help protect you against the types of HPV that most commonly cause problems in men. The HPV vaccine (Gardasil) works by preventing four common HPV types, two that cause most genital warts and two that cause cancers, including anal cancer. It protects against new HPV infections; it does not cure existing HPV infections or disease (like genital warts). It is most effective when given before a person's first sexual contact (i.e., when he or she may be exposed to HPV).

CDC recommends the HPV vaccine for all boys ages 11 or 12, and for males through age 21, who have not already received all three doses. The vaccine is also recommended for gay and bisexual men (or any man who has sex with men), and men with compromised immune systems (including HIV) through age 26, if they did not get fully vaccinated when they were younger. The vaccine is safe for all men through age 26, but it is most effective when given at younger ages.

The HPV vaccine is very safe and effective, with no serious side effects. The most common side effect is soreness in the arm. Studies show that the vaccine can protect men against genital warts and anal cancers. It is likely that this vaccine also protects men from other HPV-related cancers, like cancers of the penis and oropharynx (back of throat, including base of tongue and tonsils), but there are no vaccine studies that have evaluated these outcomes.

I just found out that my partner has HPV. What does it mean for my health?

Partners usually share HPV. If you have been with your partner for a long time, you probably have HPV already. Most sexually active adults will have HPV at some time in their lives. Although HPV is common, the health problems caused by HPV are much less common.

Condoms may lower your chances of getting HPV or developing HPV-related diseases, if used with every sex act, from start to finish. You may want to consider talking to your doctor about being vaccinated against HPV if you are 26 years or younger. But not having sex is the only sure way to avoid HPV.

If your partner has genital warts, you should avoid having sex until the warts are gone or removed. You can check for any abnormalities on your penis, such as genital warts. Also, you may want to get checked by a health care provider for genital warts and other sexually transmitted disease (STDs).

What does it mean for our relationship?

A person can have HPV for many years before it is found or causes health problems. So there is no way to know if your partner gave you HPV, or if you gave HPV to your partner. HPV should not be seen as a sign that you or your partner is having sex outside of your relationship.

I just found out I have genital warts. What does it mean for me and my partner?

Having genital warts may be hard to cope with, but they are not a threat to your health. People with genital warts can still lead normal, healthy lives.

Because genital warts may be easily passed on to sex partners, you should inform them about having genital warts and avoid sexual activity until the warts are gone or removed. There are ways to protect your partner.

You and your partner may benefit from getting screened for other STDs.

If used with every sex act, male latex condoms may lower your chances of passing genital warts. But HPV can infect areas that are not covered by a condom—so condoms may not fully protect against HPV.

It is important that sex partners discuss their health and risk for STIs. However, it is not clear if there is any health benefit to informing future sex partners about a past diagnosis of genital warts because it is not known how long a person remains contagious after warts are gone.

Section 21.3

Recurrent Respiratory Papillomatosis

"Recurrent Respiratory Papillomatosis or Laryngeal Papillomatosis," by the National Institute on Deafness and Other Communication Disorders (NIDCD, www.nidcd.nih.gov), part of the National Institutes of Health, October 2010.

Recurrent respiratory papillomatosis (RRP) is a disease in which tumors grow in the air passages leading from the nose and mouth into the lungs (respiratory tract). Although the tumors can grow anywhere in the respiratory tract, their presence in the larynx (voice box) causes the most frequent problems, a condition called laryngeal papillomatosis. The tumors may vary in size and grow very quickly. They often grow back even when removed.

What is the cause of RRP?

RRP is caused by two types of human papillomavirus (HPV), called HPV-6 and HPV-11. There are more than 150 types of HPV and they do not all have the same symptoms.

Most people who encounter HPV never develop any illness. However, many HPVs can cause small wart-like, non-cancerous tumors called papillomas. The most common illness caused by HPV-6 and HPV-11 is genital warts. Although scientists are uncertain how people are infected with HPV-6 or HPV-11, the virus is thought to be spread through sexual contact or when a mother with genital warts passes it to her baby during childbirth. HPV-6 and HPV-11 can also cause disease of the uterine cervix and, in rare cases, cervical cancer.

According to the Centers for Disease Control and Prevention, the incidence of RRP is rare. Fewer than 2,000 children get RRP each year.

Who is affected by RRP?

RRP affects adults as well as infants and small children who may have contracted the virus during childbirth. According to the RRP Foundation, there are roughly 20,000 cases in the United States. Among children, the incidence of RRP is approximately 4.3 per 100,000; among adults, it's about 1.8 per 100,000.

What are the symptoms of RRP?

Normally, voice is produced when air from the lungs is pushed past two side-by-side elastic muscles—called vocal folds or vocal cords—with sufficient pressure to cause them to vibrate. When the tumors interfere with the normal vibrations of the vocal folds, it causes hoarseness, which is the most common symptom of RRP. Eventually, the tumors may block the airway passage and cause difficulty breathing.

Because the tumors grow quickly, young children with the disease may find it difficult to breathe when sleeping, or they may experience difficulty swallowing. Adults and children may experience hoarseness, chronic coughing, or breathing problems. The symptoms tend to be more severe in children than in adults; however, some children experience some relief or remission of the disease when they begin puberty. Because of the similarity of the symptoms, RRP is sometimes misdiagnosed as asthma or chronic bronchitis.

How is RRP diagnosed?

Two routine tests for RRP are indirect and direct laryngoscopy. In an indirect laryngoscopy, an otolaryngologist—a doctor who specializes in diseases of the ear, nose, throat, head, and neck—or speech-language pathologist will typically insert a flexible fiberoptic telescope, called an endoscope, into a patient's nose or mouth and then view the larynx on a monitor. Some medical professionals use a video camera attached to a flexible tube to examine the larynx. An older, less common method is for the otolaryngologist to place a small mirror in the back of the throat and angle the mirror down toward the larynx to inspect it for tumors.

A direct laryngoscopy is conducted in the operating room with the use of general anesthesia. This method allows the otolaryngologist to view the vocal folds and other parts of the larynx under high magnification. This procedure is usually used to minimize discomfort, especially with children, or to enable the doctor to collect tissue samples from the larynx or other parts of the throat to examine them for abnormalities.

How is RRP treated?

There is no cure for RRP. Surgery is the primary method for removing tumors from the larynx or airway. Because traditional surgery can result in problems due to scarring of the larynx tissue, many surgeons are now using laser surgery, which uses an intense laser light as the surgical tool. Carbon dioxide lasers—which pass electricity through a tube containing carbon dioxide and other gases to generate light—are currently the most popular type used for this purpose. In the past 10 years, surgeons have begun using a device called a microdebrider, which uses suction to hold the tumor while a small internal rotary blade removes the growth.

Once the tumors have been removed, they have a tendency to return unpredictably. It is common for patients to require repeat surgery. With some patients, surgery may be required every few weeks in order to keep the breathing passage open, while others may require surgery only once a year. In the most extreme cases where tumor growth is aggressive, a tracheotomy may be performed. A tracheotomy is a surgical procedure in which an incision is made in the front of the patient's neck and a breathing tube (trach tube) is inserted through an opening, called a stoma, into the trachea (windpipe). Rather than breathing through the nose and mouth, the patient will now breathe through the trach tube. Although the trach tube keeps the breathing passage open, doctors try to remove it as soon as it is feasible.

Some patients may be required to keep a trach tube indefinitely in order to keep the breathing passage open. In addition, because the trach tube reroutes all or some of the exhaled air away from the vocal folds, the patient may find it difficult to speak. With the help of a voice specialist or speech-language pathologist who specializes in voice, the patient can learn how to use his or her voice.

Adjuvant therapies—therapies that are used in addition to surgery—have been used to treat more severe cases of RRP. Drug treatments may include antivirals such as interferon and cidofovir, which block the virus from making copies of itself, and indole-3-carbinol, a cancer-fighting compound found in cruciferous vegetables, such as broccoli and Brussels sprouts. To date, the results of these and other adjuvant therapies have been mixed or not yet fully proven.

Section 21.4

Pap Tests and Cervical Cancer Screening to Check for HPV

"Cervical Cancer Screening," by the Centers for Disease Control and Prevention (CDC, www.cdc.gov), November 8, 2011.

Cervical cancer is the easiest female cancer to prevent, with regular screening tests and follow-up. Two screening tests can help prevent cervical cancer or find it early:

- The Pap test (or Pap smear) looks for precancers, cell changes on the cervix that might become cervical cancer if they are not treated appropriately.

- The HPV test looks for the virus (human papillomavirus) that can cause these cell changes.

The Pap test is recommended for all women, and can be done in a doctor's office or clinic. During the Pap test, the doctor will use a plastic or metal instrument, called a speculum, to widen your vagina. This helps the doctor examine the vagina and the cervix, and collect a few cells and mucus from the cervix and the area around it. The cells are then placed on a slide or in a bottle of liquid and sent to a laboratory. The laboratory will check to be sure that the cells are normal.

If you are getting the HPV test in addition to the Pap test, the cells collected during the Pap test will be tested for HPV at the laboratory. Talk with your doctor, nurse, or other health care professional about whether the HPV test is right for you.

When you have a Pap test, the doctor may also perform a pelvic exam, checking your uterus, ovaries, and other organs to make sure there are no problems. There are times when your doctor may perform a pelvic exam without giving you a Pap test. Ask your doctor which tests you are having, if you are unsure.

If you have a low income or do not have health insurance, you may be able to get a free or low-cost Pap test through the National Breast and Cervical Cancer Early Detection Program [www.cdc.gov/cancer/nbccedp/screenings.htm].

When to Get Screened

You should start getting regular Pap tests at age 21, or within three years of the first time you have sex—whichever happens first. The Pap test, which screens for cervical cancer, is one of the most reliable and effective cancer screening tests available.

The only cancer for which the Pap test screens is cervical cancer. It does not screen for ovarian, uterine, vaginal, or vulvar cancers. So even if you have a Pap test regularly, if you notice any signs or symptoms that are unusual for you, see a doctor to find out why you're having them.

In addition to the Pap test—the main test for cervical cancer—the HPV test may also be used to screen women aged 30 years and older, or women of any age who have unclear Pap test results.

If you are 30 years old or older and your screening tests are normal, your chance of getting cervical cancer in the next few years is very low. For that reason, your doctor may tell you that you will not need another screening test for up to three years. But you should still go to the doctor regularly for a check-up that may include a pelvic exam.

It is important for you to continue getting a Pap test regularly—even if you think you are too old to have a child, or are not having sex anymore. If you are older than 65 and have had normal Pap test results for several years, or if you have had your cervix removed (during an operation called a hysterectomy), your doctor may tell you it is okay to stop getting regular Pap tests.

How to Prepare for Your Pap Test

You should not schedule your Pap test for a time when you are having your period. If you are going to have a Pap test in the next two days, adhere to the following:

- You should not douche (rinse the vagina with water or another fluid).
- You should not use a tampon.
- You should not have sex.
- You should not use a birth control foam, cream, or jelly.
- You should not use a medicine or cream in your vagina.

Pap Test Results

It can take up to three weeks to receive your Pap test results. If your test shows that something might not be normal, your doctor will contact you and figure out how best to follow up. There are many reasons why Pap test results might not be normal. It usually does not mean you have cancer.

If your Pap test results show cells that are not normal and may become cancer, your doctor will let you know if you need to be treated. In most cases, treatment prevents cervical cancer from developing. It is important to follow up with your doctor right away to learn more about your test results and receive any treatment that may be needed.

Section 21.5

Making Sense of Your HPV Test Results

Excerpted from "Making Sense of Your Pap and HPV Test Results," by the Centers for Disease Control and Prevention (CDC, www.cdc.gov), January 2012.

Getting abnormal test results does not mean that you have cervical cancer now. For specific questions about your test results, talk to your doctor.

Screening tests can find early problems before you get sick. The Pap test is a screening test for cervical cancer. It looks for abnormal cells on your cervix that could turn into cancer over time. That way, problems can be found and treated before they ever turn into cancer. An HPV test may also be used with the Pap test for women 30 years or older, as part of routine screening.

Getting regular cervical cancer screening is key to preventing this disease.

Every year in the United States, about 12,000 women get cervical cancer, but it is the most preventable type of female cancer, with both HPV vaccines and regular screening tests.

Since cervical cancer often does not cause symptoms until it is advanced, it is important to get screened even when you feel healthy.

The Pap and HPV tests look for different things. The Pap test checks your cervix for abnormal cells that could turn into cervical cancer. The HPV test checks your cervix for the virus (HPV) that can cause abnormal cells and lead to cervical cancer.

The Pap and HPV tests can find early problems that could lead to cervical cancer over time. These tests do not do the following:

- Check for early signs of other cancers

- Check your fertility (ability to get pregnant)

- Check for all HPV types (The HPV test only checks for specific HPV types that are linked to cervical cancer.)

- Check for other sexually transmitted diseases (STDs)

When should I get an HPV test?

Experts recommend HPV testing for women who are:

- age 30 or older—as part of regular screening, with a Pap test; or

- age 21 or older—for follow up of an abnormal Pap test result.

You don't need to ask your doctor for an HPV test. Your doctor should offer you an HPV test if you need it and it is available in their practice.

Why is the HPV test not recommended as part of regular screening for younger women and teens?

HPV is very common in women under age 30. But it is not useful to test women under age 30 for HPV, since most HPV that is found in these women will never cause them health problems. Most young women will fight off HPV within a few years.

HPV is less common in women over the age of 30, who are at increasing risk for cervical cancer. HPV is also more likely to signal a health problem for these women, who may have had the virus for many years. Doctors may use the HPV test with the Pap test to tell if these women are more likely to get cervical cancer in the future, and if they need to be screened more often.

Getting regular Pap tests, even without the HPV test, is still a good way to prevent cervical cancer—for both younger and older women.

What does my Pap test result mean?

Your Pap test will come back as either normal, unclear, or abnormal.

Normal: A normal result means that no cell changes were found on your cervix. This is good news. But you still need to get Pap tests in the future. New cell changes can still form on your cervix.

Unclear: It is common for test results to come back unclear. Your doctor may use other words to describe this result, like equivocal, inconclusive, or ASC-US. These all mean the same thing: that your cervical cells look like they could be abnormal. It is not clear if it's related to HPV. It could be related to life changes like pregnancy, menopause, or an infection. The HPV test can help find out if your cell changes are related to HPV.

Abnormal: An abnormal result means that cell changes were found on your cervix. This usually does not mean that you have cervical cancer.

Abnormal changes on your cervix are likely caused by HPV. The changes may be minor (low-grade) or serious (high-grade). Most of the time, minor changes go back to normal on their own. But more serious changes can turn into cancer if they are not removed. The more serious changes are often called precancer because they are not yet cancer, but they can turn into cancer over time. It is important to make sure these changes do not get worse.

In rare cases, an abnormal Pap test can show that you may have cancer. You will need other tests to be sure. The earlier you find cervical cancer, the easier it is to treat.

If your Pap test results are unclear or abnormal, you will likely need more tests so your doctor can tell if your cell changes could be related to cancer.

I see my doctor regularly for a Pap test. This year, my doctor told me the test was abnormal. He also said I have HPV. I was confused. What does this mean?

If you have an HPV test at the same time as your Pap test, it can be confusing to get both results at the same time.

Your HPV test will come back as either positive or negative:

- A negative HPV test means you do not have an HPV type that is linked to cervical cancer.

- A positive HPV test means you do have an HPV type that has been linked to cervical cancer. This does not mean you have cervical cancer now. But it could be a warning.

HPV test results are only meaningful **with** your Pap test results.

If your HPV test is negative (normal), and your Pap test is . . .

Pap test is normal

This means the following:

- Your cervical cells are normal.
- You do not have HPV.
- You have a very low chance of getting cervical cancer in the next few years.

You should:

- Wait three years before getting your next Pap and HPV test.
- Ask your doctor when to come in for your next visit.

Experts used to suggest yearly Pap tests. But now you can safely wait longer because having two tests gives you extra peace of mind.

Pap test is unclear (ASC-US)

This means the following:

- You do not have HPV, but you may have cell changes on your cervix.
- Even if you do have cell changes, it is unlikely that they are caused by HPV (or related to cervical cancer).

You should get another Pap test in one year.

Pap test is abnormal

This means the following:

- Your cervical cells are abnormal.
- You do not have HPV.

It's important to find out why the two tests are showing different things.

For minor cell changes, your doctor will take a closer look at your cervix to decide next steps.

For major cell changes, your doctor will take a closer look at your cervix and/or treat you right away.

If your HPV test is positive (abnormal), and your Pap test is . . .

Pap test is normal

This means your cervical cells are normal, but you do have HPV.

You may fight off HPV naturally and never get cell changes. Or, you may not fight off HPV, and HPV could cause cell changes in the future.

It is believed that most women fight off HPV within two years. It is not known why some women fight off HPV and others do not.

You should get another Pap test and HPV test in one year.

Cell changes happen slowly. Some time must pass before your doctor can tell if HPV will go away or cause cell changes.

Pap test is unclear (ASC-US)

This means you have HPV, and you may have cell changes on your cervix.

You doctor will take a closer look at your cervix to find out if your cells are abnormal.

Your doctor may need to remove the abnormal cells or follow up with you over time to make sure the cells do not get worse.

Pap test is abnormal

This means you have HPV and/or your cervical cells are abnormal.

This does not usually mean you have cancer.

For minor cell changes, your doctor will take a closer look at your cervix to decide next steps.

For major cell changes, your doctor will take a closer look at your cervix and/or treat you right away.

If I have HPV, do I have cervical cancer?

No, HPV is not the same as cervical cancer. HPV is the virus that can cause cervical cancer. Many women have HPV. Few of them get cervical cancer if they follow their doctor's advice for more testing and/or treatment.

What will happen if I need to come back for more testing?

Your doctor will do what's right for you, based on your test results. Your doctor may do the following:

- Your doctor may ask you to wait before giving you your next Pap and/or HPV test. This is called watchful waiting. It is common.

- Your doctor may take a closer look at your cervix. This is done using a special lens that makes your cervical cells look bigger (called a colposcopy).

- Your doctor may take a small sample of your cervix (biopsy) to study it more carefully.

- Your doctor may treat you. This involves killing or taking out the abnormal cells. These treatments may be uncomfortable, but they can be done during one visit to your doctor.

- Your doctor may refer you to a specialist. This might happen if your test results suggest that you may have cancer.

Why wait for more tests if I could have cancer?

It is possible that your cell changes will never turn into cancer. They may go back to normal on their own. But cervical cells change very slowly. Some time must pass before your doctor can tell if your cells need treatment. Since treatment can have risks and side effects, it is best to make sure you really need it. Be patient. Go back to your doctor for all appointments and testing—to make sure your cell changes do not get worse.

Remember: Many women get HPV or abnormal Pap tests. But few of them get cervical cancer—as long as they get the tests and treatments their doctor recommends. Most times, problems that are found can be treated before they ever turn into cervical cancer.

What else can I do to prevent cervical cancer?

- Keep your next doctor's appointment. Mark your calendar or post a note on your fridge, so you remember it.

- Go back for more testing or treatment if your doctor tells you to.

- Keep getting regular Pap tests—at least once every three years.

- Do not smoke. Smoking harms all of your body's cells, including your cervical cells. If you smoke and have HPV, you have higher chances of getting cervical cancer. If you smoke, ask your doctor for help quitting.

- If you are age 26 or younger, you can get vaccinated against HPV. HPV vaccines do not cure existing HPV or related problems (like abnormal cervical cells), but they can protect you from getting new HPV infections in the future.

What questions should I ask my doctor?

- How do I know if I got an HPV test?

- When and how should I expect to get my test results?

- What do my test results mean?

- What other tests or treatment will I need if my Pap or HPV test is abnormal?

- When do I need to come back for more testing or treatment?

- What should I expect during and after these tests or treatments?

- Are there risks or side effects?

- Will the testing or treatment affect my chance to get or stay pregnant?

- Will the added tests or treatment be covered by my insurance?

- Where can I get help to cover the costs?

Section 21.6

What You Should Know When You Are Diagnosed with Genital Warts

"What Patients Should Know When They Are Diagnosed with Genital Warts," by the Centers for Disease Control and Prevention (CDC, www.cdc.gov), March 2012.

Genital warts are caused by a virus called genital human papillomavirus (HPV), which is very common in sexually active men and women.

HPV is passed on through genital contact, most often during vaginal and anal sex.

Most sexually active people will get HPV at some time in their lives, though most will never know it because HPV usually has no signs or symptoms.

There are about 40 types of genital HPV. In most cases, HPV goes away on its own, without causing any health problems. It is thought that the immune system fights off HPV infection naturally.

But sometimes, HPV does not go away on its own. Some HPV types can cause genital warts. Other HPV types can cause cervical cancer and other less common genital cancers. The types of HPV that cause genital warts are different from the types that can cause cancer.

There is no treatment for HPV (a virus), but there are treatments for the conditions it can cause, including genital warts.

It is common for genital warts to recur (come back after treatment), especially in the first three months after treatment.

Treating genital warts will not necessarily lower your risk of passing HPV to a sex partner. You can still pass the virus on to sex partners, even after the warts are treated. It is not known how long a person remains contagious after warts are treated.

If you don't treat genital warts, they may go away, remain unchanged, or grow in size or number. Genital warts will not turn into cancer over time, even if they are not treated.

There is a very low risk that a pregnant woman with genital warts can pass HPV to her baby. In the rare cases where HPV is passed, the baby could develop warts in the throat or voice box. Cesarean births do not seem to prevent a mother from passing HPV to her baby.

271

All women who have ever been sexually active, including those with genital warts, should get regular Pap tests to screen for cervical cancer. This is because a person can be infected with more than one HPV type.

If you have genital warts, you may benefit from screening for other sexually transmitted diseases (STDs).

If you have questions, please write them down and ask about them during your next doctor's visit.

Talking to Your Partner

You and your partner may benefit from talking openly about your sexual health and HPV.

You and your partner should know the following:

- There is no sure way to know when you got HPV or who gave it to you.

- Genital warts can be transmitted by a person without visible signs of warts. They may appear weeks, months, or years after exposure, or they may never appear.

- Partners who have been together for a while tend to share HPV. This means that your partner likely has HPV already, even though your partner may have no signs or symptoms. It is not clear why some people with wart-causing types of HPV develop genital warts and others do not.

- Condoms may lower your risk of passing genital warts on to your sex partner(s), if used all the time and the right way. But HPV can infect genital areas that are not protected by a condom, so condoms may not fully protect against HPV.

Your current partner may benefit from seeing a health professional for counseling and getting checked for genital warts and other STDs.

It is not clear if there is any health benefit to telling future sex partners about a past diagnosis of genital warts (once warts are treated). That's because it is not known if or how long you would remain contagious after treatment.

Ways to lower your chances of getting future HPV infections include the following:

- Use condoms all the time and the right way. Condoms may also lower your chances of developing other HPV-related diseases (cervical cancer in women). But HPV can infect areas that are not covered by a condom—so condoms may not fully protect you against HPV.

- Be in a mutually faithful relationship with someone who has had no or few other sex partners.

- Limit your number of sex partners and choose partners who have had few sex partners.

Abstaining from sexual contact is the only sure way to prevent future HPV infections.

Section 21.7

Treating HPV and Related Problems

This section includes text excerpted from "Human Papillomavirus (HPV)," by the Centers for Disease Control and Prevention (CDC, www.cdc.gov), March 22, 2012. The text under the heading "HPV and Genital Warts Treatment Facts" is from "Human Papillomavirus (HPV) and Genital Warts Fact Sheet," by the Office on Women's Health (www.womenshealth.gov), part of the U.S. Department of Health and Human Services, January 1, 2009.

HPV Treatment

There is no treatment for HPV itself, but there are treatments for the problems that HPV can cause:

- Visible genital warts can be removed by the patient with medications. They can also be treated by a health care provider. Some people choose not to treat warts, but to see if they disappear on their own. No one treatment is better than another.

- Abnormal cervical cells (found on a Pap test) often become normal over time, but they can sometimes turn into cancer. If they remain abnormal, these cells can usually be treated to prevent cervical cancer from developing. This may depend on the severity of the cell changes, the woman's age and past medical history, and other test results. It is critical to follow up with testing and treatment, as recommended by a doctor.

- Cervical cancer is most treatable when it is diagnosed and treated early. Problems found can usually be treated, depending on their severity and on the woman's age, past medical history, and other test results. Most women who get routine cervical cancer screening and follow up as told by their provider can find problems before cancer even develops. Prevention is always better than treatment.

- Other HPV-related cancers are also more treatable when diagnosed and treated early.

- Recurrent respiratory papillomatosis (RRP), a rare condition in which warts grow in the throat, can be treated with surgery or medicines. It can sometimes take many treatments or surgeries over a period of years.

HPV and Genital Warts Treatment Facts

Can HPV be cured?

No. There is no cure for the virus HPV. But there are treatments for the changes HPV can cause on the cervix. Genital warts can also be treated. Sometimes, the virus goes away on its own.

What treatments are used to get rid of abnormal cells on the cervix?

If you have abnormal cells on the cervix, follow up with your doctor. If the problem is mild, your doctor may wait to see if the cells heal on their own. Or your doctor may suggest taking out the abnormal tissue. Treatment options include the following:

- Cryosurgery, when abnormal tissue is frozen off

- Loop electrosurgical excision procedure (LEEP), where tissue is removed using a hot wire loop

- Laser treatment, which uses a beam of light to destroy abnormal tissue

- Cone biopsy, where a cone-shaped sample of abnormal tissue is removed from the cervix and looked at under the microscope for signs of cancer

Cone biopsy also can serve as a treatment if all the abnormal tissue is removed.

After these treatments, you may have the following:

- Vaginal bleeding

- Cramping

- Brownish-black discharge

- Watery discharge

After treatment, follow up with your doctor to see if any abnormal cells come back.

How are genital warts treated?

Genital warts can be treated or not treated.

Some people may want warts taken off if they cause itching, burning, and discomfort. Others may want to clear up warts you can see with the eye.

If you decide to have warts removed, do not use over-the-counter medicines meant for other kinds of warts. There are special treatments for genital warts. Your doctor may treat the warts by putting on a chemical in the office. Or your doctor may prescribe a cream you can apply at home. Surgery is also an option. Your doctor may also do the following:

- Use an electric current to burn off the warts

- Use a light/laser to destroy warts

- Freeze off the warts

- Cut the warts out

Even when warts are treated, the HPV virus may remain. This is why warts can come back after treatment. It isn't clear if treating genital warts lowers a person's chance of giving HPV to a sex partner. It is not fully known why low-risk HPV causes genital warts in some cases and not in others.

If left untreated, genital warts may do the following:

- Go away

- Remain unchanged

- Increase in size or number

The warts will not turn into cancer.

Section 21.8

HPV Infection and Cancer

This section includes text from "HPV-Associated Cancers Statistics," by the Centers for Disease Control and Prevention (CDC, www.cdc.gov), April 30, 2012, and text excerpted from "Human Papillomaviruses and Cancer," by the National Cancer Institute (NCI, www.cancer.gov), part of the National Institutes of Health, September 7, 2011.

HPV-Associated Cancers Statistics

A large study that covered 83% of the U.S. population during 1998–2003 estimated that about 24,900 HPV [human papillomavirus]-associated cancers occur each year.

More than 17,300 HPV-associated cancers occur yearly in women, and almost 7,600 occur yearly in men. Cervical cancer is the most common HPV-associated cancer among women, and head and neck (oral cavity and oropharyngeal) cancers are the most common HPV-associated cancers among men. The following statistics are from this study.

Because these numbers are based on 83% of the U.S. population, they may under-represent the actual number of cancers diagnosed during this time period. Also, this study used cancer registry data to estimate the amount of potentially HPV-associated cancer in the United States by examining cancer in parts of the body and cancer cell types that are more likely to be caused by HPV. Cancer registries do not collect data on the presence or absence of HPV in cancer tissue at the time of diagnosis.

Although nearly all cervical cancers are caused by HPV, cancer in some other areas of the body are often, but not always, caused by HPV. In general, HPV is thought to be responsible for about 90% of anal cancers; 65% of vaginal cancers; 50% of vulvar cancers; and 35% of penile cancers.

Recent studies show that about 60% of oropharyngeal cancers (cancers of the back of the throat, including the base of the tongue and tonsils) are linked to HPV.

Human Papillomaviruses and Cancer

HPVs, also called human papillomaviruses, are a group of more than 150 related viruses. More than 40 of these viruses can be easily spread through direct skin-to-skin contact during vaginal, anal, and oral sex.

HPV infections are the most common sexually transmitted infections in the United States. In fact, more than half of sexually active people are infected with one or more HPV types at some point in their lives. Recent research indicates that, at any point in time, 42.5 percent of women have genital HPV infections, whereas less than 7 percent of adults have oral HPV infections.

Sexually transmitted HPVs fall into two categories:

- One category is low-risk HPVs, which do not cause cancer but can cause skin warts (technically known as condylomata acuminata) on or around the genitals or anus. For example, HPV types 6 and 11 cause 90 percent of all genital warts.

- The other category is high-risk or oncogenic HPVs, which can cause cancer. At least a dozen high-risk HPV types have been identified. Two of these, HPV types 16 and 18, are responsible for the majority of HPV-caused cancers.

What is the association between HPV infection and cancer?

High-risk HPV infection accounts for approximately five percent of all cancers worldwide. However, most high-risk HPV infections occur without any symptoms, go away within one to two years, and do not cause cancer. These transient infections may cause cytologic abnormalities, or abnormal cell changes, that go away on their own.

Some HPV infections, however, can persist for many years. Persistent infections with high-risk HPV types can lead to more serious cytologic abnormalities or lesions that, if untreated, may progress to cancer.

Which cancers are caused by HPVs?

Virtually all cervical cancers are caused by HPV infections, with just two HPV types, 16 and 18, responsible for about 70 percent of all cases. HPV also causes anal cancer, with about 85 percent of all cases caused by HPV-16. HPV types 16 and 18 have also been found to cause close to half of vaginal, vulvar, and penile cancers.

Most recently, HPV infections have been found to cause cancer of the oropharynx, which is the middle part of the throat including the soft palate, the base of the tongue, and the tonsils. In the United States, more than half of the cancers diagnosed in the oropharynx are linked to HPV-16.

The incidence of HPV-associated oropharyngeal cancer has increased during the past 20 years, especially among men. It has been estimated that, by 2020, HPV will cause more oropharyngeal cancers than cervical cancers in the United States.

Other factors may increase the risk of developing cancer following a high-risk HPV infection. These other factors include the following:

- Smoking

- Having a weakened immune system

- Having many children (for increased risk of cervical cancer)

- Long-term oral contraceptive use (for increased risk of cervical cancer)

- Poor oral hygiene (for increased risk of oropharyngeal cancer)

- Chronic inflammation

Can HPV infection be prevented?

The most reliable way to prevent infection with either a high-risk or a low-risk HPV is to avoid any skin-to-skin oral, anal, or genital contact with another person. For those who are sexually active, a long-term, mutually monogamous relationship with an uninfected partner is the strategy most likely to prevent HPV infection. However, because of the lack of symptoms it is hard to know whether a partner who has been sexually active in the past is currently infected with HPV.

Research has shown that correct and consistent use of condoms can reduce the transmission of HPVs between sexual partners. Areas not covered by a condom can be infected with the virus, though, so condoms are unlikely to provide complete protection against virus spread.

The Food and Drug Administration (FDA) has approved two HPV vaccines: Gardasil for the prevention of cervical, anal, vulvar, and vaginal cancer, as well as precancerous lesions in these tissues and genital warts caused by HPV infection; and Cervarix for the prevention of cervical cancer and precancerous cervical lesions caused by HPV infection. Both vaccines are highly effective in preventing infections with HPV types 16 and 18. Gardasil also prevents infection with HPV types 6 and 11. These vaccines have not been approved for prevention of penile or oropharyngeal cancer.

How are HPV infections detected?

HPV infections can be detected by testing a sample of cells to see if they contain viral DNA [deoxyribonucleic acid] or RNA [ribonucleic acid].

The most common test detects DNA from several high-risk HPV types, but it cannot identify the type(s) that are present. Another test is specific for DNA from HPV types 16 and 18, the two types that cause most HPV-associated cancers. A third test can detect DNA from several high-risk HPV types and can indicate whether HPV-16 or HPV-18 is present. A fourth test detects RNA from the most common high-risk HPV types. These tests can detect HPV infections before cell abnormalities are evident.

Theoretically, the HPV DNA and RNA tests could be used to identify HPV infections in cells taken from any part of the body. However, the tests are approved by the FDA for only two indications: for follow-up testing of women who seem to have abnormal Pap test results and for cervical cancer screening in combination with a Pap test among women over age 30.

There are no FDA-approved tests to detect HPV infections in men. There are also no currently recommended screening methods similar to a Pap test for detecting cell changes caused by HPV infection in anal, vulvar, vaginal, penile, or oropharyngeal tissues. However, this is an area of ongoing research.

What are treatment options for HPV-infected individuals?

There is currently no medical treatment for HPV infections. However, the genital warts and precancerous lesions resulting from HPV infections can be treated.

Methods commonly used to treat precancerous cervical lesions include cryosurgery (freezing that destroys tissue), LEEP (loop electrosurgical excision procedure, or the removal of cervical tissue using a hot wire loop), surgical conization (surgery with a scalpel, a laser, or both to remove a cone-shaped piece of tissue from the cervix and cervical canal), and laser vaporization conization (use of a laser to destroy cervical tissue).

Treatments for other types of precancerous lesions caused by HPV (vaginal, vulvar, penile, and anal lesions) and genital warts include topical chemicals or drugs, excisional surgery, cryosurgery, electrosurgery, and laser surgery.

HPV-infected individuals who develop cancer generally receive the same treatment as patients whose tumors do not harbor HPV infections, according to the type and stage of their tumors. However, people who are diagnosed with HPV-positive oropharyngeal cancer may be treated differently than people with oropharyngeal cancers that are HPV-negative. Recent research has shown that patients with HPV-positive oropharyngeal tumors have a better prognosis and may do just as well on less intense treatment.

How do high-risk HPVs cause cancer?

HPVs infect epithelial cells. These cells, which are organized in layers, cover the inside and outside surfaces of the body, including the skin, the throat, the genital tract, and the anus. Because HPVs are not thought to enter the bloodstream, having an HPV infection in one part of the body should not cause an infection in another part of the body.

Once an HPV enters an epithelial cell, the virus begins to make proteins. Two of the proteins made by high-risk HPVs interfere with normal functions in the cell, enabling the cell to grow in an uncontrolled manner and to avoid cell death.

Many times these infected cells are recognized by the immune system and eliminated. Sometimes, however, these infected cells are not destroyed, and a persistent infection results. As the persistently infected cells continue to grow, they may develop mutations that promote even more cell growth, leading to the formation of a high-grade lesion and, ultimately, a tumor.

Researchers believe that it can take between 10 and 20 years from the time of an initial HPV infection until a tumor forms. However, even high-grade lesions do not always lead to cancer. The percentage of high-grade cervical lesions that progress to invasive cervical cancer has been estimated to be 50 percent or less.

Chapter 22

Lymphogranuloma Venereum

What is LGV?

LGV (Lymphogranuloma venereum) is a sexually transmitted disease (STD) caused by three strains of the bacterium *Chlamydia trachomatis*. The visual signs include genital papule(s) (e.g., raised surface or bumps) and or ulcers, and swelling of the lymph glands in the genital area. LGV may also produce rectal ulcers, bleeding, pain, and discharge, especially among those who practice receptive anal intercourse. Genital lesions caused by LGV can be mistaken for other ulcerative STDs such as syphilis, genital herpes, and chancroid. Complications of untreated LGV may include enlargement and ulcerations of the external genitalia and lymphatic obstruction, which may lead to elephantiasis of the genitalia.

How common is LGV?

Signs and symptoms associated with rectal infection can be mistakenly thought to be caused by ulcerative colitis. While the frequency of LGV infection is thought to be rare in industrialized countries, its identification is not always obvious, so the number of cases of LGV in the United States is unknown. However, outbreaks in the Netherlands and other European countries among men who have sex with men (MSM) have raised concerns about cases of LGV in the United States.

"Lymphogranuloma Venereum (LGV)—CDC Fact Sheet," by the Centers for Disease Control and Prevention (CDC, www.cdc.gov), February 23, 2011.

How do people get LGV?

LGV is passed from person to person through direct contact with lesions, ulcers, or other areas where the bacteria are located. Transmission of the organism occurs during sexual penetration (vaginal, oral, or anal) and may also occur via skin-to-skin contact. The likelihood of LGV infection following an exposure is unknown, but it is considered less infectious than some other STDs. A person who has had sexual contact with an LGV-infected partner within 60 days of symptom onset should be examined, tested for urethral or cervical chlamydial infection, and treated with doxycycline, twice daily for 7 days.

What are the signs and symptoms of LGV?

LGV can be difficult to diagnose. Typically, the primary lesion produced by LGV is a small genital or rectal lesion, which can ulcerate at the site of transmission after an incubation period of 3–30 days. These ulcers may remain undetected within the urethra, vagina, or rectum. As with other STDs that cause ulcers, LGV may facilitate transmission and acquisition of HIV.

How is LGV diagnosed?

Because of limitations in a commercially available test, diagnosis is primarily based on clinical findings. Direct identification of the bacteria from a lesion or site of the infection may be possible through testing for chlamydia but, this would not indicate if the chlamydia infection is LGV. However, the usual chlamydia tests that are available have not been FDA [U.S. Food and Drug Administration] approved for testing rectal specimens. In a patient with rectal signs or symptoms suspicious for LGV, a health care provider can collect a specimen and send the sample to his/her state health department for referral to CDC, which is working with state and local health departments to test specimens and validate diagnostic methods for LGV.

What is the treatment for LGV?

There is no vaccine against the bacteria. LGV can be treated with three weeks of antibiotics. CDC STD Treatment Guidelines recommend the use of doxycycline, twice a day for 21 days. An alternative treatment is erythromycin base or azithromycin. The health care provider will determine which is best.

If you have been treated for LGV, you should notify any sex partners you had sex with within 60 days of the symptom onset so they can be evaluated and treated. This will reduce the risk that your partners will develop symptoms and/or serious complications of LGV. It will reduce your risk of becoming reinfected as well as reduce the risk of ongoing transmission in the community. You and all of your sex partners should avoid sex until you have completed treatment for the infection and your symptoms and your partners' symptoms have disappeared.

Note: Doxycycline is not recommended for use in pregnant women. Pregnant and lactating women should be treated with erythromycin. Azithromycin may prove useful for treatment of LGV in pregnancy, but no published data are available regarding its safety and efficacy. A health care provider (like a doctor or nurse) can discuss treatment options with patients.

Persons with both LGV and HIV infection should receive the same LGV treatment as those who are HIV-negative. Prolonged therapy may be required, and delay in resolution of symptoms may occur among persons with HIV.

How can LGV be prevented?

The surest way to avoid transmission of sexually transmitted diseases is to abstain from sexual contact, or to be in a long-term mutually monogamous relationship with a partner who has been tested and is asymptomatic and uninfected.

Male latex condoms, when used consistently and correctly, may reduce the risk of LGV transmission. Genital ulcer diseases can occur in male or female genital areas that may or may not be covered (protected by the condom).

Having had LGV and completing treatment does not prevent reinfection. Effective treatment is available and it is important that persons suspected of having LGV be treated as if they have it. Persons who are treated for LGV treatment should abstain from sexual contact until the infection is cleared.

Chapter 23

Syphilis

Chapter Contents

Section 23.1—What Is Syphilis? 286

Section 23.2—Treating Syphilis... 289

Section 23.1

What Is Syphilis?

"Syphilis—CDC Fact Sheet," by the Centers for Disease Control
and Prevention (CDC, www.cdc.gov), September 16, 2010.

What is syphilis?

Syphilis is a sexually transmitted disease (STD) caused by the bacterium *Treponema pallidum*. It has often been called "the great imitator" because so many of the signs and symptoms are indistinguishable from those of other diseases.

How common is syphilis?

In the United States, health officials reported over 36,000 cases of syphilis in 2006, including 9,756 cases of primary and secondary (P&S) syphilis. In 2006, half of all P&S syphilis cases were reported from 20 counties and 2 cities; and most P&S syphilis cases occurred in persons 20 to 39 years of age. The incidence of P&S syphilis was highest in women 20 to 24 years of age and in men 35 to 39 years of age. Reported cases of congenital syphilis in newborns increased from 2005 to 2006, with 339 new cases reported in 2005 compared to 349 cases in 2006.

Between 2005 and 2006, the number of reported P&S syphilis cases increased 11.8 percent. P&S rates have increased in males each year between 2000 and 2006 from 2.6 to 5.7 and among females between 2004 and 2006. In 2006, 64% of the reported P&S syphilis cases were among men who have sex with men (MSM).

How do people get syphilis?

Syphilis is passed from person to person through direct contact with a syphilis sore. Sores occur mainly on the external genitals, vagina, anus, or in the rectum. Sores also can occur on the lips and in the mouth. Transmission of the organism occurs during vaginal, anal, or oral sex. Pregnant women with the disease can pass it to the babies they are carrying. Syphilis cannot be spread through contact with toilet seats, doorknobs, swimming pools, hot tubs, bathtubs, shared clothing, or eating utensils.

What are the signs and symptoms in adults?

Many people infected with syphilis do not have any symptoms for years, yet remain at risk for late complications if they are not treated. Although transmission occurs from persons with sores who are in the primary or secondary stage, many of these sores are unrecognized. Thus, transmission may occur from persons who are unaware of their infection.

Primary stage: The primary stage of syphilis is usually marked by the appearance of a single sore (called a chancre), but there may be multiple sores. The time between infection with syphilis and the start of the first symptom can range from 10 to 90 days (average 21 days). The chancre is usually firm, round, small, and painless. It appears at the spot where syphilis entered the body. The chancre lasts three to six weeks, and it heals without treatment. However, if adequate treatment is not administered, the infection progresses to the secondary stage.

Secondary stage: Skin rash and mucous membrane lesions characterize the secondary stage. This stage typically starts with the development of a rash on one or more areas of the body. The rash usually does not cause itching. Rashes associated with secondary syphilis can appear as the chancre is healing or several weeks after the chancre has healed. The characteristic rash of secondary syphilis may appear as rough, red, or reddish brown spots both on the palms of the hands and the bottoms of the feet. However, rashes with a different appearance may occur on other parts of the body, sometimes resembling rashes caused by other diseases. Sometimes rashes associated with secondary syphilis are so faint that they are not noticed. In addition to rashes, symptoms of secondary syphilis may include fever, swollen lymph glands, sore throat, patchy hair loss, headaches, weight loss, muscle aches, and fatigue. The signs and symptoms of secondary syphilis will resolve with or without treatment, but without treatment, the infection will progress to the latent and possibly late stages of disease.

Late and latent stages: The latent (hidden) stage of syphilis begins when primary and secondary symptoms disappear. Without treatment, the infected person will continue to have syphilis even though there are no signs or symptoms; infection remains in the body. This latent stage can last for years. The late stages of syphilis can develop in about 15% of people who have not been treated for syphilis, and can appear 10–20 years after infection was first acquired. In the late stages of syphilis, the disease may subsequently damage the internal organs, including the brain, nerves, eyes, heart, blood vessels, liver, bones, and joints. Signs and symptoms of the late stage of syphilis include difficulty coordinating muscle movements, paralysis, numbness, gradual blindness, and dementia. This damage may be serious enough to cause death.

How does syphilis affect a pregnant woman and her baby?

The syphilis bacterium can infect the baby of a woman during her pregnancy. Depending on how long a pregnant woman has been infected, she may have a high risk of having a stillbirth (a baby born dead) or of giving birth to a baby who dies shortly after birth. An infected baby may be born without signs or symptoms of disease. However, if not treated immediately, the baby may develop serious problems within a few weeks. Untreated babies may become developmentally delayed, have seizures, or die.

How is syphilis diagnosed?

Some health care providers can diagnose syphilis by examining material from a chancre (infectious sore) using a special microscope called a dark-field microscope. If syphilis bacteria are present in the sore, they will show up when observed through the microscope.

A blood test is another way to determine whether someone has syphilis. Shortly after infection occurs, the body produces syphilis antibodies that can be detected by an accurate, safe, and inexpensive blood test. A low level of antibodies will likely stay in the blood for months or years even after the disease has been successfully treated. Because untreated syphilis in a pregnant woman can infect and possibly kill her developing baby, every pregnant woman should have a blood test for syphilis.

What is the link between syphilis and HIV?

Genital sores (chancres) caused by syphilis make it easier to transmit and acquire HIV (human immunodeficiency virus) infection sexually. There is an estimated two- to five-fold increased risk of acquiring HIV if exposed to that infection when syphilis is present.

Ulcerative STDs that cause sores, ulcers, or breaks in the skin or mucous membranes, such as syphilis, disrupt barriers that provide protection against infections. The genital ulcers caused by syphilis can bleed easily, and when they come into contact with oral and rectal mucosa during sex, increase the infectiousness of and susceptibility to HIV. Having other STDs is also an important predictor for becoming HIV infected because STDs are a marker for behaviors associated with HIV transmission.

Will syphilis recur?

Having syphilis once does not protect a person from getting it again. Following successful treatment, people can still be susceptible to reinfection. Only laboratory tests can confirm whether someone has syphilis. Because syphilis sores can be hidden in the vagina, rectum, or mouth, it may not be obvious that a sex partner has syphilis. Talking with a health care provider will help to determine the need to be retested for syphilis after being treated.

Section 23.2

Treating Syphilis

"Syphilis: Treatment," by the National Institute of Allergy and Infectious Diseases (NIAID, www.niaid.nih.gov), part of the National Institutes of Health, December 17, 2010.

Syphilis is easy to cure in its early stages. Penicillin, an antibiotic, injected into the muscle, is the best treatment for syphilis. If you are allergic to penicillin, your healthcare provider may give you another antibiotic to take by mouth.

If you have neurosyphilis, you may need to get daily doses of penicillin intravenously (in the vein) and you may need to be treated in the hospital.

If you have late syphilis, damage done to your body organs cannot be reversed.

While you are being treated, you should abstain from sex until any sores are completely healed. You should also notify your sex partners so they can be tested for syphilis and treated if necessary.

Can there be complications?

Pregnancy: Syphilis can cause miscarriages, premature births, or stillbirths. It can also cause death of newborn babies. Some infants with congenital syphilis have symptoms at birth, but most develop symptoms later.

Untreated babies with congenital syphilis can have deformities, delays in development, or seizures, along with many other problems such as rash, fever, swollen liver and spleen, anemia, and jaundice. Sores on infected babies are infectious. Rarely, the symptoms of syphilis may go unseen in infants and they develop the symptoms of late-stage syphilis, including damage to their bones, teeth, eyes, ears, and brains.

HIV (human immunodeficiency virus) infection: People infected with syphilis have a two- to five-fold increased risk of getting infected with HIV. Strong evidence shows the increased odds of getting and transmitting HIV in the presence of sexually transmitted diseases (STDs). You should discuss this and other STDs with your healthcare provider.

How do I prevent syphilis?

To prevent getting syphilis, you must avoid contact with infected tissue (a group of cells) and body fluids of an infected person. However, syphilis is usually transmitted by people who have no rashes or sores that can be seen and who do not know they are infected.

If you aren't infected with syphilis and are sexually active, having mutually monogamous sex with an uninfected partner is the best way to prevent syphilis.

Using condoms properly and consistently during sex reduces your risk of getting syphilis.

Washing or douching after sex won't prevent syphilis.

Even if you have been treated for syphilis and cured, you can be reinfected by having sex with an infected partner.

The risk of a mother transmitting syphilis to her unborn baby during pregnancy declines with time but persists during latent syphilis. To prevent passing congenital syphilis to their unborn babies, all pregnant women should be tested for syphilis.

Chapter 24

Trichomoniasis

What is trichomoniasis?

Trichomoniasis (or trich) is a very common sexually transmitted disease (STD) that is caused by infection with a protozoan parasite called *Trichomonas vaginalis*. Although symptoms of the disease vary, most women and men who have the parasite cannot tell they are infected.

How common is trichomoniasis?

Trichomoniasis is considered the most common curable STD. In the United States, an estimated 3.7 million people have the infection, but only about 30% develop any symptoms of trichomoniasis. Infection is more common in women than in men, and older women are more likely than younger women to have been infected.

How do people get trichomoniasis?

The parasite is passed from an infected person to an uninfected person during sex. In women, the most commonly infected part of the body is the lower genital tract (vulva, vagina, or urethra), and in men, the most commonly infected body part is the inside of the penis (urethra). During sex, the parasite is usually transmitted from a penis to a vagina, or from a vagina to a penis, but it can also be passed

"Trichomoniasis—CDC Fact Sheet," by the Centers for Disease Control and Prevention (CDC, www.cdc.gov), November 30, 2011.

from a vagina to another vagina. It is not common for the parasite to infect other body parts, like the hands, mouth, or anus. It is unclear why some people with the infection get symptoms while others do not, but it probably depends on factors like the person's age and overall health. Infected people without symptoms can still pass the infection on to others.

What are the signs and symptoms of trichomoniasis?

About 70% of infected people do not have any signs or symptoms. When trichomoniasis does cause symptoms, they can range from mild irritation to severe inflammation. Some people with symptoms get them within 5 to 28 days after being infected, but others do not develop symptoms until much later. Symptoms can come and go.

Men with trichomoniasis may feel itching or irritation inside the penis, burning after urination or ejaculation, or some discharge from the penis.

Women with trichomoniasis may notice itching, burning, redness or soreness of the genitals, discomfort with urination, or a thin discharge with an unusual smell that can be clear, white, yellowish, or greenish.

Having trichomoniasis can make it feel unpleasant to have sex. Without treatment, the infection can last for months or even years.

What are the complications of trichomoniasis?

Trichomoniasis can increase the risk of getting or spreading other sexually transmitted infections. For example, trichomoniasis can cause genital inflammation that makes it easier to get infected with HIV [human immunodeficiency virus] or to pass HIV on to a sex partner.

How does trichomoniasis affect a pregnant woman and her baby?

Pregnant women with trichomoniasis are more likely to have their babies too early (preterm delivery). Also, babies born to infected mothers are more likely to have an officially low birth weight (less than 5.5 pounds).

How is trichomoniasis diagnosed?

It is not possible to diagnose trichomoniasis based on symptoms alone. For both men and women, your primary care doctor or another trusted health care provider must do a check and a laboratory test to diagnose trichomoniasis.

What is the treatment for trichomoniasis?

Trichomoniasis can be cured with a single dose of prescription antibiotic medication (either metronidazole or tinidazole), pills which can be taken by mouth. It is okay for pregnant women to take this medication. Some people who drink alcohol within 24 hours after taking this kind of antibiotic can have uncomfortable side effects.

People who have been treated for trichomoniasis can get it again. About one in five people get infected again within three months after treatment. To avoid getting reinfected, make sure that all of your sex partners get treated too, and wait to have sex again until all of your symptoms go away (about a week). Get checked again if your symptoms come back.

How can trichomoniasis be prevented?

Using latex condoms correctly every time you have sex will help reduce the risk of getting or spreading trichomoniasis. However, condoms don't cover everything, and it is possible to get or spread this infection even when using a condom.

The only sure way to prevent sexually transmitted infections is to avoid having sex entirely. Another approach is to talk about these kinds of infections before you have sex with a new partner, so that you can make informed choices about the level of risk you are comfortable taking with your sex life.

If you or someone you know has questions about trichomoniasis or any other STD, especially with symptoms like unusual discharge, burning during urination, or a sore in the genital area, check in with a health care provider and get some answers.

Part Three

Complications
That May Accompany
STD Infection

Chapter 25

Infections and Syndromes That Develop after Sexual Contact

Chapter Contents

Section 25.1—Bacterial Vaginosis 298

Section 25.2—Cytomegalovirus 302

Section 25.3—Fungal (Yeast) Infection 305

Section 25.4—Intestinal Parasites 309

Section 25.5—Molluscum Contagiosum 311

Section 25.6—Proctitis, Proctocolitis, and Enteritis: Sexually Transmitted Gastrointestinal Syndromes 314

Section 25.7—Pubic Lice 316

Section 25.8—Scabies 320

Section 25.1

Bacterial Vaginosis

"Bacterial Vaginosis Fact Sheet," by the Office on Women's
Health (www.womenshealth.gov), part of the U.S. Department
of Health and Human Services, September 1, 2008.

What is bacterial vaginosis (BV)?

The vagina normally has a balance of mostly "good" bacteria and
fewer "harmful" bacteria.

Bacterial vaginosis, known as BV, develops when the balance changes. With BV, there is an increase in harmful bacteria and a decrease in good bacteria.

BV is the most common vaginal infection in women of childbearing age.

What causes BV?

Not much is known about how women get BV. Any woman can get BV. But there are certain things that can upset the normal balance of bacteria in the vagina, raising your risk of BV:

- Having a new sex partner or multiple sex partners

- Douching

- Using an intrauterine device (IUD) for birth control

- Not using a condom

BV is more common among women who are sexually active, but it is not clear how sex changes the balance of bacteria. You cannot get BV from the following:

- Toilet seats

- Bedding

- Swimming pools

- Touching objects around you

What are the signs of BV?

Women with BV may have an abnormal vaginal discharge with an unpleasant odor. Some women report a strong fish-like odor, especially after sex. The discharge can be white (milky) or gray. It may also be foamy or watery. Other symptoms may include burning when urinating, itching around the outside of the vagina, and irritation. These symptoms may also be caused by another type of infection, so it is important to see a doctor. Some women with BV have no symptoms at all.

How can I find out if I have BV?

There is a test to find out if you have BV. Your doctor takes a sample of fluid from your vagina and has it tested. Your doctor may also see signs of BV during an examination of the vagina. To help your doctor find the signs of BV or other infections, do the following:

- Schedule the exam when you do not have your period.

- Don't douche for at least 24 hours before seeing your doctor. Experts suggest that women do not douche at all.

- Don't use vaginal deodorant sprays. They might cover odors that are important for diagnosis. It may also lead to irritation.

- Don't have sex or put objects, such as a tampon, in your vagina for at least 24 hours before going to the doctor.

How is BV treated?

BV is treated with antibiotic medicines prescribed by your doctor. Your doctor may give you either metronidazole or clindamycin. Generally, male sex partners of women with BV don't need to be treated. However, BV can be spread to female partners. If your current partner is female, talk to her about treatment. You can get BV again even after being treated.

Is it safe to treat pregnant women who have BV?

All pregnant women with symptoms of BV should be tested and treated if they have it. This is especially important for pregnant women who have had a premature delivery or low birth weight baby in the past. There are treatments available at any stage of your pregnancy. Be sure to talk to your doctor about what is right for you.

Can BV cause health problems?

In most cases, BV doesn't cause any problems. But some problems can arise if BV is untreated.

- Pregnancy problems: BV can cause premature delivery and low birth weight babies (less than five pounds).

- PID: Pelvic inflammatory disease or PID is an infection that can affect a woman's uterus, ovaries, and fallopian tubes. Having BV increases the risk of getting PID after a surgical procedure, such as a hysterectomy or an abortion.

- Higher risk of getting HIV (human immunodeficiency virus) and other sexually transmitted infections (STIs): Having BV can raise your risk of HIV, chlamydia, and gonorrhea. Women with HIV who get BV are also more likely to pass HIV to a sexual partner.

How can I lower my risk of BV?

Experts are still figuring out the best way to prevent BV. But there are steps you can take to lower your risk.

- Help keep your vaginal bacteria balanced. Wash your vagina and anus every day with mild soap. When you go to the bathroom, wipe from your vagina to your anus. Keep the area cool by wearing cotton or cotton-lined underpants. Avoid tight pants and skip the pantyhose in summer.

- Don't douche. Douching removes some of the normal bacteria in the vagina that protects you from infection. This may raise your risk of BV. It may also make it easier to get BV again after treatment.

- Have regular pelvic exams. Talk with your doctor about how often you need exams, as well as STI tests.

- Finish your medicine. If you have BV, finish all the medicine your doctor gives you to treat it. Even if the symptoms go away, you still need to finish all of the medicine.

Practicing safe sex is also very important. Below are ways to help protect yourself.

- Don't have sex. The best way to prevent any STI is to not have vaginal, oral, or anal sex.

- Be faithful. Having sex with just one partner can also lower your risk. Be faithful to each other. That means that you only have sex with each other and no one else.

- Use condoms. Protect yourself with a condom every time you have vaginal, anal, or oral sex. Condoms should be used for any type of sex with every partner. For vaginal sex, use a latex male condom or a female polyurethane condom. For anal sex, use a latex male condom. For oral sex, use a condom or a dental dam. A dental dam is a rubbery material that can be placed over the anus or the vagina before sexual contact.

- Talk with your sex partner(s) about STIs and using condoms. It's up to you to make sure you are protected. Remember, it's your body. For more information, call the Centers for Disease Control and Prevention at 800-232-4636.

- Talk frankly with your doctor or nurse and your sex partner(s) about any STIs you or your partner(s) have or had. Talk about any discharge in the genital area. Try not to be embarrassed.

Section 25.2

Cytomegalovirus

Cytomegalovirus at a Glance

- CMV stands for cytomegalovirus.

- [It] often has no symptoms.

- [It has] no cure, but treatment is available for the symptoms.

- [It] can be spread during sex play.

- Condoms reduce your risk of infection.

- Want to get tested for cytomegalovirus? Find a health center.

We all want to protect ourselves and each other from infections like cytomegalovirus (CMV). Learning more about CMV is an important first step.

Here are some of the most common questions we hear people ask about CMV. We hope you find the answers helpful, whether you think you may have CMV, have been diagnosed with it, or are just curious about it.

What Is CMV?

You may have heard of cytomegalovirus or CMV, but many people are not sure what it is. Cytomegalovirus (sigh-tow-MEG-a-low-VI-rus) is a virus that is transmitted through many bodily fluids. It is usually spread during casual contact, and it can also be transmitted during sex.

CMV is quite common. About 4 out of every 10 Americans get CMV by the time they reach puberty, mainly through contact with other children's saliva. Adults, however, usually become reinfected through sexual activity.

Like many other viruses, CMV remains in the body for life.

What Are the Symptoms of CMV?

There are usually no symptoms with the first infection with cytomegalovirus. Rarely, reinfection with CMV, or having a weakened immune system, may reactivate the virus and cause symptoms to appear.

When symptoms do appear, they may include:

* swollen glands, fatigue, fever, and general weakness;

* irritations of the digestive tract, nausea, diarrhea;

* jaundice (yellowing of the skin or eyes).

CMV can be very dangerous for people with weakened immune systems. In addition to the symptoms listed above, it can cause blindness and mental disorders.

How Can I Know If I Have CMV?

Your health care provider can do a blood test to see if you have cytomegalovirus (CMV).

Is There a Treatment for CMV?

There is no cure. But when symptoms of cytomegalovirus (CMV) are present, they may be managed with medicine.

Where Can I Get a Test or Treatment for CMV?

Staff at your local Planned Parenthood health center, many other clinics, health departments, and private health care providers can diagnose cytomegalovirus (CMV) and help you get any treatment you may need.

Want to get tested for cytomegalovirus? Find a health center [http://www.plannedparenthood.org/health-center.]

How Is CMV Spread?

Cytomegalovirus (CMV) can be in saliva, semen, blood, cervical and vaginal secretions, urine, and breast milk. It can be spread through:

* close personal contact;

- vaginal and anal intercourse;

- oral sex;

- blood transfusion and sharing IV [intravenous] drug equipment;

- pregnancy, childbirth, and breastfeeding.

CMV and Pregnancy

CMV is the most common infection in the United States that is spread from a woman to her developing fetus. CMV can be passed during pregnancy, childbirth, or breastfeeding. The risk of infection is greatest when a woman gets CMV for the first time during pregnancy.

About one out of every 100 babies born in the United States has CMV. Most babies born with CMV have no problems from the virus. But about 1–2 out every 10 of them develop serious health problems. These problems can include hearing or vision loss, developmental and learning disabilities, and liver problems. In rare cases the problems can be fatal.

If you have CMV, talk with your health care provider if you are planning to get pregnant or are already pregnant.

How Can I Prevent Getting or Spreading CMV?

There are several ways to help prevent getting cytomegalovirus (CMV) or spreading it to other people.

- You can abstain from vaginal and anal intercourse and oral sex.

- If you choose to have vaginal or anal intercourse or oral sex, use female or latex condoms every time. Condoms and other barriers may reduce the risk of CMV, but kissing and other intimate touching can spread the virus.

- Careful hand washing can reduce the risk of infection from casual contact.

Section 25.3

Fungal (Yeast) Infection

"Vaginal Yeast Infections Fact Sheet," by the Office on Women's Health (www.womenshealth.gov), part of the U.S. Department of Health and Human Services, September 23, 2008.

What is a vaginal yeast infection?

A vaginal yeast infection is irritation of the vagina and the area around it called the vulva.

Yeast is a type of fungus. Yeast infections are caused by overgrowth of the fungus *Candida albicans*. Small amounts of yeast are always in the vagina. But when too much yeast grows, you can get an infection.

Yeast infections are very common. About 75 percent of women have one during their lives. And almost half of women have two or more vaginal yeast infections.

What are the signs of a vaginal yeast infection?

The most common symptom of a yeast infection is extreme itchiness in and around the vagina.

Other symptoms include the following:

- Burning, redness, and swelling of the vagina and the vulva

- Pain when passing urine

- Pain during sex

- Soreness

- A thick, white vaginal discharge that looks like cottage cheese and does not have a bad smell

- A rash on the vagina

You may only have a few of these symptoms. They may be mild or severe.

305

Should I call my doctor if I think I have a yeast infection?

Yes, you need to see your doctor to find out for sure if you have a yeast infection. The signs of a yeast infection are much like those of sexually transmitted infections (STIs) like chlamydia and gonorrhea. So, it's hard to be sure you have a yeast infection and not something more serious.

If you've had vaginal yeast infections before, talk to your doctor about using over-the-counter medicines.

How is a vaginal yeast infection diagnosed?

Your doctor will do a pelvic exam to look for swelling and discharge. Your doctor may also use a swab to take a fluid sample from your vagina. A quick look with a microscope or a lab test will show if yeast is causing the problem.

Why did I get a yeast infection?

Many things can raise your risk of a vaginal yeast infection, such as the following:

- Stress

- Lack of sleep

- Illness

- Poor eating habits, including eating extreme amounts of sugary foods

- Pregnancy

- Having your period

- Taking certain medicines, including birth control pills, antibiotics, and steroids

- Diseases such as poorly controlled diabetes and HIV/AIDS [human immunodeficiency virus/acquired immunodeficiency syndrome]

- Hormonal changes during your periods

Can I get a yeast infection from having sex?

Yes, but it is rare. Most often, women don't get yeast infections from sex. The most common cause is a weak immune system.

How are yeast infections treated?

Yeast infections can be cured with antifungal medicines that come as creams, tablets, and ointments or suppositories that are inserted into the vagina.

These products can be bought over the counter at the drug store or grocery store. Your doctor can also prescribe you a single dose of oral fluconazole. But do not use this drug if you are pregnant.

Infections that don't respond to these medicines are starting to be more common. Using antifungal medicines when you don't really have a yeast infection can raise your risk of getting a hard-to-treat infection in the future.

Is it safe to use over-the-counter medicines for yeast infections?

Yes, but always talk with your doctor before treating yourself for a vaginal yeast infection if you are pregnant, have never been diagnosed with a yeast infection, or keep getting yeast infections.

Studies show that two thirds of women who buy these products don't really have a yeast infection. Using these medicines the wrong way may lead to a hard-to-treat infection. Plus, treating yourself for a yeast infection when you really have something else may worsen the problem. Certain STIs that go untreated can cause cancer, infertility, pregnancy problems, and other health problems.

If you decide to use these over-the-counter medicines, read and follow the directions carefully. Some creams and inserts may weaken condoms and diaphragms.

If I have a yeast infection, does my sexual partner need to be treated?

Yeast infections are not STIs, and health experts don't know for sure if they are transmitted sexually. About 12 to 15 percent of men get an itchy rash on the penis if they have unprotected sex with an infected woman. If this happens to your partner, he should see a doctor. Men who haven't been circumcised are at higher risk.

Lesbians may be at risk for spreading yeast infections to their partner(s). Research is still being done to know for sure. If your female partner has any symptoms, she should also be tested and treated.

How can I avoid getting another yeast infection?

To help prevent vaginal yeast infections, you can do the following:

- Avoid douches.

- Avoid scented hygiene products like bubble bath, sprays, pads, and tampons.

- Change tampons and pads often during your period.

- Avoid tight underwear or clothes made of synthetic fibers.

- Wear cotton underwear and pantyhose with a cotton crotch.

- Change out of wet swimsuits and exercise clothes as soon as you can.

- Avoid hot tubs and very hot baths.

If you keep getting yeast infections, be sure and talk with your doctor.

What should I do if I get repeat yeast infections?

Call your doctor. About 5 percent of women get four or more vaginal yeast infections in one year. This is called recurrent vulvovaginal candidiasis (RVVC). RVVC is more common in women with diabetes or weak immune systems. Doctors most often treat this problem with antifungal medicine for up to six months.

Section 25.4

Intestinal Parasites

Intestinal Parasites at a Glance

- [It is] an infection of the intestines.

- [It] often has no symptoms.

- Treatment is available.

- [It] can be spread during sex play.

- There are ways to reduce your risk of infection.

- Want to get tested for intestinal parasites? Find a health center.

We all want to protect ourselves and each other from infections like intestinal parasites. Learning more about intestinal parasites is an important first step.

Here are some of the most common questions we hear people ask about intestinal parasites. We hope you find the answers helpful, whether you think you may have intestinal parasites, have been diagnosed with them, or are just curious about them.

What Are Intestinal Parasites?

You may have heard of intestinal parasites, but many people are not sure what they are. Intestinal parasites are microscopic, one-cell animals called protozoa. They infect the intestines.

Intestinal parasites are often transmitted by contaminated food and water and during nonsexual, intimate contact. They may also be transmitted sexually. They are most common in places with poor hygiene and sanitation.

Millions of Americans have intestinal parasites. For people with weakened immune systems, such as people with HIV [human immunodeficiency virus], intestinal parasites can be very serious—even life threatening.

What Are the Symptoms of Intestinal Parasites?

Often there are no intestinal parasites symptoms. When there are symptoms, they may include:

- diarrhea, which may become severe and chronic;
- abdominal pain;
- bloating;
- nausea and vomiting.

How Can I Know If I Have Intestinal Parasites?

A health care provider can do tests to see if you have intestinal parasites, even if you do not have intestinal parasite symptoms. Your health care provider will examine your stool (feces). Other tests are sometimes needed, such as proctoscopy—a test that involves a health care provider inserting a thin tube that has a light into the rectum.

Is There a Treatment for Intestinal Parasites?

Yes, medicines are available for treatment. Pregnant women cannot take some of them. And treatments may not be as effective for people with weakened immune systems.

Where Can I Get a Test or Treatment for Intestinal Parasites?

Staff at your local Planned Parenthood health center, many other clinics, health departments, and private health care providers can diagnose intestinal parasites and help you get any treatment you may need.

Want to get tested for intestinal parasites? Find a health center [http://www.plannedparenthood.org/health-center].

How Are Intestinal Parasites Spread?

Intestinal parasites are spread when fecal matter—bits of feces—gets into the mouth. This can happen through:

- contaminated food or water;

- oral and anal sex play, or nonsexual intimate contact, such as diaper changing.

How Can I Prevent Getting or Spreading Intestinal Parasites?

There are a few things you can do to prevent getting intestinal parasites:

- Observe strict rules of day-to-day hygiene, like careful hand washing.
- Use a Sheer Glyde dam, dental dam, or piece of plastic wrap during oral/anal sex play.

Section 25.5

Molluscum Contagiosum

"Molluscum Contagiosum," by the National Center for Emerging and Zoonotic Infectious Diseases (NCEZID), part of the Centers for Disease Control (CDC, www.cdc.gov), January 13, 2011.

Molluscum contagiosum is a common skin disease that is caused by a virus. The disease is generally mild and should not be a reason for concern or worry.

Molluscum infection causes small white, pink, or flesh-colored bumps or growths with a dimple or pit in the center. The bumps are usually smooth and firm and can appear anywhere on the body. They may become sore, red, and swollen but are usually painless. The bumps normally disappear within 6 to 12 months without treatment and without leaving scars. In people with weakened immune systems, molluscum growths may grow very large, spread more easily to other parts of the body, and may be harder to cure.

How It Spreads

People with this skin disease can cause the bumps to spread to different parts of their body. This is called autoinoculation. Such spread can occur by touching or scratching a bump and then touching another part of the body.

311

The virus can also be spread from person to person. This can happen if the growths on one person are touched by another person. It can also happen if the virus gets on an object that is touched by other people. Examples of such objects are towels, clothing, and toys. Molluscum can also be spread from one person to another by sexual contact. Anyone who develops bumps in the genital area (on or near the penis, vulva, vagina, or anus) should see a health care provider. Bumps in these areas sometimes mean that molluscum or some other disease was spread through sexual contact.

How to Prevent the Spread of Molluscum

Wash Your Hands

There are ways to prevent the spread of molluscum contagiosum. The best way is to follow good hygiene (cleanliness) habits. Keeping your hands clean is the best way to avoid molluscum infection, as well as many other infections. Hand washing removes germs that may have been picked up from other people or from surfaces that have germs on them.

Don't Scratch or Pick at Molluscum Bumps

It is important not to touch, pick, or scratch skin that has bumps or blisters—that includes not only your own skin but anyone else's. Picking and scratching can spread the virus to other parts of the body and makes it easier to spread the disease to other people, too.

Keep Molluscum Bumps Covered

It is important to keep the area with molluscum growths clean and covered with clothing or a bandage so that others do not touch the bumps and become infected with molluscum. Do remember to keep the affected skin clean and dry.

However, when there is no risk of others coming into contact with your skin, such as at night when you sleep, uncover the bumps to help keep your skin healthy.

Sports and Activities to Avoid or Be Careful with When You Have Molluscum

To prevent spread of the infection to other people, people with molluscum should not take part in contact sports unless all growths can be covered by clothing or bandages. Wrestling, basketball, and football are examples of contact sports.

Activities that use shared gear should also be avoided unless all bumps can be covered. Helmets, baseball gloves, and balls are examples of shared gear.

Swimming should also be avoided unless all growths can be covered by watertight bandages. Personal items (such as towels, goggles, and swimsuits) should not be shared. Other items and equipment (such as kickboards and water toys) should be used only when all bumps are covered by clothing or watertight bandages.

Other Ways to Avoid Sharing Your Infection

- Other personal items that may spread the virus should not be shared by people with molluscum. Some examples of personal items are unwashed clothes, hair brushes, wrist watches, and bar soap.

- People with molluscum should not shave or have electrolysis performed on body areas that have growths.

- People who have bumps in the genital area (on or near the penis, vulva, vagina, or anus) should avoid sexual contact until they have seen a health care provider.

Treating Molluscum

Some treatments exist for molluscum that may prevent spread of the infection to other parts of the body and to other people. A health care provider can remove the growths with surgery or laser therapy. A health care provider may also prescribe a cream to apply on the bumps or a medicine to take by mouth.

However, treatment is not usually required because the bumps disappear on their own within six months. However, they may not go away completely for up to four years. In addition, not all treatments are successful for all people. For example, it is more difficult to treat persons who have a weak immune system. This includes people who are infected with HIV (human immunodeficiency syndrome) or who are receiving drugs to treat cancer.

Some molluscum treatments that are advertised on the Internet are not effective and may even be harmful. Therefore, always discuss any therapy with a health care provider before using it.

Section 25.6

Proctitis, Proctocolitis, and Enteritis: Sexually Transmitted Gastrointestinal Syndromes

From the Centers for Disease Control and Prevention (CDC, www.cdc.gov), part of the National Institutes of Health, January 28, 2011.

Sexually transmitted gastrointestinal syndromes include proctitis, proctocolitis, and enteritis. Evaluation for these syndromes should include appropriate diagnostic procedures (e.g., anoscopy or sigmoidoscopy, stool examination, and culture).

Proctitis is inflammation of the rectum (i.e., the distal 10–12 cm) that can be associated with anorectal pain, tenesmus, or rectal discharge. *N. gonorrhoeae* [gonorrhea], *C. trachomatis* ([chlamydia] including LGV [lymphogranuloma venereum] serovars), *T. pallidum* [syphilis], and HSV [herpes simplex virus] are the most common sexually transmitted pathogens involved. In patients coinfected with HIV [human immunodeficiency virus], herpes proctitis can be especially severe. Proctitis occurs predominantly among persons who participate in receptive anal intercourse.

Proctocolitis is associated with symptoms of proctitis, diarrhea or abdominal cramps, and inflammation of the colonic mucosa extending to 12 cm above the anus. Fecal leukocytes might be detected on stool examination, depending on the pathogen. Pathogenic organisms include *Campylobacter* sp., *Shigella* sp., *Entamoeba histolytica*, and LGV serovars of *C. trachomatis*. CMV [cytomegalovirus] or other opportunistic agents can be involved in immunosuppressed HIV-infected patients.

Proctocolitis can be acquired by the oral route or by oral-anal contact, depending on the pathogen.

Enteritis usually results in diarrhea and abdominal cramping without signs of proctitis or proctocolitis; it occurs among persons whose sexual practices include oral-anal contact. In otherwise healthy persons, *Giardia lamblia* is most frequently implicated. When outbreaks of gastrointestinal illness occur among social or sexual networks of MSM [men who have sex with men], clinicians should consider sexual transmission as a mode of spread and provide counseling accordingly. Among HIV-infected patients, gastrointestinal illness can be caused by other infections that usually are not sexually transmitted, including CMV, *Mycobacterium avium–intracellulare, Salmonella* sp., *Campylobacter* sp., *Shigella* sp., *Cryptosporidium, Microsporidium,* and *Isospora.* Multiple stool examinations might be necessary to detect *Giardia,* and special stool preparations are required to diagnose cryptosporidiosis and microsporidiosis. In addition, enteritis can be directly caused by HIV infection.

When laboratory diagnostic capabilities are available, treatment decisions should be based on the specific diagnosis. Diagnostic and treatment recommendations for all enteric infections are beyond the scope of this text.

Treatment

Acute proctitis of recent onset among persons who have recently practiced receptive anal intercourse is usually sexually acquired. Such patients should be examined by anoscopy and should be evaluated for infection with HSV, *N. gonorrhoeae, C. trachomatis,* and *T. pallidum.* If an anorectal exudate is detected on examination or if polymorphonuclear leukocytes are detected on a Gram-stained smear of anorectal secretions, the following therapy should be prescribed while awaiting additional laboratory tests. The recommended regimen is ceftriaxone 250 mg IM [intramuscular] plus doxycycline 100 mg orally twice a day for seven days.

Patients with suspected or documented herpes proctitis should be managed in the same manner as those with genital herpes. If painful perianal ulcers are present or mucosal ulcers are detected on anoscopy, presumptive therapy should include a regimen for genital herpes and LGV. Appropriate diagnostic testing for LGV should be conducted in accordance with state or federal guidelines, and doxycycline therapy should be administered 100 mg orally twice daily for three weeks.

For MSM, treatment for LGV proctitis/proctocolitis with three weeks of doxycycline in those with anorectal chlamydia and either 1) proctitis (as detected by proctoscopic examination and the presence of >10 white-blood cells upon high-power field examination of an anorectal smear specimen) or 2) HIV infection can be considered.

Follow-Up

Follow-up should be based on specific etiology and severity of clinical symptoms. Reinfection might be difficult to distinguish from treatment failure.

Management of Sex Partners

Partners of persons with sexually transmitted enteric infections should be evaluated for any diseases diagnosed in the index patient.

Section 25.7

Pubic Lice

"Pubic Lice Frequently Asked Questions" and
"Pubic Lice Treatment," by the Centers for Disease Control and
Prevention (CDC, www.cdc.gov), November 2, 2010.

What are pubic lice?

Also called crab lice or crabs, pubic lice are parasitic insects found primarily in the pubic or genital area of humans. Pubic lice infestation is found worldwide and occurs in all races, ethnic groups, and levels of society.

What do pubic lice look like?

Pubic lice have three forms: The egg (also called a nit), the nymph, and the adult.

- **Nit:** Nits are lice eggs. They can be hard to see and are found firmly attached to the hair shaft. They are oval and usually yellow to white. Pubic lice nits take about 6–10 days to hatch.

- **Nymph:** The nymph is an immature louse that hatches from the nit (egg). A nymph looks like an adult pubic louse but it is smaller. Pubic lice nymphs take about two to three weeks after hatching to mature into adults capable of reproducing. To live, a nymph must feed on blood.

- **Adult:** The adult pubic louse resembles a miniature crab when viewed through a strong magnifying glass. Pubic lice have six legs; their two front legs are very large and look like the pincher claws of a crab. This is how they got the nickname crabs. Pubic lice are tan to grayish-white in color. Females lay nits and are

316

usually larger than males. To live, lice must feed on blood. If the louse falls off a person, it dies within one to two days.

Where are pubic lice found?

Pubic lice usually are found in the genital area on pubic hair; but they may occasionally be found on other coarse body hair, such as hair on the legs, armpits, mustache, beard, eyebrows, or eyelashes. Pubic lice on the eyebrows or eyelashes of children may be a sign of sexual exposure or abuse. Lice found on the head generally are head lice, not pubic lice.

Animals do not get or spread pubic lice.

What are the signs and symptoms of pubic lice?

Signs and symptoms of pubic lice include the following:

* Itching in the genital area
* Visible nits (lice eggs) or crawling lice

How did I get pubic lice?

Pubic lice usually are spread through sexual contact and are most common in adults. Pubic lice found on children may be a sign of sexual exposure or abuse. Occasionally, pubic lice may be spread by close personal contact or contact with articles such as clothing, bed linens, or towels that have been used by a person with pubic lice. A common misconception is that pubic lice are spread easily by sitting on a toilet seat. This would be extremely rare because lice cannot live long away from a warm human body and they do not have feet designed to hold onto or walk on smooth surfaces such as toilet seats.

People with pubic lice should be examined for the presence of other sexually transmitted diseases.

How is a pubic lice infestation diagnosed?

A pubic lice infestation is diagnosed by finding a "crab" louse or egg (nit) on hair in the pubic region or, less commonly, elsewhere on the body (eyebrows, eyelashes, beard, mustache, armpit, perianal area, groin, trunk, scalp). Pubic lice may be difficult to find because there may be only a few. Pubic lice often attach themselves to more than one hair and generally do not crawl as quickly as head and body lice. If crawling lice are not seen, finding nits in the pubic area strongly suggests that a person is infested and should be treated. If you are

317

unsure about infestation or if treatment is not successful, see a health care provider for a diagnosis. Persons infested with pubic lice should be investigated for the presence of other sexually transmitted diseases.

Although pubic lice and nits can be large enough to be seen with the naked eye, a magnifying lens may be necessary to find lice or eggs.

How is a pubic lice infestation treated?

A lice-killing lotion containing 1% permethrin or a mousse containing pyrethrins and piperonyl butoxide can be used to treat pubic (crab) lice. These products are available over the counter without a prescription at a local drug store or pharmacy. These medications are safe and effective when used exactly according to the instructions in the package or on the label.

Lindane shampoo is a prescription medication that can kill lice and lice eggs. However, lindane is not recommended as a first-line therapy. Lindane can be toxic to the brain and other parts of the nervous system; its use should be restricted to patients who have failed treatment with or cannot tolerate other medications that pose less risk. Lindane should not be used to treat premature infants, persons with a seizure disorder, women who are pregnant or breastfeeding, persons who have very irritated skin or sores where the lindane will be applied, infants, children, the elderly, and persons who weigh less than 110 pounds.

Malathion lotion 0.5% (Ovide) is a prescription medication that can kill lice and some lice eggs; however, malathion lotion (Ovide) currently has not been approved by the U.S. Food and Drug Administration (FDA) for treatment of pubic (crab) lice.

Ivermectin has been used successfully to treat lice; however, ivermectin currently has not been approved by the U.S. Food and Drug Administration (FDA) for treatment of lice.

How to treat pubic lice infestations: (Warning: See special instructions for treatment of lice and nits on eyebrows or eyelashes. The lice medications described in this section should not be used near the eyes.)

1. Wash the infested area; towel dry.

2. Carefully follow the instructions in the package or on the label. Thoroughly saturate the pubic hair and other infested areas with lice medication. Leave medication on hair for the time recommended in the instructions. After waiting the recommended time, remove the medication by following carefully the instructions on the label or in the box.

3. Following treatment, most nits will still be attached to hair shafts. Nits may be removed with fingernails or by using a fine-toothed comb.

4. Put on clean underwear and clothing after treatment.

5. To kill any lice or nits remaining on clothing, towels, or bedding, machine-wash and machine-dry those items that the person with pubic lice used during the two to three days before treatment. Use hot water (at least 130 degrees Fahrenheit) and the hot dryer cycle.

6. Items that cannot be laundered can be dry cleaned or stored in a sealed plastic bag for two weeks.

7. All sex partners from within the previous month should be informed that they are at risk for infestation and should be treated.

8. Persons should avoid sexual contact with their sex partner(s) until both they and their partners have been successfully treated and reevaluated to rule out persistent infestation.

9. Repeat treatment in 9–10 days if live lice are still found.

10. Persons with pubic lice should be evaluated for other sexually transmitted diseases (STDs).

Special instructions for treatment of lice and nits found on eyebrows or eyelashes:

- If only a few live lice and nits are present, it may be possible to remove these with fingernails or a nit comb.

- If additional treatment is needed for lice or nits on the eyelashes, careful application of ophthalmic-grade petrolatum ointment (only available by prescription) to the eyelid margins 2–4 times a day for 10 days is effective. Regular petrolatum (e.g., Vaseline) should not be used because it can irritate the eyes if applied.

Section 25.8

Scabies

"Scabies Frequently Asked Questions,"
by the Centers for Disease Control and Prevention
(CDC, www.cdc.gov), November 2, 2010.

What is scabies?

Scabies is an infestation of the skin by the human itch mite (*Sarcoptes scabiei var. hominis*). The microscopic scabies mite burrows into the upper layer of the skin where it lives and lays its eggs. The most common symptoms of scabies are intense itching and a pimple-like skin rash. The scabies mite usually is spread by direct, prolonged, skin-to-skin contact with a person who has scabies.

Scabies is found worldwide and affects people of all races and social classes. Scabies can spread rapidly under crowded conditions where close body and skin contact is frequent. Institutions such as nursing homes, extended-care facilities, and prisons are often sites of scabies outbreaks. Child care facilities also are a common site of scabies infestations.

What is crusted (Norwegian) scabies?

Crusted scabies is a severe form of scabies that can occur in some persons who are immunocompromised (have a weak immune system), elderly, disabled, or debilitated. It is also called Norwegian scabies. Persons with crusted scabies have thick crusts of skin that contain large numbers of scabies mites and eggs. Persons with crusted scabies are very contagious to other persons and can spread the infestation easily both by direct skin-to-skin contact and by contamination of items such as their clothing, bedding, and furniture. Persons with crusted scabies may not show the usual signs and symptoms of scabies such as the characteristic rash or itching (pruritus). Persons with crusted scabies should receive quick and aggressive medical treatment for their infestation to prevent outbreaks of scabies.

How soon after infestation do symptoms of scabies begin?

If a person has never had scabies before, symptoms may take as long as four to six weeks to begin. It is important to remember that an infested person can spread scabies during this time, even if he/she does not have symptoms yet.

In a person who has had scabies before, symptoms usually appear much sooner (one to four days) after exposure.

What are the signs and symptoms of scabies infestation?

The most common signs and symptoms of scabies are intense itching (pruritus), especially at night, and a pimple-like (papular) itchy rash. The itching and rash each may affect much of the body or be limited to common sites such as the wrist, elbow, armpit, webbing between the fingers, nipple, penis, waist, belt-line, and buttocks. The rash also can include tiny blisters (vesicles) and scales. Scratching the rash can cause skin sores; sometimes these sores become infected by bacteria.

Tiny burrows sometimes are seen on the skin; these are caused by the female scabies mite tunneling just beneath the surface of the skin. These burrows appear as tiny raised and crooked (serpiginous) grayish-white or skin-colored lines on the skin surface. Because mites are often few in number (only 10–15 mites per person), these burrows may be difficult to find. They are found most often in the webbing between the fingers, in the skin folds on the wrist, elbow, or knee, and on the penis, breast, or shoulder blades.

The head, face, neck, palms, and soles often are involved in infants and very young children, but usually not adults and older children.

Persons with crusted scabies may not show the usual signs and symptoms of scabies such as the characteristic rash or itching (pruritus).

How did I get scabies?

Scabies usually is spread by direct, prolonged, skin-to-skin contact with a person who has scabies. Contact generally must be prolonged; a quick handshake or hug usually will not spread scabies. Scabies is spread easily to sexual partners and household members. Scabies in adults frequently is sexually acquired. Scabies sometimes is spread indirectly by sharing articles such as clothing, towels, or bedding used by an infested person; however, such indirect spread can occur much more easily when the infested person has crusted scabies.

How is scabies infestation diagnosed?

Diagnosis of a scabies infestation usually is made based on the customary appearance and distribution of the rash and the presence of burrows. Whenever possible, the diagnosis of scabies should be confirmed by identifying the mite, mite eggs, or mite fecal matter (scybala). This can be done by carefully removing a mite from the end of its burrow using the tip of a needle or by obtaining skin scraping to examine under a microscope for mites, eggs, or mite fecal matter. It is important to remember that a person can still be infested even if mites, eggs, or fecal matter cannot be found; typically fewer than 10–15 mites can be present on the entire body of an infested person who is otherwise healthy. However, persons with crusted scabies can be infested with thousands of mites and should be considered highly contagious.

How long can scabies mites live?

On a person, scabies mites can live for as long as one to two months. Off a person, scabies mites usually do not survive more than 48–72 hours. Scabies mites will die if exposed to a temperature of 50 degrees Celsius (122 degrees Fahrenheit) for 10 minutes.

Can scabies be treated?

Yes. Products used to treat scabies are called scabicides because they kill scabies mites; some also kill eggs. Scabicides to treat human scabies are available only with a doctor's prescription; no "over-the-counter" (non-prescription) products have been tested and approved for humans.

Always follow carefully the instructions provided by the doctor and pharmacist, as well as those contained in the box or printed on the label. When treating adults and older children, scabicide cream or lotion is applied to all areas of the body from the neck down to the feet and toes; when treating infants and young children, the cream or lotion also is applied to the head and neck. The medication should be left on the body for the recommended time before it is washed off. Clean clothes should be worn after treatment.

In addition to the infested person, treatment also is recommended for household members and sexual contacts, particularly those who have had prolonged skin-to-skin contact with the infested person. All persons should be treated at the same time in order to prevent reinfestation. Retreatment may be necessary if itching continues more than two to four weeks after treatment or if new burrows or rash continue to appear.

Never use a scabicide intended for veterinary or agricultural use to treat humans.

Who should be treated for scabies?

Anyone who is diagnosed with scabies, as well as his or her sexual partners and other contacts who have had prolonged skin-to-skin contact with the infested person, should be treated. Treatment is recommended for members of the same household as the person with scabies, particularly those persons who have had prolonged skin-to-skin contact with the infested person. All persons should be treated at the same time to prevent reinfestation.

Retreatment may be necessary if itching continues more than two to four weeks after treatment or if new burrows or rash continue to appear.

How soon after treatment will I feel better?

If itching continues more than two to four weeks after initial treatment or if new burrows or rash continue to appear (if initial treatment includes more than one application or dose, then the two- to four-week time period begins after the last application or dose), retreatment with scabicide may be necessary; seek the advice of a physician.

Did I get scabies from my pet?

No. Animals do not spread human scabies. Pets can become infested with a different kind of scabies mite that does not survive or reproduce on humans but causes mange in animals. If an animal with mange has close contact with a person, the animal mite can get under the person's skin and cause temporary itching and skin irritation. However, the animal mite cannot reproduce on a person and will die on its own in a couple of days. Although the person does not need to be treated, the animal should be treated because its mites can continue to burrow into the person's skin and cause symptoms until the animal has been treated successfully.

Can scabies be spread by swimming in a public pool?

Scabies is spread by prolonged skin-to-skin contact with a person who has scabies. Scabies sometimes also can be spread by contact with items such as clothing, bedding, or towels that have been used by a person with scabies, but such spread is very uncommon unless the infested person has crusted scabies.

Scabies is very unlikely to be spread by water in a swimming pool. Except for a person with crusted scabies, only about 10–15 scabies mites are present on an infested person; it is extremely unlikely that any would emerge from under wet skin.

Although uncommon, scabies can be spread by sharing a towel or item of clothing that has been used by a person with scabies.

How can I remove scabies mites from my house or carpet?

Scabies mites do not survive more than two to three days away from human skin. Items such as bedding, clothing, and towels used by a person with scabies can be decontaminated by machine-washing in hot water and drying using the hot cycle or by dry cleaning. Items that cannot be washed or dry cleaned can be decontaminated by removing from any body contact for at least 72 hours.

Because persons with crusted scabies are considered very infectious, careful vacuuming of furniture and carpets in rooms used by these persons is recommended.

Fumigation of living areas is unnecessary.

How can I remove scabies mites from my clothes?

Scabies mites do not survive more than two to three days away from human skin. Items such as bedding, clothing, and towels used by a person with scabies can be decontaminated by machine washing in hot water and drying using the hot cycle or by dry cleaning. Items that cannot be washed or dry cleaned can be decontaminated by removing from any body contact for at least 72 hours.

My spouse and I were diagnosed with scabies. After several treatments, he/she still has symptoms while I am cured. Why?

The rash and itching of scabies can persist for several weeks to a month after treatment, even if the treatment was successful and all the mites and eggs have been killed. Your health care provider may prescribe additional medication to relieve itching if it is severe. Symptoms that persist for longer than two weeks after treatment can be due to a number of reasons, including the following:

- Incorrect diagnosis of scabies: Many drug reactions can mimic the symptoms of scabies and cause a skin rash and itching; the diagnosis of scabies should be confirmed by a skin scraping that includes observing the mite, eggs, or mite feces (scybala) under a microscope. If you are sleeping in the same bed with your spouse and have not become reinfested, and you have not retreated yourself for at least 30 days, then it is unlikely that your spouse has scabies.

- Reinfestation with scabies from a family member or other infested person if all patients and their contacts are not treated at the same time; infested persons and their contacts must be treated at the same time to prevent reinfestation.

- Treatment failure caused by resistance to medication, by faulty application of topical scabicides, or by failure to do a second application when necessary; no new burrows should appear 24–48 hours after effective treatment.

- Treatment failure of crusted scabies because of poor penetration of scabicide into thick scaly skin containing large numbers of scabies mites; repeated treatment with a combination of both topical and oral medication may be necessary to treat crusted scabies successfully.

- Reinfestation from items (fomites) such as clothing, bedding, or towels that were not appropriately washed or dry cleaned (this is mainly of concern for items used by persons with crusted scabies); potentially contaminated items (fomites) should be machine washed in hot water and dried using the hot temperature cycle, dry cleaned, or removed from skin contact for at least 72 hours.

Persistent symptoms may also be due to an allergic skin rash (dermatitis) or exposure to household mites that cause symptoms to persist because of cross-reactivity between mite antigens.

If itching continues more than two to four weeks or if new burrows or rash continue to appear, seek the advice of a physician; retreatment with the same or a different scabicide may be necessary.

If I come in contact with a person who has scabies, should I treat myself?

No. If a person thinks he or she might have scabies, he/she should contact a doctor. The doctor can examine the person, confirm the diagnosis of scabies, and prescribe an appropriate treatment. Products used to treat scabies in humans are available only with a doctor's prescription.

Sleeping with or having sex with any scabies infested person presents a high risk for transmission. The longer a person has skin-to-skin exposure, the greater is the likelihood for transmission to occur. Although briefly shaking hands with a person who has non-crusted scabies could be considered as presenting a relatively low risk, holding the hand of a person with scabies for 5–10 minutes could be considered to present a relatively high risk of transmission. However, transmission can occur even after brief skin-to-skin contact, such as a handshake, with a person who has crusted scabies. In general, a person who has skin-to-skin contact with a person who has crusted scabies would be considered a good candidate for treatment.

To determine when prophylactic treatment should be given to reduce the risk of transmission, early consultation should be sought with a health care provider who understands the following:

1. The type of scabies (i.e., non-crusted vs crusted) to which a person has been exposed

2. The degree and duration of skin exposure that a person has had to the infested patient

3. Whether the exposure occurred before or after the patient was treated for scabies

4. Whether the exposed person works in an environment where he/she would be likely to expose other people during the asymptomatic incubation period. For example, a nurse or caretaker who works in a nursing home or hospital often would be treated prophylactically to reduce the risk of further scabies transmission in the facility.

Chapter 26

Cervicitis

Cervicitis is swelling (inflammation) of the end of the uterus (cervix).

Causes

Cervicitis is most often caused by an infection, usually caught during sexual activity. Sexually transmitted diseases (STDs) that can cause cervicitis include:

- chlamydia;
- gonorrhea;
- herpes virus (genital herpes);
- human papillomavirus (genital warts);
- trichomoniasis.

However, in a few cases it may be due to:

- a device inserted into the pelvic area such as [a]:
  - cervical cap,
  - device to support the uterus (pessary),
  - diaphragm;
- an allergy to spermicides used for birth control or to latex in condoms;

"Cervicitis," © 2012 A.D.A.M., Inc. Reprinted with permission.

- exposure to a chemical.

Cervicitis is very common, affecting more than half of all women at some point during their adult life. Risks include:

- high-risk sexual behavior;
- history of STDs;
- many sexual partners;
- sex (intercourse) at an early age;
- sexual partners who have engaged in high-risk sexual behavior or have had an STD.

Bacteria (such as staphylococcus and streptococcus) and too much growth of normal bacteria in the vagina (bacterial vaginosis) can also cause cervicitis.

Symptoms

- Abnormal vaginal bleeding
  - After intercourse
  - After menopause
  - Between periods
- Unusual vaginal discharge
  - Does not go away
  - Gray, white, or yellow color
  - May have an odor
- Painful sexual intercourse
- Pain in the vagina
- Pressure or heaviness in the pelvis

Note: There may be no symptoms, so it is recommended that certain women be tested for chlamydia, even if they do not have symptoms.

Exams and Tests

A pelvic examination may show:

- discharge from the cervix;
- redness of the cervix;

- swelling (inflammation) of the walls of the vagina.

Tests:

- Inspection of the discharge under a microscope (may show candidiasis, trichomoniasis, or bacterial vaginosis)
- Pap smear
- Tests for gonorrhea or chlamydia

Rarely, colposcopy and biopsy of the cervix is necessary.

Treatment

Antibiotics are used to treat bacterial infections, such as chlamydia, gonorrhea, and others. Drugs called antivirals may be used to treat herpes infections.

Hormonal therapy (with estrogen or progesterone) may be used in women who have reached menopause (postmenopausal).

When these treatments have not worked or when cervicitis has been present for a long time, treatment may include:

- cryosurgery (freezing);
- electrocauterization;
- laser therapy.

Outlook (Prognosis)

Simple cervicitis usually heals with treatment if the cause is found and there is a treatment for that cause.

Possible Complications

Cervicitis may last for months to years. Cervicitis may lead to pain with intercourse (dyspareunia).

When to Contact a Medical Professional

Call your health care provider if you have symptoms of cervicitis.

Prevention

Ways to reduce the risk of cervicitis include [the following]:

- Avoid chemical irritants such as douches and deodorant tampons.

- Make sure that any foreign objects you insert into your vagina (such as tampons) are placed properly. Be sure to follow the guidelines on how long to leave the object inside, how often to change it, or how often to clean it.

- Not having sexual intercourse (abstinence) is the only absolute method of preventing sexually transmitted cervicitis. A monogamous sexual relationship with someone who is known to be free of any STD can reduce the risk. Monogamous means you and your partner do not have sex with any other people.

- You can greatly lower your risk of catching an STD by using a condom every time you have sex. Condoms are available for both men and women, but are most commonly worn by the man. A condom must be used properly every time.

Alternative Names

Cervical inflammation; Inflammation—cervix

References

Eckert LO, Lentz GM. Infections of the lower genital tract: Vulva, vagina, cervix, toxic shock syndrome, HIV infections. In: Katz VL, Lentz GM, Lobo RA, Gershenson DM, eds. *Comprehensive Gynecology*. 5th ed. Philadelphia, Pa: Mosby Elsevier; 2007:chap 2.

Zeimet A, McBride DR, Basilan R, Roland WE, McCrary D, Hoonmo K. Infectious diseases. In: Rakel RE, ed. *Textbook of Family Medicine*. 8th ed. Philadelphia, Pa: Saunders Elsevier; 2011:chap 16.

Centers for Disease Control and Prevention. Sexually Transmitted Diseases Treatment Guidelines, 2010. *MMWR* 2010;59(No. RR-12).

Chapter 27

Epididymitis

Epididymitis is swelling (inflammation) of the epididymis, the tube that connects the testicle with the vas deferens.

Causes

Epididymitis is most common in young men ages 19–35. It is a major cause of hospital admissions in the military.

Epididymitis is usually caused by the spread of a bacterial infection from the urethra or the bladder. The most common infections that cause this condition in young heterosexual men are gonorrhea and chlamydia. In children and older men, *E. coli* and similar infections are much more common. This is also true in homosexual men.

Mycobacterium tuberculosis (TB) can occur as epididymitis. Other bacteria (such as *Ureaplasma*) may also cause the condition.

Another cause of epididymitis is the use of a medication called amiodarone, which prevents abnormal heart rhythms.

The following increase the risk for epididymitis:

- Being uncircumcised

- Recent surgery or a history of structural problems in the urinary tract

- Regular use of a urethral catheter

- Sexual intercourse with more than one partner and not using condoms

Symptoms

Epididymitis may begin with a low-grade fever, chills, and a heavy sensation in the testicle area. The area becomes more and more sensitive to pressure.

Other symptoms include:

- blood in the semen;
- discharge from the urethra (the opening at the end of the penis);
- discomfort in the lower abdomen or pelvis;
- fever;
- groin pain;
- lump in the testicle;
- pain during ejaculation;
- pain or burning during urination;
- painful scrotal swelling (epididymis is enlarged);
- tender, swollen groin area on affected side;
- testicle pain that gets worse during a bowel movement.

Exams and Tests

Physical examination shows a red, tender, and sometimes swollen lump (mass) on the affected side of the scrotum. Tenderness is usually in a small area of the testicle where the epididymis is attached.

There may be enlarged lymph nodes in the groin area (inguinal nodes), and a discharge from the penis. A rectal examination may show an enlarged or tender prostate.

These tests may be performed:

- Complete blood count (CBC)
- Doppler ultrasound
- Testicular scan (nuclear medicine scan)
- Urinalysis and culture (you may need to give several specimens, including initial stream, mid-stream, and after a prostate massage)
- Tests for chlamydia and gonorrhea

It is important to distinguish this condition from testicular torsion. Testicular torsion is an emergency and should be treated with surgery as soon as possible.

Treatment

Your health care provider will prescribe medications to treat the infection. Sexually transmitted infections require specific antibiotics. Your sexual partners should also be treated. You may need pain medications and anti-inflammatory medications.

The treatment for epididymitis caused by the medication amiodarone is a lower dose or change in the medication.

Bed rest, while elevating the scrotum and applying ice packs to the area, is recommended. It is very important to have a follow-up visit with your health care provider to find out whether the infection has gone away completely.

Outlook (Prognosis)

Epididymitis usually gets better with antibiotic treatment. There usually is no reduction in sexual or reproductive abilities. However, the condition may return.

If not treated, or in some other cases, the condition can become long-term (chronic). In chronic cases, there is usually no swelling, but there is pain.

Possible Complications

Complications include:

- abscess in the scrotum;
- chronic epididymitis;
- fistula on the skin of the scrotum (cutaneous scrotal fistula);
- death of testicular tissue due to lack of blood (testicular infarction);
- infertility.

Acute pain in the scrotum is a medical emergency. It needs to be checked out by a health care provider immediately.

When to Contact a Medical Professional

Call your health care provider if you develop symptoms of epididymitis. Go to the emergency room or call the local emergency number (such as 911) if you have severe testicle pain suddenly or after an injury.

Prevention

You can prevent complications from epididymitis by getting diagnosed early, and by treating any infections.

Your doctor may prescribe antibiotics before a surgery that increases the risk for epididymitis. Practicing safe sex (having intercourse with only one partner at a time, using condoms) may help prevent epididymitis caused by sexually transmitted diseases.

Chapter 28

Infertility Linked to STD Infection

What is infertility?

Infertility means not being able to get pregnant after one year of trying (or six months if a woman is 35 or older). Women who can get pregnant but are unable to stay pregnant may also be infertile.

Pregnancy is the result of a process that has many steps. To get pregnant, the following must occur:

- A woman's body must release an egg from one of her ovaries (ovulation).

- The egg must go through a fallopian tube toward the uterus (womb).

- A man's sperm must join with (fertilize) the egg along the way.

- The fertilized egg must attach to the inside of the uterus (implantation).

Infertility can happen if there are problems with any of these steps.

Is infertility a common problem?

Yes. About 10 percent of women (6.1 million) in the United States ages 15–44 have difficulty getting pregnant or staying pregnant, according to the Centers for Disease Control and Prevention (CDC).

Excerpted from "Infertility Fact Sheet," by the Office on Women's Health (www.womenshealth.gov), part of the U.S. Department of Health and Human Services, July 2009.

Is infertility just a woman's problem?

No, infertility is not always a woman's problem. Both women and men can have problems that cause infertility. About one-third of infertility cases are caused by women's problems. Another one third of fertility problems are due to the man. The other cases are caused by a mixture of male and female problems or by unknown problems.

What causes infertility in women?

Most cases of female infertility are caused by problems with ovulation. Without ovulation, there are no eggs to be fertilized. Some signs that a woman is not ovulating normally include irregular or absent menstrual periods.

Ovulation problems are often caused by polycystic ovarian syndrome (PCOS). PCOS is a hormone imbalance problem that can interfere with normal ovulation. PCOS is the most common cause of female infertility. Primary ovarian insufficiency (POI) is another cause of ovulation problems. POI occurs when a woman's ovaries stop working normally before she is 40. POI is not the same as early menopause.

Less common causes of fertility problems in women include the following:

- Blocked fallopian tubes due to pelvic inflammatory disease, endometriosis, or surgery for an ectopic pregnancy

- Physical problems with the uterus

- Uterine fibroids, which are non-cancerous clumps of tissue and muscle on the walls of the uterus

What things increase a woman's risk of infertility?

Many things can change a woman's ability to have a baby. These include the following:

- Age
- Smoking
- Excess alcohol use
- Stress
- Poor diet
- Athletic training
- Being overweight or underweight

- Sexually transmitted diseases (STDs)

- Health problems that cause hormonal changes, such as polycystic ovarian syndrome and primary ovarian insufficiency

How do doctors treat infertility?

Infertility can be treated with medicine, surgery, artificial insemination, or assisted reproductive technology. Many times these treatments are combined. In most cases infertility is treated with drugs or surgery.

Doctors recommend specific treatments for infertility based on the following:

- Test results

- How long the couple has been trying to get pregnant

- The age of both the man and woman

- The overall health of the partners

- Preference of the partners

Doctors often treat infertility in men in the following ways:

- Sexual problems: Doctors can help men deal with impotence or premature ejaculation. Behavioral therapy and/or medicines can be used in these cases.

- Too few sperm: Sometimes surgery can correct the cause of the problem. In other cases, doctors surgically remove sperm directly from the male reproductive tract. Antibiotics can also be used to clear up infections affecting sperm count.

- Sperm movement: Sometimes semen has no sperm because of a block in the man's system. In some cases, surgery can correct the problem.

In women, some physical problems can also be corrected with surgery.

A number of fertility medicines are used to treat women with ovulation problems. It is important to talk with your doctor about the pros and cons of these medicines. You should understand the possible dangers, benefits, and side effects.

Chapter 29

Neurosyphilis

Neurosyphilis is a disease of the coverings of the brain, the brain itself, or the spinal cord. It can occur in people with syphilis, especially if they are left untreated. Neurosyphilis is different from syphilis because it affects the nervous system, whereas syphilis is a sexually transmitted disease with different signs and symptoms. There are five types of neurosyphilis:

- Asymptomatic neurosyphilis
- Meningeal neurosyphilis
- Meningovascular neurosyphilis
- General paresis
- Tabes dorsalis

Asymptomatic neurosyphilis means that neurosyphilis is present, but the individual reports no symptoms and does not feel sick. Meningeal syphilis can occur between the first few weeks to the first few years of getting syphilis. Individuals with meningeal syphilis can have headache, stiff neck, nausea, and vomiting. Sometimes there can also be loss of vision or hearing. Meningovascular syphilis causes the same symptoms as meningeal syphilis but affected individuals also

"Neurosyphilis," by the National Institute of Neurological Disorders and Stroke (NINDS, www.ninds.nih.gov), part of the National Institutes of Health, October 29, 2009.

have strokes. This form of neurosyphilis can occur within the first few months to several years after infection. General paresis can occur between 3–30 years after getting syphilis. People with general paresis can have personality or mood changes. Tabes dorsalis is characterized by pains in the limbs or abdomen, failure of muscle coordination, and bladder disturbances. Other signs include vision loss, loss of reflexes and loss of sense of vibration, poor gait, and impaired balance. Tabes dorsalis can occur anywhere from 5–50 years after initial syphilis infection. General paresis and tabes dorsalis are now less common than the other forms of neurosyphilis because of advances made in prevention, screening, and treatment. People with HIV/AIDS (human immunodeficiency virus/acquired immunodeficiency syndrome) are at higher risk of having neurosyphilis.

Treatment

Penicillin, an antibiotic, is used to treat syphilis. Individuals with neurosyphilis can be treated with penicillin given by vein, or by daily intramuscular injections for 10–14 days. If they are treated with daily penicillin injections, individuals must also take probenecid by mouth four times a day. Some medical professionals recommend another antibiotic called ceftriaxone for neurosyphilis treatment. This drug is usually given daily by vein, but it can also be given by intramuscular injection. Individuals who receive ceftriaxone are also treated for 10–14 days. People with HIV/AIDS who get treated for neurosyphilis may have different outcomes than individuals without HIV/AIDS.

Prognosis

Prognosis can change based on the type of neurosyphilis and how early in the course of the disease people with neurosyphilis get diagnosed and treated. Individuals with asymptomatic neurosyphilis or meningeal neurosyphilis usually return to normal health. People with meningovascular syphilis, general paresis, or tabes dorsalis usually do not return to normal health, although they may get much better. Individuals who receive treatment many years after they have been infected have a worse prognosis. Treatment outcome is different for every person.

Research

The National Institute of Neurological Disorders and Stroke supports and conducts research on neurodegenerative disorders, such as neurosyphilis, in an effort to find ways to prevent, treat, and ultimately cure these disorders.

NIH Patient Recruitment for Neurosyphilis Clinical Trials

- At NIH Clinical Center [http://patientinfo.ninds.nih.gov]

- Throughout the U.S. and Worldwide [http://clinicaltrials.gov/search/term=Neurosyphilis]

- NINDS Clinical Trials [http://www.ninds.nih.gov/disorders/clinical_trials/index_all.htm#Neurosyphilis]

Organizations That Provide Information about Syphilis

Centers for Disease Control and Prevention
1600 Clifton Road
Atlanta, GA 30333
Toll-Free: 800-CDC-INFO (800-232-4636)
Toll-Free TTY: 888-232-6348
Phone: 404-639-3311
Websites: www.cdc.gov
E-mail: cdcinfo@cdc.gov

National Institute of Allergy and Infectious Diseases
6610 Rockledge Drive, MSC 6612
Bethesda, MD 20892-6612
Toll-Free: 866-284-4107
Toll-Free TDD: 800-877-8339
Phone: 301-496-5717
Fax: 301-402-3573
Website: www.niaid.nih.gov
E-mail: ocpostoffice@niaid.nih.gov

National Institute of Neurological Disorders and Stroke
PO Box 5801
Bethesda, MD 20824
Toll-Free: 800-352-9424
Phone: 301-496-5751
TTY: 301-468-5981
Website: www.ninds.nih.gov

Chapter 30

Pelvic Inflammatory Disease

What is pelvic inflammatory disease (PID)?

Pelvic inflammatory disease (PID) is an infection of a woman's pelvic organs. The pelvic organs include the uterus (womb), fallopian tubes, ovaries, and cervix.

What causes PID?

A woman can get PID if bacteria (germs) move up from her vagina and infect her pelvic organs. Many different types of bacteria can cause PID. But most cases of PID are caused by bacteria that cause two common sexually transmitted diseases (STDs)—gonorrhea and chlamydia. It can take from a few days to a few months for an infection to travel up from the vagina to the pelvic organs.

You can get PID without having an STD. Normal bacteria found in the vagina and on the cervix can sometimes cause PID. No one is sure why this happens.

How common is PID?

Each year in the United States, more than 1 million women have an episode of PID. More than 100,000 women become infertile each

"Pelvic Inflammatory Disease Fact Sheet," by the Office on Women's Health (www.womenshealth.gov), part of the U.S. Department of Health and Human Services, May 18, 2010.

year because of PID. Also, many ectopic pregnancies that occur are due to problems from PID.

Are some women more likely to get PID?

Yes. You're more likely to get PID if the following are true:

- You have had an STD.

- You are under 25 years of age and are having sex.

- You have more than one sex partner.

- You douche. Douching can push bacteria into the pelvic organs and cause infection. It can also hide the signs of an infection.

- You have an intrauterine device (IUD). You should get tested and treated for any infections before getting an IUD. This will lower your risk of getting PID.

How do I know if I have PID?

Many women don't know they have PID because they don't have any symptoms. For women who have them, symptoms can range from mild to severe. The most common symptom of PID is pain in your lower abdomen (stomach area). Other symptoms include the following:

- Fever (100.4 degrees Fahrenheit or higher)

- Vaginal discharge that may smell foul

- Painful sex

- Painful urination

- Irregular periods (monthly bleeding)

- Pain in the upper right abdomen

PID can come on fast with extreme pain and fever, especially if it's caused by gonorrhea.

Are there any tests for PID?

If you think that you may have PID, see a doctor right away. If you have pain in your lower abdomen (stomach area), your doctor will perform a physical exam. This will include a pelvic (internal) exam. Your doctor will check for the following:

- Abnormal discharge from your vagina or cervix

- Lumps called abscesses near your ovaries and tubes

- Tenderness or pain in your pelvic organs

Your doctor will also test you for STDs, including HIV [human immunodeficiency virus] and syphilis, urinary tract infection, and if needed, pregnancy. If needed, your doctor may do other tests, such as the following.

- Ultrasound is a test that uses sound waves to take pictures of the pelvic area.

- Endometrial (uterine) biopsy is when the doctor removes and tests a small piece of the endometrium (the inside lining of the womb).

- Laparoscopy is when the doctor inserts a small, lighted tube through your abdomen (stomach area) to look at your pelvic organs.

These tests will help your doctor find out if you have PID, or if you have a different problem that looks like PID.

How is PID treated?

PID can be cured with antibiotics (drugs that kill bacteria). Most of the time, at least two antibiotics are used that work against a wide range of bacteria. Your doctor will work with you to find the best treatment for you. You must take all your medicine, even if your symptoms go away. This helps to make sure your infection is fully cured. You should see your doctor again two to three days after starting treatment to make sure the antibiotics are working.

Without treatment, PID can lead to severe problems like infertility, ectopic pregnancy, and chronic pelvic pain.

Any damage done to your pelvic organs before you start treatment likely cannot be undone. Still, don't put off getting treatment. If you do, you may not be able to have children. If you think you may have PID, see a doctor right away.

Your doctor may suggest going into the hospital to treat your PID if the following are true:

- You are very sick.

- You are pregnant.

- You don't respond to or cannot swallow pills. If this is the case, you will need intravenous (in the vein or IV) antibiotics.

- You have an abscess (sore) in a tube or ovary.

If you still have symptoms or if the abscess doesn't go away after treatment, you may need surgery. Problems caused by PID, such as constant pelvic pain and scarring, are often hard to treat. But, sometimes they get better after surgery.

What if my partner is infected?

Even if your sex partner doesn't have any symptoms, she or he could still be infected with bacteria that can cause PID. Take steps to protect yourself from being infected again.

- Encourage your sex partner(s) to get treated, even if she or he doesn't have symptoms.

- Don't have sex with a partner who hasn't been treated.

My friend was told she can't get pregnant because she has PID. Is this true?

The more times you have PID, the more likely it is that you won't be able to get pregnant. When you have PID, bacteria infect the tubes or cause inflammation of the tubes. This turns normal tissue into scar tissue. Scar tissue can block your tubes and make it harder to get pregnant. Even having just a little scar tissue can keep you from getting pregnant without infertility treatment.

How can I keep myself from getting PID?

PID is most often caused by an STD that hasn't been treated. You can keep from getting PID by not getting an STD.

- The best way to prevent an STD is to not have sex of any kind.

- Have sex with one partner who doesn't have any STDs.

- Use condoms every time you have vaginal, anal, or oral sex. Read and follow the directions on the package. Condoms, when used the right way, can lower your chances of getting an STD.

- Don't douche. Douching removes some of the normal bacteria in the vagina that protect you from infection. This makes it easier for you to get an STD.

- If you're having sex, ask your doctor to test you for STDs. STDs are easier to treat if they are found early.

- Learn the common symptoms of STDs. If you think you might have an STD, see your doctor right away.

What should I do if I think I have an STD?

If you think you may have an STD, see a doctor right away. You may feel scared or shy about asking for information or help. Keep in mind, the sooner you seek treatment, the less likely the STD will cause you severe harm. And the sooner you tell your sex partner(s) that you have an STD, the less likely they are to infect you again or spread the disease to others.

To learn about STDs or get tested, contact your doctor, local health department, or an STD and family planning clinic. The American Social Health Association (ASHA) keeps lists of clinics and doctors who provide treatment for STDs.

Chapter 31

Pregnancy Complications and STDs

Can pregnant women become infected with STDs?

Yes, women who are pregnant can become infected with the same sexually transmitted diseases (STDs) as women who are not pregnant. Pregnancy does not provide women or their babies any protection against STDs. The consequences of an STD can be significantly more serious, even life threatening, for a woman and her baby if the woman becomes infected with an STD while pregnant. It is important that women be aware of the harmful effects of STDs and know how to protect themselves and their children against infection.

How common are STDs in pregnant women in the United States?

Some STDs, such as genital herpes and bacterial vaginosis, are quite common in pregnant women in the United States. Other STDs, notably HIV [human immunodeficiency virus] and syphilis, are much less common in pregnant women. Table 31.1 shows the estimated number of pregnant women in the United States who are infected with specific STDs each year.

"STD and Pregnancy," by the Centers for Disease Control and Prevention (CDC, www.cdc.gov), March 25, 2011.

Table 31.1. Pregnant Women in the United States Infected with Specific STDs

STDs	Estimated Number of Pregnant Women
Bacterial vaginosis	1,080,000
Herpes simplex virus 2	880,000
Chlamydia	100,000
Trichomoniasis	124,000
Gonorrhea	13,200
Hepatitis B	16,000
HIV	6,400
Syphilis	<1,000

How do STDs affect a pregnant woman and her baby?

STDs can have many of the same consequences for pregnant women as women who are not pregnant. STDs can cause cervical and other cancers, chronic hepatitis, pelvic inflammatory disease, infertility, and other complications. Many STDs in women are silent; that is, without signs or symptoms.

STDs can be passed from a pregnant woman to the baby before, during, or after the baby's birth. Some STDs (like syphilis) cross the placenta and infect the baby while it is in the uterus (womb). Other STDs (like gonorrhea, chlamydia, hepatitis B, and genital herpes) can be transmitted from the mother to the baby during delivery as the baby passes through the birth canal. HIV can cross the placenta during pregnancy, infect the baby during the birth process, and unlike most other STDs, can infect the baby through breastfeeding.

A pregnant woman with an STD may also have early onset of labor, premature rupture of the membranes surrounding the baby in the uterus, and uterine infection after delivery.

The harmful effects of STDs in babies may include stillbirth (a baby that is born dead), low birth weight (less than five pounds), conjunctivitis (eye infection), pneumonia, neonatal sepsis (infection in the baby's bloodstream), neurologic damage, blindness, deafness, acute hepatitis, meningitis, chronic liver disease, and cirrhosis. Most of these problems can be prevented if the mother receives routine prenatal care, which includes screening tests for STDs starting early in pregnancy and repeated close to delivery, if necessary. Other problems can be treated if the infection is found at birth.

Should pregnant women be tested for STDs?

Yes, STDs affect women of every socioeconomic and educational level, age, race, ethnicity, and religion. The CDC 2010 Sexually Transmitted Diseases Treatment Guidelines recommend that pregnant women be screened on their first prenatal visit for STDs, which may include the following:

- Chlamydia

- Gonorrhea

- Hepatitis B

- HIV

- Syphilis

Pregnant women should ask their doctors about getting tested for these STDs, since some doctors do not routinely perform these tests. New and increasingly accurate tests continue to become available. Even if a woman has been tested in the past, she should be tested again when she becomes pregnant.

Can STDs be treated during pregnancy?

Chlamydia, gonorrhea, syphilis, trichomoniasis, and bacterial vaginosis (BV) can be treated and cured with antibiotics during pregnancy. There is no cure for viral STDs, such as genital herpes and HIV, but antiviral medication may be appropriate for pregnant women with herpes and definitely is for those with HIV. For women who have active genital herpes lesions at the time of delivery, a cesarean delivery (C-section) may be performed to protect the newborn against infection. C-section is also an option for some HIV-infected women. Women who test negative for hepatitis B may receive the hepatitis B vaccine during pregnancy.

How can pregnant women protect themselves against infection?

The surest way to avoid transmission of sexually transmitted diseases is to abstain from sexual contact, or to be in a long-term mutually monogamous relationship with a partner who has been tested and is known to be uninfected.

Latex condoms, when used consistently and correctly, are highly effective in preventing transmission of HIV, the virus that causes AIDS [acquired immunodeficiency virus]. Latex condoms, when used consistently and correctly, can reduce the risk of transmission of gonorrhea, chlamydia, and trichomoniasis. Correct and consistent use of latex condoms can reduce the risk of genital herpes, syphilis, and chancroid only when the infected area or site of potential exposure is protected by the condom. Correct and consistent use of latex condoms may reduce the risk for genital human papillomavirus (HPV) and associated diseases (e.g., warts and cervical cancer).

Chapter 32

Vaginitis

Vaginitis is described medically as irritation and/or inflammation of the vagina. Vaginitis is a very common disease affecting millions of women each year. The three most common vaginal infections are bacterial vaginosis (BV), candida vaginitis (yeast infection), and trichomonas vaginitis ("trich").

What are the signs or symptoms of vaginitis?

Vaginal infections can produce a variety of symptoms, such as abnormal or increased discharge, itching, fishy odor, irritation, painful urination or vaginal bleeding. When you have vaginitis, you may have some or all of these symptoms. If you have any of these symptoms, discuss them with you doctor or nurse so that you can be tested.

What causes vaginitis and how common is it?

Vaginitis has various causes. It may result from bacterial infections, fungal infection, protozoan infection, contact dermatitis, or even an allergic reaction. Vaginitis affects millions of women and is one of the primary reasons women visit their doctor. Trichomonas is sexually transmitted, but other vaginitis infections are not usually sexually transmitted.

"Vaginitis," reprinted with permission from the Illinois Department of Public Health (http://www.idph.state.il.us). © 2012 State of Illinois.

What is the difference between the three types of vaginitis?

- **Bacterial:** This type of infection is caused when healthy vaginal organisms are replaced by bacteria. It is referred to as bacterial vaginosis and is the most common type of vaginitis.

- **Yeast:** This type of infection is called candidiasis. It is caused by a fungus and is the second most common type of vaginitis.

- **Protozoan:** This type of infection is called trichomoniasis and it is considered a sexually transmitted disease (STD). It is the least common and comprises 3% to 5% of all vaginitis infections.

What causes bacterial vaginosis?

Bacterial vaginosis is when the natural balance of organisms in the vagina is changed. The healthy vagina normally contains a variety of bacteria. One type of "good" bacteria, *Lactobacillus*, is particularly important. *Lactobacillus* keeps the vagina slightly acidic to reduce the growth of potentially harmful organisms. When *Lactobacilli* are replaced with different kinds of "bad" bacteria called anaerobic bacteria, an unpleasant vaginal odor develops and an infection (vaginitis) occurs.

Are there any complications associated with vaginitis?

Yes, there may be, especially from bacterial vaginosis. If left untreated, BV may result in increased risk of pelvic inflammatory disease (PID), infertility, pre-term birth, premature rupture of membranes, low birth weight, intra-amniotic infections, endometritis, cervical intra-epithelial neoplasia (CIN), post-gynecological surgery infections, and increased risk of sexually transmitted diseases.

Will my Pap smear diagnose a vaginal infection?

Although your annual Pap smear is a very important test, it is not typically used as a test for vaginitis.

How can my doctor tell if I have an infection?

The tests for vaginitis are simple and can be done right in your doctor's office. Your doctor will examine your vagina and use a swab to get a sample of the discharge. Vaginitis is identified by checking vaginal fluid appearance, vaginal pH, the presence of volatile amines (the odor causing gas), and the microscopic detection of clue cells. New tests are now available to aid the physician in his or her diagnosis.

How do I address the subject with my healthcare provider?

First, do not be embarrassed. Vaginal infections occur in millions of women of all ages and backgrounds. Regular check-ups and open discussions regarding your symptoms will go a long way toward maintaining good vaginal health. Your healthcare provider can perform simple tests to determine the type of vaginal infection and provide you with the best treatment.

How is vaginitis treated?

There are several ways to treat vaginitis, depending upon the cause of the infection: Bacterial vaginosis can be treated orally or intra-vaginally with a prescription for medication; a yeast infection can be treated orally or intra-vaginally with either prescription or over-the-counter antifungal medications; and a trichomonas infection is usually treated with a prescribed oral antibiotic.

What can I do to prevent initial infections or recurrences?

In order to minimize the risk of developing vaginitis, here are some general suggestions for good vaginal health:

- Practice good hygiene by keeping the vaginal area clean using a mild soap and dry area well.
- Avoid douching and irritating agents such as harsh soaps and feminine hygiene sprays. Douches can disrupt the normal balance of vaginal organisms and should be avoided.
- Avoid spreading bacteria from the rectum to the vagina by wiping front to back after going to the bathroom.
- Avoid tight jeans, panty hose without a cotton crotch, and other clothing that can trap moisture.
- Practice abstinence or safe sex and avoid multiple partners. Latex condoms, when used consistently and correctly, can reduce the risk of transmission of STDs.
- Studies have shown that stress can also be a contributing factor.

Can vaginitis affect my baby?

Yes it can. Premature delivery and low birth weight of the baby are more common in women with bacterial vaginosis. Early diagnosis and treatment is important.

Does my partner need to be tested?

Ask your healthcare provider. Some types of vaginitis can be transmitted from one person to another during sexual intercourse. It depends upon what type of vaginitis you have.

Can I also be infected with something else?

Yes. You can be infected with a sexually transmitted disease and also have vaginitis. Each infection needs to be treated with different medications so it is important to visit your doctor to determine if you have more than one type of infection.

For answers to other questions, please speak with your doctor or nurse.

Part Four

STD Testing and Treatment Concerns

Chapter 33

Frequently Asked Questions about STD and HIV Testing

Who should be tested for STDs?

In the past, the Centers for Disease Control (CDC) recommended HIV testing for people felt to be at high risk for HIV. In 2006, the CDC revised their recommendations to the following:

- All patients aged 13–64 years should be screened.

- All pregnant women should be screened.

- Persons at high risk for HIV should be screened at least annually.

- All patients initiating treatment for tuberculosis should be screened.

- All patients seeking treatment for STDs should be screened.

The CDC recommends that patients be informed that they will be tested unless they decline screening (opt out). They recommend that no one should be tested against their will or without their knowledge.

Excerpted from "Frequently Asked Questions," by the National Prevention Information Network (NPIN, www.cdcnpin.org), a service of the Centers for Disease Control and Prevention (CDC). This document is undated. Reviewed and revised by David A. Cooke, MD, FACP, July 10, 2012.

How long after a possible exposure should I wait to get tested for HIV?

Most HIV tests are antibody tests that measure the antibodies your body makes against HIV. It can take some time for the immune system to produce enough antibodies for the antibody test to detect and this time period can vary from person to person. This time period is commonly referred to as the "window period." Most people will develop detectable antibodies within two to eight weeks (the average is 25 days). Even so, there is a chance that some individuals will take longer to develop detectable antibodies. Therefore, if the initial negative HIV test was conducted within the first three months after possible exposure, repeat testing should be considered more than three months after the exposure occurred to account for the possibility of a false-negative result. Ninety seven percent will develop antibodies in the first three months following the time of their infection. In very rare cases, it can take up to six months to develop antibodies to HIV.

Another type of test is an RNA [ribonucleic acid] test, which detects the HIV virus directly. The time between HIV infection and RNA detection is 9–11 days. These tests, which are more costly and used less often than antibody tests, are used in some parts of the United States.

For information on HIV testing, you can talk to your health care provider or you can find the location of the HIV testing site nearest to you by calling CDC-INFO 24 Hours/Day at 800-CDC-INFO (800-232-4636) or 888-232-6348 (TTY). Both of these resources are confidential.

How do HIV tests work?

Once HIV enters the body, the immune system starts to produce antibodies—(chemicals that are part of the immune system that recognize invaders like bacteria and viruses and mobilize the body's attempt to fight infection). In the case of HIV, these antibodies cannot fight off the infection, but their presence is used to tell whether a person has HIV in his or her body. In other words, most HIV tests look for the HIV antibodies rather than looking for HIV itself. There are tests that look for HIV's genetic material directly, but these are not in widespread use.

The most common HIV tests use blood to detect HIV infection. Tests using saliva or urine are also available. Some tests take a few days for results, but rapid HIV tests can give results in about 20 minutes. All positive HIV tests must be followed up by another test to confirm the positive result. Results of this confirmatory test can take a few days to a few weeks.

What are the different HIV screening tests available in the United States?

In most cases the EIA (enzyme immunoassay), used on blood drawn from a vein, is the most common screening test used to look for antibodies to HIV. A positive (reactive) EIA must be used with a follow-up (confirmatory) test such as the Western blot to make a positive diagnosis. There are EIA tests that use other body fluids to look for antibodies to HIV. These include the following:

- **Oral fluid tests:** These tests use oral fluid (not saliva) that is collected from the mouth using a special collection device. This is an EIA antibody test similar to the standard blood EIA test. A follow-up confirmatory Western Blot uses the same oral fluid sample.

- **Urine tests:** These tests use urine instead of blood. The sensitivity and specificity (accuracy) are somewhat less than that of the blood and oral fluid tests. This is also an EIA antibody test similar to blood EIA tests and requires a follow-up confirmatory Western Blot using the same urine sample.

- **Rapid tests:** A rapid test is a screening test that produces very quick results, in approximately 20 minutes. Rapid tests use blood from a vein or from a finger stick, or oral fluid to look for the presence of antibodies to HIV. As is true for all screening tests, a reactive rapid HIV test result must be confirmed with a follow-up confirmatory test before a final diagnosis of infection can be made. These tests have similar accuracy rates as traditional EIA screening tests.

- **Home testing kits:** Consumer-controlled test kits (popularly known as "home testing kits") were first licensed in 1997. Although home HIV tests are sometimes advertised through the Internet, only the Home Access HIV-1 Test System and the OraQuick Advance HIV Test are approved by the Food and Drug Administration. (The accuracy of other home test kits cannot be verified).

  - The Home Access HIV-1 Test System can be found at most local drug stores. It is not a true home test, but a home collection kit. The testing procedure involves pricking a finger with a special device, placing drops of blood on a specially treated card, and then mailing the card in to be tested at a licensed laboratory. Customers are given an identification number to use when phoning in for the results. Callers

361

may speak to a counselor before taking the test, while waiting for the test result, and when the results are given. All individuals receiving a positive test result are provided referrals for a follow-up confirmatory test, as well as information and resources on treatment and support services.

- The OraQuick Advance HIV home test was approved by the Food and Drug Administration in July 2012 and is expected to be available by October 2012. It resembles and is read similarly to a home pregnancy test, but uses an oral swab instead of a urine sample. The test provides results in 20–40 minutes.

- **RNA tests:** RNA tests look for genetic material of the virus and can be used in screening the blood supply and for detection of very early infection in rare cases when antibody tests are unable to detect antibodies to HIV.

If I test HIV negative, does that mean that my sex partner is HIV negative also?

No. Your HIV test result reveals only your HIV status. Your negative test result does not indicate whether your partner has HIV. HIV is not necessarily transmitted every time you have sex. Therefore, taking an HIV test should not be seen as a method to find out if your partner is infected.

Ask your partner if he or she has been tested for HIV and what risk behaviors he or she has engaged in, both currently and in the past. Think about getting tested together.

It is important to take steps to reduce your risk of getting HIV. Not having (abstaining from) sex is the most effective way to avoid HIV. If you choose to be sexually active, having sex with one person who only has sex with you and who is uninfected is also effective. If you are not sure that both you and your partner are HIV negative, use a latex condom to help protect both you and your partner from HIV and other STDs. Studies have shown that latex condoms are very effective, though not 100%, in preventing HIV transmission when used correctly and consistently. If either partner is allergic to latex, plastic (polyurethane) condoms for either the male or female can be used.

What if I test positive for HIV?

If you test positive for HIV, the sooner you take steps to protect your health, the better. Early medical treatment and a healthy lifestyle can help you stay well. Prompt medical care may delay the onset of AIDS [acquired immunodeficiency syndrome] and prevent some life-threatening conditions. There are a number of important steps you can take immediately to protect your health:

- See a licensed health care provider, even if you do not feel sick. Try to find a health care provider who has experience treating HIV. There are now many medications to treat HIV infection and help you maintain your health. It is never too early to start thinking about treatment possibilities.

- Have a TB (tuberculosis) test. You may be infected with TB and not know it. Undetected TB can cause serious illness, but it can be successfully treated if caught early.

- Smoking cigarettes, drinking too much alcohol, or using illegal drugs (such as methamphetamines) can weaken your immune system. There are programs available that can help you stop or reduce your use of these substances.

- Get screened for other sexually transmitted diseases. Undetected STDs can cause serious health problems. It is also important to practice safe-sex behaviors so you can avoid getting STDs.

There is much you can do to stay healthy. Learn all that you can about maintaining good health.

Not having (abstaining from) sex is the most effective way to avoid transmitting HIV to others. If you choose to have sex, use a latex condom to help protect your partner from HIV and other STDs. Studies have shown that latex condoms are very effective, though not 100%, in preventing HIV transmission when used correctly and consistently. If either partner is allergic to latex, plastic (polyurethane) condoms for either the male or female can be used.

Why does CDC recommend HIV screening for all pregnant women?

HIV testing during pregnancy is important because antiviral therapy can improve the mother's health and greatly lower the chance that an HIV-infected pregnant woman will pass HIV to her infant before, during, or after birth. The treatment is most effective for babies when started as early as possible during pregnancy. However, there are still great health benefits to beginning treatment even during labor or shortly after the baby is born.

CDC recommends HIV screening for all pregnant women because risk-based testing (when the health care provider offers an HIV test based on the provider's assessment of the pregnant woman's risk) misses many women who are infected with HIV. CDC does recommend providing information on HIV and, for women with risk factors, referrals to prevention counseling.

HIV testing provides an opportunity for infected women to find out that they are infected and to gain access to medical treatment that may help improve their own health. It also allows them to make informed choices that can prevent transmission to their infant. For some uninfected women with risks for HIV, the prenatal care period could be an ideal opportunity for HIV prevention and subsequent behavior change to reduce risk for acquiring HIV infection.

Chapter 34

Talking to Your Health Care Professional about STDs

Chapter Contents

Section 34.1—Talking about Your Health 366

Section 34.2—Questions to Ask Your Health Care
            Professional about STDs..................................... 370

Section 34.3—For Teens: How Do I Discuss Embarrassing
            Things with My Doctor?..................................... 372

Section 34.1

Talking about Your Health

"Questions Are the Answer," by the Agency for Healthcare Research and Quality (www.ahrq.gov). The date of this document is unknown. Reviewed by David A. Cooke, MD, FACP, July 10, 2012.

Your health depends on good communication. Asking questions and providing information to your doctor and other care providers can improve your care. Talking with your doctor builds trust and leads to better results, quality, safety, and satisfaction.

Quality health care is a team effort. You play an important role. One of the best ways to communicate with your doctor and health care team is by asking questions. Because time is limited during medical appointments, you will feel less rushed if you prepare your questions before your appointment.

Your Doctor Wants Your Questions

Doctors know a lot about a lot of things, but they don't always know everything about you or what is best for you.

Your questions give your doctor and health care team important information about you, such as your most important health care concerns.

That is why they need you to speak up.

Ten Questions You Should Know

A simple question can help you feel better, let you take better care of yourself, or save your life. The questions below can get you started.

1. What is the test for?

2. How many times have you done this procedure?

3. When will I get the results?

4. Why do I need this treatment?

5. Are there any alternatives?

6. What are the possible complications?

7. Which hospital is best for my needs?

8. How do you spell the name of that drug?

9. Are there any side effects?

10. Will this medicine interact with medicines that I'm already taking?

Before Your Appointment

You can make sure you get the best possible care by being an active member of your health care team. Being involved means being prepared and asking questions.

Asking questions about your diagnoses, treatments, and medicines can improve the quality, safety, and effectiveness of your health care.

Taking steps before your medical appointments will help you to make the most of your time with your doctor and health care team.

Time is limited during doctor visits. Prepare for your appointment by thinking about what you want to do during your next visit.

- Do you want to talk about a health problem?

- Do you want to get or change a medicine?

- Do you want to get medical tests?

- Do you want to talk about surgery or treatment options?

Write down your questions or make a list of questions to bring to your appointment.

The answers can help you make better decisions, get good care, and feel better about your health care.

During Your Appointment

During your appointment, make sure to ask the questions you prepared before your appointment. Start by asking the ones that are most important to you.

To get the most from your visit, tell the nurse or person at the front desk that you have questions for your doctor. If your doctor does not ask you if you have questions, ask your doctor when the best time would be to ask them.

Asking questions is important but so is making sure you hear—and understand—the answers you get. Take notes. Or bring someone to your appointment to help you understand and remember what you heard. If you don't understand or are confused, ask your doctor to explain the answer again.

It is very important to understand the plan or next steps that your doctor recommends. Ask questions to make sure you understand what your doctor wants you to do.

The questions you may want to ask will depend on whether your doctor gives you a diagnosis; recommends a treatment, medical test, or surgery; or gives you a prescription for medicine.

Questions could include the following:

- What is my diagnosis?

- What are my treatment options? What are the benefits of each option? What are the side effects?

- Will I need a test? What is the test for? What will the results tell me?

- What will the medicine you are prescribing do? How do I take it? Are there any side effects?

- Why do I need surgery? Are there other ways to treat my condition? How often do you perform this surgery?

- Do I need to change my daily routine?

Find out what you are to do next. Ask for written instructions, brochures, videos, or websites that may help you learn more.

After Your Appointment

After you meet with your doctor, you will need to follow his or her instructions to keep your health on track.

Your doctor may have you fill a prescription or make another appointment for tests, lab work, or a follow-up visit. It is important for you to follow your doctor's instructions.

It also is important to call your doctor if you are unclear about any instructions or have more questions.

Create a list of follow-up questions if the following apply to you:

- You have a health problem.

- You need to get or change a medicine.

- You need a medical test.

- You need to have surgery.

There are other times when you should follow up on your care and call your doctor. Call your doctor if the following are true:

- If you experience any side effects or other problems with your medicines

- If your symptoms get worse after seeing the doctor

- If you receive any new prescriptions or start taking any over-the-counter medicines

- To get results of any tests you've had (Do not assume that no news is good news.)

- To ask about test results you do not understand

Your questions help your doctor and health care team learn more about you. Your doctor's answers to your questions can help you make better decisions, receive a higher level of care, avoid medical harm, and feel better about your health care. Your questions can also lead to better results for your health.

Section 34.2

Questions to Ask Your Health Care Professional about STDs

Excerpted from "Questions to Ask Your Health Care Professional," by the National Library of Medicine (NLM, www.nlm.nih.gov), part of the National Institutes of Health, September 2008.

More than 19 million men and women in this country are affected by sexually transmitted diseases (STDs) every year, according to the Centers for Disease Control and Prevention. Once called venereal diseases, STDs are among the most common infections in the United States today. The annual medical costs of STDs in the United States are estimated to be up to $14 billion.

Understanding the basic facts about STDs—the ways in which they are spread, their common symptoms, and how they can be treated—is the first step toward preventing them.

Symptoms

The symptoms vary among the different types of STDs. Some examples of common symptoms include the following:

- Unusual discharge from the penis or vagina
- Sores or warts on the genital area
- Burning while urinating
- Itching and redness in the genital area
- Anal itching, soreness, or bleeding

Diagnosis

Talk with your doctor or nurse about getting tested for STDs. She or he can tell you how to test for each STD.

An exam will include a thorough look at your genital area, oral cavity, and rectum. Swabs from open sores or discharges may be taken. Women will have a pelvic exam. You will also have urine and blood tests.

Many symptoms of STDs come and go. Just because your symptoms disappear, it does not mean you are cured without medical treatment.

Treatment

The treatment depends on the type of STD. For some STDs, treatment may involve taking drugs or getting a shot. For other STDs that can't be cured, like herpes, there is treatment to relieve the symptoms.

Prevention

The only way to ensure that you won't get infected is to not have sex. This means avoiding all types of intimate sexual contact.

If you are sexually active, you can reduce your risk of getting STDs by practicing "safe sex." This means using a condom for vaginal, oral, and anal intercourse—every time; knowing your partner and his/her STD status and health; and having regular medical check-ups, especially if you have more than one sexual partner.

Questions to Ask Your Health Care Professional

- How can I prevent getting an STD?

- If I already have an STD, what should I do so I don't spread the disease?

- What long-term health effects will there be with an STD?

Section 34.3

For Teens: How Do I Discuss Embarrassing Things with My Doctor?

"Talking to Your Doctor," July 2009, reprinted with permission from www.kidshealth.org. This information was provided by KidsHealth®, one of the largest resources online for medically reviewed health information written for parents, kids, and teens. For more articles like this, visit www.KidsHealth.org, or www.TeensHealth.org. Copyright © 1995–2012 The Nemours Foundation. All rights reserved.

Let's face it, life can get way more complex when you're a teen. On top of all of the emotional and physical changes you go through, there are more choices and decisions to make and more stresses from school, sports, jobs, family, and even friends.

So who can you talk to about your physical and emotional concerns? Sometimes friends or parents can be helpful, but you can always talk to your doctor, too.

Why Do I Need to Talk with My Doctor?

When you were a little kid, your parents took care of things like scheduling your doctors' appointments, getting your prescriptions, and making sure you took your medicine. If you had a pain or a worry, your parents were the ones to take care of it. But now that you're getting older, you may want—or be expected—to take on more responsibility for your health. It's all part of becoming an adult and taking charge.

As you get older, the issues you face can get more complicated and personal. Health issues that might have been simpler before now can include concerns about things such as sexual development, emotions, or weight problems. It's important to find someone to talk to who is both knowledgeable and someone you can trust.

Many teens are comfortable talking with their parents about almost any topic, at any time. But let's face it—not everyone is. Some teens— even though they have a fairly open relationship with their parents— just aren't comfortable talking about certain topics with their mother or father. What are they supposed to do?

Of course, they can always ask a friend—or go to the internet. Sometimes, those places can be a good start. But friends might not really know the answers you're looking for—and not every website is accurate or up-to-date.

That's where your doctor or nurse can help out.

Doctors and nurses are trained to help you with your health and emotional concerns. You can talk with them, they can ask you questions, and they can check out what worries you. That's their job.

Even if you feel embarrassed at first about raising personal subjects (like physical development or sexual health), it's helpful to know that doctors deal with those concerns—and all sorts of things—every day. And sometimes ignoring the risks of not talking to your doctor can outweigh the few moments of discomfort you may feel in raising sensitive health concerns.

Special Concerns for Teens

Maybe you're developing later or earlier than your friends and want to know what's going on. There might be times you feel more depressed or angry than you used to. New sexual feelings and behaviors can be confusing, too. Topics you never had to think about before, such as sexually transmitted diseases (STDs) and pregnancy, may suddenly be on your radar.

How Do I Discuss Embarrassing Things?

It's perfectly normal to feel nervous when talking with your doctor about things like sex, drugs, eating problems, weight concerns, depression, suicidal thoughts, and even body odor. You should be able to talk to your doctor about everything, but we all know that's easier said than done. Being examined and questioned about your body can also be intimidating, especially when the doctor needs to examine you in places you have always considered private, such as your genitals or breasts.

But there are things you can bear in mind to make it easier:

- Your doctor's seen it before. Most experienced doctors have cared for hundreds or even thousands of patients, so chances are they've heard, seen, and even smelled just about everything before. No matter how troubling something might be to you, it probably won't surprise your doctor.

- Your doctor is there to help, not judge or punish. If you've been going to the same doctor all your life, you may wonder if the doctor will be disappointed in you when you want to talk about sex or personal things that may be bothering you. That's what doctors do all the time, though. Your doctor is interested in keeping you healthy, not judging you for something you have or haven't done. For this reason, a person who is concerned about a sensitive topic, such as having an STD, shouldn't avoid going to the doctor because he or she is ashamed or worried about what the doctor might think. Not having things like STDs checked might only make a condition worse and may even result in a permanent health problem, such as infertility. A doctor's role is to listen respectfully, examine, educate, and treat people, not criticize them. If you think your doctor is judging or preaching to you, talk to your parents about finding someone with whom you're more comfortable.

• It's your job to talk openly about your symptoms and concerns. A doctor can't help you unless you tell the whole story. Even if you're uncomfortable, being open and honest will only benefit you. Most doctors realize that people can feel uncomfortable about raising sensitive issues, and they try to be good listeners. If you feel you can't put your concerns into words, try showing up for your appointment with a written list to give to the doctor. It can include your problems, symptoms, questions, and concerns. This approach can jump-start the communication process and help put you at ease. Many people find that once they've brought the subject up and gotten past those first nervous moments, they feel a lot more comfortable talking openly.

Do My Parents Have to Be Involved?

Lots of teens feel comfortable talking to their parents about all of their medical issues, but others prefer to keep certain aspects of their health private. Because parents usually need to stay involved in certain aspects of their child's medical care until that person reaches 18, it can help to find a "middle ground" that allows you to meet your privacy concerns and your parents' needs.

Here are some ideas on approaching your parents about taking charge of your medical care:

• Express your interest in taking an active role in your medical care. Start by talking with your parents about things you'd like to handle by yourself, like making appointments, calling your doctor with questions, and seeing the doctor alone for part of the time. Most doctors will allow a teen to go to an appointment alone if a parent calls and gives permission for treatment.

- Balance your needs with your parents' needs. Parents are not only interested in ensuring you get the best medical care available, they may need to stay involved in your health care for other reasons, like insurance. Most states require that doctors have a parent's permission before providing some types of medical tests and treatment (there are some things that you should be able to keep confidential from your folks if you want to, though—more on that later). Some doctors suggest that both you and a parent meet with the doctor together for the first part of the appointment. Parents can often help by providing information on your (and your family's) medical history. At that point, if you prefer, the doctor can ask your parent to leave so you can talk and be examined in private. If you have private questions or concerns that you want to discuss with your doctor without your parent being in the room, this is a good time to bring these things up.

Sometimes you need to talk to a doctor ahead of time, not just after a problem has developed. For example, if you're considering becoming sexually active, going on a special diet, or treating yourself with medication, you need to talk openly and honestly with medical experts you trust.

Ask a parent to help you find a new doctor if you need one. It's your right to have a doctor who makes you feel comfortable and treats you with respect. Of course the doctor you've had since you were a little kid knows your medical history better than anyone, but if you're not comfortable talking with him or her for any reason, what do you do? Ask your parents about finding another doctor both you and they can trust. Sometimes it helps to tell your parents you'd like to find a doctor who has lots of experience treating teens.

Ideally it's best to involve your parents in your health care because their advice and input can help you make the decision that's best for you. Plus, if you're still in your early teens, parents may feel more inclined to oversee your medical care than they might if you were older. But many people find it difficult to talk with their parents about certain medical or emotional concerns, even if they don't mind talking about most of their medical care. That's where confidentiality comes in.

Can I Keep My Visit Private?

It's a good idea to talk to your parents first about these types of issues, and many people do. Your health is the most important thing.

375

If talking to a parent or other responsible adult in your family isn't possible, you still need to get good care for yourself. That's where confidentiality comes in.

Confidential care means that your medical treatment stays between you and your doctor—you don't have to get a parent's permission. Confidentiality helps to ensure honesty and openness between a patient and a doctor. Most states ensure that teens can get confidential care for some sensitive medical matters, such as sexual health education and treatment, mental health issues like suicide and depression, and drug abuse. Sexual health education and treatment includes counseling, birth control, pregnancy care, and examinations and treatment for STDs.

So where can you get these services? Many family doctors will agree to treat their teen patients confidentially, so you may be able to approach your own family doctor and ask if he or she will do so. If you're not sure whether your treatment will be confidential, ask beforehand: Some doctors will treat their teen patients confidentially only when they have a parent's approval to do so. Most doctors agree to keep things confidential unless they feel their patient is either in danger or is a danger to others—in these cases, the doctor is obligated to inform the teen's parents.

Some schools offer health clinics to students during school hours. A teen also can visit a health clinic like Planned Parenthood or a gynecologist (a doctor who specializes in reproductive health) at a public health clinic to receive confidential advice and treatment on matters involving sexual health. If you don't want your parents to know and can't use their insurance, these clinics usually offer cheaper services or make it easy for teens to pay. Most school clinics and public health clinics that treat teens are very careful to maintain confidentiality.

Many parents are happy to have their teens see a doctor if they need to. Discuss with your parents the idea that you can see a doctor privately when you need to. Your doctor's office may need to call you with confidential test results. Let the doctor know the best way to reach you confidentially, such as a personal cell phone if you have one. Because the doctor's bill will need to be paid, talk with your parents and the doctor about how that can happen and still keep the visit confidential.

The more you know your body, the more you can be in control of your own health. Finding a doctor you can respect and who respects you, someone you can be open with, puts you on a great path to taking charge of your health for the rest of your life.

Chapter 35

Confidentiality Issues Associated with STD Testing

Chapter Contents

Section 35.1—Anonymous Testing for STDs Like HIV............. 378

Section 35.2—Confidentiality for Adolescents Who Seek
STD Testing and Care... 380

Section 35.3—At-Home/Mail Order STD Tests Protect
Patient Confidentiality 381

Section 35.1

Anonymous Testing for STDs Like HIV

"Confidential and Anonymous Testing,"
by AIDS.gov, part of the U.S. Department of Health
and Human Services, June 8, 2010.

HIV Test Results and Privacy Issues

HIV [human immunodeficiency virus] test results fall under the same privacy rules as all of your medical information. Information about your HIV test cannot be released without your permission. The Health Insurance Portability and Accountability Act of 1996 (HIPAA) ensures that the privacy of individuals' health information is protected while ensuring access to care. However it is important to note that not all HIV testing sites are bound by HIPAA regulations. Before you get tested be sure to inquire about the privacy rules of the HIV test site as well those surrounding your test results.

Available Testing Services

HIV tests can be taken either confidentially or anonymously. Most states offer both anonymous and confidential testing; however, some states only offer confidential testing services.

- Confidential testing means that your name and other identifying information will be attached to your test results. The results will go in your medical record and may be shared with your health-care providers and your insurance company. Otherwise, the results are protected by state and federal privacy laws.

- Anonymous testing means that nothing ties your test results to you. When you take an anonymous HIV test, you get a unique identifier that allows you to get your test results. Not all HIV test sites offer anonymous testing. Contact your local health department or 800-CDC-INFO (800-232-4636) to see if there are anonymous test sites in your area.

Names-Based Reporting

Since the beginning of the epidemic, AIDS [acquired immunodeficiency syndrome] cases have been reported to state health departments using name-based reporting. This is now also true for HIV cases. This means, if you test positive for HIV or another STD, the test result and your name will be reported to the state and local health department for the purposes of public health surveillance. Only public health personnel have access to this information at the state level and use this information to get better estimates of the rates of HIV in the state. The state health department will then remove all personal information about you (name, address, etc.) and share the remaining non-identifying information with the CDC so they can best track national public health trends. The CDC does not share this information with anyone else, including insurance companies.

If you have concerns regarding who can have access to your tests results, it is important to ask your testing center about their privacy policies and who they are required to report a positive result to.

Section 35.2

Confidentiality for Adolescents Who Seek STD Testing and Care

Excerpted from "Special Populations," part of the *Sexually Transmitted Diseases Treatment Guidelines, 2010*, by the Centers for Disease Control and Prevention (CDC, www.cdc.gov), March 4, 2011.

In the United States, prevalence rates of many sexually acquired infections are highest among adolescents. For example, the reported rates of chlamydia and gonorrhea are highest among females aged 15–19 years, and many persons acquire HPV infection during their adolescent years.

Persons who initiate sex early in adolescence are at higher risk for STDs, along with persons residing in detention facilities, attending STD clinics, young men having sex with men (YMSM), and youth who use injection drugs. Factors contributing to this increased risk during adolescence include having multiple sexual partners concurrently, having sequential sexual partnerships of limited duration, failing to use barrier protection consistently and correctly, having increased biologic susceptibility to infection, and experiencing multiple obstacles to accessing health care.

All 50 states and the District of Columbia explicitly allow minors to consent for their own health services for STDs. No state requires parental consent for STD care or requires that providers notify parents that an adolescent minor has received STD services, except in limited or unusual circumstances.

Protecting confidentiality for such care, particularly for adolescents enrolled in private health insurance plans, presents multiple problems. After a claim has been reported, many states mandate that health plans provide a written statement to a beneficiary indicating the benefits and charges covered or not covered by the health plan (i.e., explanation of benefit [EOB]). In addition, federal laws obligate notices to beneficiaries when claims are denied, including alerting consumers who need to pay for care until the allowable deductible is reached. For STD detection- and treatment-related care, an EOB or medical bill that is received by a parent might disclose services provided and list any laboratory tests performed. This type of mandated notification breeches confidentiality, and at a minimum, could prompt parents and guardians to question the costs and reasons for service provision.

Despite the high rates of infections documented in the adolescent population, providers frequently fail to inquire about sexual behaviors, assess STD risks, provide risk reduction counseling, and ultimately, fail to screen for asymptomatic infections during clinical encounters. Sexual health discussions should be appropriate for the patient's developmental level and should be aimed at identifying risk behaviors (e.g., unprotected oral, anal, or vaginal sex and drug-use behaviors). Careful, nonjudgmental, and thorough counseling is particularly vital for adolescents who might not feel comfortable acknowledging their engagement in behaviors that place them at high risk for STDs.

Section 35.3

At-Home/Mail Order STD Tests Protect Patient Confidentiality

"Free Web-Based Ordering of Home Test Kits for Sexually Transmitted Infections Proves Popular and Effective with Teens and Young Adults," © Johns Hopkins Medicine, February 11, 2011. Reprinted with permission.

Infectious disease experts at Johns Hopkins say new research clearly shows that screening teens and young adults for sexually transmitted infections (STIs) may best be achieved by making free, confidential home-kit testing available over the Internet. From a public health standpoint, the project is a clear winner, the experts say.

Reporting in the February [2011] issue of *Sexually Transmitted Diseases,* the Johns Hopkins team describes the success of the program started in Baltimore in 2004 that lets men and women in their 20s or teens order home-testing kits for the most common STIs over the Internet at www.iwantthekit.org.

The Johns Hopkins group designed the website, accessible now in several states, to track new and recurrent infections by providing private, confidential testing for *Chlamydia trachomatis, Neisseria gonorrhoeae,* and *Trichomonas vaginalis.* The project also facilitates treatment for those who test positive.

"Our results are repeatedly showing us that we have to go online if we want young people to be screened for sexually transmitted infections, especially young people in harder-to-reach, urban-poor minority groups," says infectious disease specialist Charlotte Gaydos, MS, DrPH, senior study investigator. She says the website now routinely gets 100,000 monthly hits.

As of January 1 [2011], some 3,500 young people, half under the age of 23, and many from low-income households, have gotten their test kit for free via the website, some more than once. Initially, kits were also offered at local pharmacies and in public health clinics, but 9 of 10 who used the kit ordered it online. "The Internet is by far the most popular means of getting tested among this sexually active group, and at a time when they are most at risk of becoming infected."

The program, which Gaydos says "could readily be introduced to all 50 states and overseas," has grown increasingly popular since its debut, when only test kits for women were offered. Kits for both sexes can be ordered by anyone in Maryland, the District of Columbia, West Virginia and parts of Illinois, and in Denver and Philadelphia.

Gaydos and her team expect an influx of orders after federally funded newspaper and radio ads to promote the website appear in Washington, DC, throughout Maryland and in Philadelphia during April, national sexually transmitted infections awareness month.

Each home test kit comes with instructions, a unique identification number, and a prepaid return envelope to return self-collected vaginal, penile, or rectal swabs in specially sealed test tubes to Gaydos' lab at Johns Hopkins. The kits are mailed in plain, brown paper envelopes and contain a detailed questionnaire that allows researchers to gather important information about who used the kit and why. Within two weeks of sending the test to the lab, people can call a toll-free number, provide their identification number and a secret password chosen when they ordered, and get their test results.

So far, 444 women and girls, some as young as 15, and 192 men and boys, for whom screening started in 2006, have tested positive for one or more bacterial or protozoon infections. All but four women and one man who tested positive sought subsequent treatment. For those who test positive, referrals are offered to nearby public health clinics.

"Using the Web is a very safe, private, secure, and practical forum for young people to deal with sexually transmitted infections," says Gaydos, a professor at the Johns Hopkins University School of

Medicine. "People can order a kit any time of day, without having to leave school or work, and can get tested with a level of anonymity that minimizes any fear of stigma or self-conscious feelings that may come with talking to a parent, school counselor, or health professional about a sex-related health problem."

The latest study results focused on women and showed that over a five-year period in Maryland, the iwantthekit.org screening program detected more cases of chlamydia infection among young females than regular screening programs available at traditional family planning clinics. Infection rates for chlamydia, which if left untreated can lead to so-called pelvic inflammatory disease and infertility in women, ranged from 3.3 percent to 5.5 percent in local clinics to 4.4 percent to 15.2 percent with the Internet service, statistics that Gaydos says demonstrate the online program's potentially greater reach.

"A lot of these young women are poor with little to no health insurance, and seldom see a physician or undergo a health check-up, so this is a free means of getting them tested and cared for quickly and before they potentially pass the infection on to someone else," says Gaydos, who notes that at least four in five people infected show no symptoms, so the chances of them unknowingly spreading infections are high.

Overall, Gaydos says the program, funded by a grant from the U.S. Centers for Disease Control and Prevention (CDC), is also highly effective in promoting retesting, noting that 17 percent of users feel comfortable enough with the system to use it again and almost half of these people have been screened multiple times, even if they test negative at first.

Gaydos stresses that people who have been infected once are 10 percent more likely to get re-infected. This is why, she says, the CDC recommends that all sexually active women age 25 or younger get screened for chlamydia at least once a year, with women who have tested positive getting retested within three months of their initial infection. Gaydos says 6 percent of repeat kit-users have tested positive before, while her other research has shown a 25 percent chlamydia re-infection rate among young women in the Baltimore area alone.

The need for repeat testing applies equally to sexually active males, says Gaydos, whose team reported in December in *Sexually Transmitted Diseases* that among 501 tested, some as young as 14, many did not practice safe sex. Only 13 percent used condoms. Even more were at risk of re-infection, with 34 percent having already had an infection and 29 percent having had sex with someone who had previously been infected.

Fortunately, Gaydos adds, 89 percent of males tested said they would use the iwantthekit.org screening program again, citing how easy it was to simply mail in a penile swab.

As part of the April campaign, run under the slogan "GYT," text speak for get yourself tested, Gaydos plans to distribute iwantthekit.org flyers and brochures at shopping malls, recreation centers, and libraries—all gathering spots for young people. She also plans to supply handouts to municipal public health departments and family planning clinics throughout the region.

To make kit-ordering easier, the Johns Hopkins team has incorporated product bar coding in its brochures and advertisements that can be read by standard computer apps, which are also free. People can take a picture of the bar code with their cell phone, open the app and be taken, automatically, to the ordering page of the iwantthekit.org website. This is very important for reaching underprivileged youth, says Gaydos, especially many Hispanic and black teens and other young adults who cannot afford a home computer and whose access to the Internet is mainly through their smart phones. Home test kits can also be ordered through the website's Facebook page.

The Johns Hopkins team launched the iwantthekit.org program in Baltimore, Maryland, in part because of the city's high infection rates.

Baltimore consistently ranks among the top 10 U.S. cities for newly acquired cases of chlamydia. According to previous CDC biannual surveys of risky youth behaviors in the United States, 32 percent of students are sexually active by the ninth grade.

Besides Gaydos, other Johns Hopkins University researchers involved in these studies were Shua Chai, MD, MPH; Mathilda Barnes, MS; Bulbul Aumakhan MD, MPH, PhD; Mary Jett-Goheen, BS; Nicole Quinn, BS; Patricia Agreda, MS; and M. Terry Hogan, MPH. Additional research support was provided by Catherine Wright, MPH, at the Family Planning Clinics, in Philadelphia; Wiley Jenkins, PhD, at the Department of Family and Community Medicine, at the Southern Illinois University School of Medicine in Carbondale, Illinois; Cornelius Rietmeijer, MD, PhD, at the Denver Public Health Department and the Colorado School of Public Health, at the University of Colorado in Denver; and Pamela Whittle, BS, at the Baltimore City Health Department.

Chapter 36

Testing for STDs

Chapter Contents

Section 36.1—Where to Go and How It Works.......................... 386

Section 36.2—Diagnostic Laparoscopy: A Way to
Test for STD Complications 390

Section 36.1

Where to Go and How It Works

STD Testing at a Glance

You must ask for an STD test if you want to be tested.

- STD tests are easy to get.

- Consider testing if you have had unprotected sex, even if you don't have symptoms.

- There are different tests for different STDs.

You might be wondering if you need a test for sexually transmitted diseases (STDs). You might be wondering if your partner needs one. Or you may simply be interested in learning more about STD testing. Whatever the reason, the more information you have, the better you can protect your sexual health.

If you think you may have been exposed to an infection, getting tested for STDs is a great way to protect your sexual health. It's also a great way to protect the health of your sex partners.

Should I Get Tested for STDs?

If you have symptoms of an STD, it's important to be tested. Some common symptoms of STDs include sores on the genitals, discharge from the penis or vagina, itching, and burning during urination.

But remember, many infections often do not cause any symptoms. Many people have sexually transmitted infections and never know it. Many people get or spread infections without ever having symptoms.

If you've had sex play with another person and did not use a condom, female condom, dental dam, or other barrier, it's a good idea to talk to your health care provider about STD testing. Getting tested can put your mind at ease or get you (and your partner) needed treatment.

It's also important to learn about ways you and your partner can protect yourselves in the future through safer sex.

How Do I Get Tested for STDs?

You must ask your health care provider to give you an STD test.

Some people assume they will be tested for STDs when they have an exam for another reason, such as when a woman has a Pap test or when a man has a physical. This is not true—you will not automatically be tested for STDs.

If you are seeing your health care provider for another reason, and are not sure if you need an STD test, just ask. Your provider can help you decide if you need any tests, and which one(s) you may need.

Where Can I Get an STD Test?

Your local Planned Parenthood health center, many other clinics, private health care providers, and health departments offer STD tests.

Which STD Tests Do I Need?

There is no single test for every sexually transmitted disease—tests are specific to each infection. And some infections can be found using different kinds of tests.

You and your health care provider will decide what STD tests make the most sense for you. In most cases, your provider will first ask you questions about:

- your sexual practices—such as how many partners you have, whether you use condoms or other barrier methods, and what body parts are used during sex play;

- whether you have symptoms—and to describe the symptoms if you do have any;

- whether you have had symptoms in the past;

- whether you've ever had any STDs;

- whether you have used over-the-counter medications to treat your symptoms;

- whether your partner(s) have any STDs or symptoms of STDs;

- any drug allergies you may have;

- your last period, if you're a woman—to see if you could you be pregnant.

It is important to be honest with your health care provider. Your provider will be helping you make important decisions about what test(s) you may need.

How Are STD Tests Done?

It depends on which infection you may have. And some infections can be tested for in more than one way. Your test may include a:

- physical exam—your health care provider may look at your genitals and/or your anus for any signs of an infection, such as a rash, discharge, sores, or warts. For women, this exam can be similar to a pelvic exam.

- blood sample—your provider may take a blood sample, either with a needle or by pricking the skin to draw drops of blood.

- urine sample—you may be asked to urinate into a special cup.

- discharge, tissue, cell, or saliva sample—your provider will use a swab to collect samples that will be looked at under a microscope.

See Table 36.1 for more information on the tests used for specific STDs.

Sometimes a diagnosis can be made based on your symptoms and/ or a physical exam. Treatment could be prescribed right away. Other times, your health care provider may need to send a sample to a lab to be tested. In that case, the results may not be available for several days or weeks.

Do People under 18 Need Their Parents' Permission for STD Testing?

In general, parental permission is not needed for STD testing. However, there may be certain locations where, for one reason or another, a health care provider will require parental permission or may notify a parent about testing.

Planned Parenthood's policy is to protect confidentiality to the extent the law allows. Laws vary from state to state.

Whether you come to a Planned Parenthood health center or go somewhere else for testing, if you concerned about confidentiality, ask your health care provider about your local laws and policies.

Table 36.1. STD Testing Quick Reference Guide

Which STD is being tested?	What's the test?
HIV/acquired immuno-deficiency syndrome (AIDS)	Blood test; oral swab test—a special tool is used to test cells from inside the mouth; urine test (rarely used)
Bacterial vaginosis (BV) (affects only women)	Pelvic exam; test of vaginal discharge
Chlamydia	Physical exam; test of discharge from the anus, urethra, or vagina; test of a cell sample—cells from the cervix, penis, vagina, or anus; urine test
Cytomegalovirus	Blood test
Genital warts	Physical exam—some warts can be seen by the naked eye during a pelvic exam. A special tool called a colpo-scope may be used to detect warts that are too small to be seen by the naked eye.
Gonorrhea	Test of discharge from the anus, urethra, or vagina; test of a cell sample—cells from the cervix, penis, anus, or throat; urine test
Hepatitis B	Blood test
Herpes	Blood test; test of fluid taken from a herpes sore
High-risk human papil-lomavirus (HPV)	No HPV test for men; test of cell samples from the cervix
Intestinal parasites	Test of a stool (feces) sample; proctoscopy may be needed—a test that involves a health care provider in-serting a thin lighted tube into the rectum
Molluscum contagio-sum	Physical exam; test of a cell sample
Pelvic inflammatory disease (affects only women)	Pelvic exam; blood test; test of discharge from the cervix or vagina; laparoscopy—a special instrument is inserted through a small cut in the navel to look at the reproductive organs
Pubic lice	Physical exam; may be self-diagnosed based on symp-toms
Scabies	Physical exam; may be self-diagnosed based on symp-toms; test of a cell sample; biopsy may be necessary
Syphilis	Blood test; test of fluid taken from a syphilis sore
Trichomoniasis	Test of discharge from the vagina or urethra

Section 36.2

Diagnostic Laparoscopy: A Way to Test for STD Complications

"Diagnostic Laparoscopy," © 2012 A.D.A.M., Inc.
Reprinted with permission.

Diagnostic laparoscopy is a procedure that allows a health care provider to look directly at the contents of a patient's abdomen or pelvis, including the fallopian tubes, ovaries, uterus, small bowel, large bowel, appendix, liver, and gallbladder.

How the Test Is Performed

The procedure is usually done in the hospital or outpatient surgical center under general anesthesia (while the patient is unconscious and pain-free). However, very rarely, this procedure may also be done using local anesthesia, which numbs only the area affected by the surgery and allows you to stay awake.

A surgeon makes a small cut below the belly button (navel) and inserts a needle into the area. Carbon dioxide gas is passed into the area to help move the abdominal wall and any organs out of the way, creating a larger space to work in. This helps the surgeon see the area better.

A tube is placed through the cut in your abdominal area. A tiny video camera (laparoscope) goes through this tube and is used to see the inside of your pelvis and abdomen. Additional small cuts may be made if other instruments are needed to get a better view of certain organs.

In the case of gynecologic laparoscopy, dye may be injected into your cervix area so the surgeon can better see your fallopian tubes.

After the exam, the laparoscope and instruments are removed, and the cuts are closed. You will have bandages over those areas.

How to Prepare for the Test

Do not eat or drink anything for eight hours before the test. You must sign a consent form.

How the Test Will Feel

If you are given general anesthesia, you will feel no pain during the procedure, although the surgical cuts may throb and be slightly painful afterward. Your doctor may prescribe medicine to relieve pain.

With local anesthesia, you may feel a prick and a burning sensation when the local anesthetic is given. The laparoscope may cause pressure, but there should be no pain during the procedure. Afterward, you may also feel soreness at the site of the surgical cut. A pain reliever may be prescribed by your doctor.

You may also have shoulder pain for a few days, because the gas used during the procedure can irritate the diaphragm, which shares some of the same nerves as the shoulder. You may also have an increased urge to urinate, since the gas can put pressure on the bladder.

Why the Test Is Performed

The examination helps identify the cause of pain in the abdomen and pelvic area. It is done after other, noninvasive tests.

Laparoscopy may detect or diagnose the following conditions:

- Appendicitis

- Cancer, such as ovarian cancer

- Ectopic pregnancy

- Endometriosis

- Inflammation of the gallbladder (cholecystitis)

- Pelvic inflammatory disease

The procedure may also be done instead of open surgery after an accident to see if there is any injury to the abdomen.

Major procedures to treat cancer, such as surgery to remove an organ, may begin with laparoscopy to rule out the presence of cancer spread (metastatic disease), which would change the course of treatment.

Normal Results

There is no blood in the abdomen, no hernias, no intestinal obstruction, and no cancer in any visible organs. The uterus, fallopian tubes, and ovaries are of normal size, shape, and color. The liver is normal.

What Abnormal Results Mean

Abnormal results may be due to a number of different conditions, including:

- adhesions;
- appendicitis;
- cholecystitis;
- endometriosis;
- ovarian cysts;
- pelvic inflammatory disease;
- signs of injury;
- spread of cancer;
- tumors;
- uterine fibroids.

Risks

There is some risk of infection. Antibiotics may be given to prevent this complication.

There is a risk of puncturing an organ, which could cause leakage of intestinal contents, or bleeding into the abdominal cavity. Such a complication could lead to immediate open surgery (laparotomy).

Chapter 37

Understanding Antibiotic Resistance and STD Treatment

Antibiotics are drugs used for treating infections caused by bacteria. Also known as antimicrobial drugs, antibiotics have saved countless lives.

Misuse and overuse of these drugs, however, have contributed to a phenomenon known as antibiotic resistance. This resistance develops when potentially harmful bacteria change in a way that reduces or eliminates the effectiveness of antibiotics.

A Public Health Issue

Antibiotic resistance is a growing public health concern worldwide. When a person is infected with an antibiotic-resistant bacterium, not only is treatment of that patient more difficult, but the antibiotic-resistant bacterium may spread to other people.

When antibiotics don't work, the result can be:

- longer illnesses;

- more complicated illnesses;

- more doctor visits;

- the use of stronger and more expensive drugs;

- more deaths caused by bacterial infections.

"Combating Antibiotic Resistance," by the U.S. Food and Drug Administration (FDA, www.fda.gov), December 8, 2011.

Examples of the types of bacteria that have become resistant to antibiotics include the species that cause skin infections, meningitis, sexually transmitted diseases, and respiratory tract infections such as pneumonia.

Antibiotics Fight Bacteria, Not Viruses

Antibiotics are meant to be used against bacterial infections. For example, they are used to treat strep throat, which is caused by streptococcal bacteria, and skin infections caused by staphylococcal bacteria.

Although antibiotics kill bacteria, they are not effective against viruses. Therefore, they will not be effective against viral infections such as colds, most coughs, many types of sore throat, and influenza (flu).

Using antibiotics against viral infections:

• will not cure the infection;

• will not keep other individuals from catching the virus;

• will not help a person feel better;

• may cause unnecessary, harmful side effects;

• may contribute to the development of antibiotic-resistant bacteria.

Patients and health care professionals alike can play an important role in combating antibiotic resistance. Patients should not demand antibiotics when a health care professional says the drugs are not needed. Health care professionals should prescribe antibiotics only for infections they believe to be caused by bacteria.

As a patient, your best approach is to ask your health care professional whether an antibiotic is likely to be effective for your condition. Also, ask what else you can do to relieve your symptoms.

So how do you know if you have a bad cold or a bacterial infection?

Joseph Toerner, MD, MPH, a medical officer in the U.S. Food and Drug Administration's Center for Drug Evaluation and Research, says that the symptoms of a cold or flu generally lessen over the course of a week. But if you have a fever and other symptoms that persist and worsen with the passage of days, you may have a bacterial infection and should consult your health care provider.

Follow Directions for Proper Use

When you are prescribed an antibiotic to treat a bacterial infection, it's important to take the medication exactly as directed. Here are more tips to promote proper use of antibiotics.

- Complete the full course of the drug. It's important to take all of the medication, even if you are feeling better. If treatment stops too soon, the drug may not kill all the bacteria. You may become sick again, and the remaining bacteria may become resistant to the antibiotic that you've taken.

- Do not skip doses. Antibiotics are most effective when they are taken regularly.

- Do not save antibiotics. You might think that you can save an antibiotic for the next time you get sick, but an antibiotic is meant for your particular infection at the time. Never take left-over medicine. Taking the wrong medicine can delay getting the appropriate treatment and may allow your condition to worsen.

- Do not take antibiotics prescribed for someone else. These may not be appropriate for your illness, may delay correct treatment, and may allow your condition to worsen.

- Talk with your health care professional. Ask questions, especially if you are uncertain about when an antibiotic is appropriate or how to take it.

It's important that you let your health care professional know of any troublesome side effects.

Chapter 38

Unproven STD Treatment Products

Beware of Bogus STD Products

Federal regulators say some companies are selling products that make unproven claims to treat sexually transmitted diseases (STDs)—claims that could pose a threat to public health.

The Food and Drug Administration (FDA) says only prescription medicines and diagnostic tools available through a health care professional are effective for STD diagnosis and treatment.

FDA and the Federal Trade Commission (FTC) are warning manufacturers and distributors that they could face legal action if the products aren't removed from the market. The agencies say at least 15 products claim to treat, prevent, or cure STDs and are being sold online and at some retail outlets.

The products—some of which are sold as dietary supplements—claim to treat a range of sexually transmitted diseases, including herpes, chlamydia, genital warts, HIV [human immunodeficiency virus], and AIDS [acquired immunodeficiency syndrome]. Specific brand names being targeted by FDA and FTC include: Medavir, Herpaflor, and Viruxo.

FDA expert Debbie Birnkrant, MD, says she's concerned that someone with an STD will waste precious time using a product that doesn't

This chapter contains text from "FDA Warns: Beware of Bogus STD Products," by the U.S. Food and Drug Administration (FDA, www.fda.gov), May 3, 2011, and text from "Questions and Answers: Fraudulent STD Products Initiative," by the U.S. Food and Drug Administration (FDA, www.fda.gov), May 3, 2011.

work, leading to a delay in medical treatment and possible spread of the infection.

"If you aren't treating your STD with an FDA-approved medication, you're not just putting your own health at risk—you could be endangering your partner," she says.

Birnkrant says there are no non-prescription drugs or dietary supplements that can treat, cure, or prevent sexually transmitted disease. Condoms are the only non-prescription product that can prevent STDs by reducing the chance that an infected person will pass on the disease. STDs can only be diagnosed and treated under the supervision of a health care professional.

Some STDs have symptoms that include sores or a discharge, but the majority of infected people have no symptoms at all. Because of this, Birnkrant says people who are sexually active, have had unprotected sex, or have been exposed to a sexually transmitted disease should get medical attention, especially if they have these symptoms:

- Burning sensation with urination

- Pelvic pain

- Discharge from the penis or vagina

- Blisters

- Sores

There are FDA-approved medications available to treat many sexually transmitted diseases. These products have met federal standards for safety, effectiveness, and quality—and they're available only by prescription, Birnkrant says.

To learn more about sexually transmitted diseases and to learn where you can be tested, go to www.hivtest.org/STDTesting.aspx.

Questions and Answers

What are fraudulent STD products?

Fraudulent STD products are products that make unproven claims to prevent, cure, and/or treat sexually transmitted diseases (STDs). Some of the products are marketed as dietary supplements and others are marketed as drugs. Currently there are no FDA-approved drugs or dietary supplements available over-the-counter (OTC) that can prevent, cure, and/or treat STDs. Condoms are the only products cleared by FDA to help prevent sexually transmitted infections. FDA-approved drugs and vaccines for the treatment and prevention of STDs can only be obtained by prescription through a licensed healthcare professional.

Fraudulent STD products are being sold primarily over the internet, but some are also available in local retail stores.

Marketers of fraudulent STD products are in violation of the Federal Food, Drug, and Cosmetic Act. These products have not been evaluated by the FDA for safety and effectiveness and may pose health risks to consumers who are misled to believe they are receiving safe, effective treatment. In addition, marketers making scientifically unsupported claims that their products can effectively prevent, cure, or treat STDs are in violation of the Federal Trade Commission Act.

Why is FDA concerned about the use of fraudulent STD products?

FDA is concerned about the use of fraudulent STD products because they have not been evaluated by the agency for safety and effectiveness. Consumers who use fraudulent STD products may not seek the medical attention they need, delaying appropriate and effective treatment, and potentially spreading infections to sexual partners because they falsely believe they are being treated for their disease.

How can consumers identify fraudulent STD products?

Consumers should know that there are no FDA-approved drugs, vaccines, or dietary supplements available over-the-counter (OTC) that can prevent, cure, and/or treat sexually transmitted diseases (STDs). FDA-approved products for the treatment and prevention of STDs can only be obtained by prescription through a licensed healthcare professional. Some fraudulent STD products that have been identified include H-Stop Dx, H-Guard Dx, Wart Dx, Molluscum Dx, EverCLR3, Herpeset, C-Cure, Viruxo, Medavir, and Wartrol. Table 38.1 provides several manufacturers of these products, but this list is not all inclusive.

What should consumers do if they are currently using a fraudulent STD product or have used one in the past?

FDA advises consumers who believe they might have used or are currently using a fraudulent STD product to stop using and discard the product, and see a licensed health care professional since they might be at risk for having an STD. Correct diagnosis and treatment of an STD requires the supervision of a trained healthcare professional. FDA recommends consumers contact a healthcare professional if they have symptoms of an STD, believe they may have been exposed to an STD, and/or are using OTC products to treat symptoms of an STD.

Symptoms of common STDs include pain or burning sensation during urination, pain during sexual intercourse, abdominal pain, abnormal discharge from the vagina or penis, abnormal vaginal bleeding, genital itching, genital warts, and/or blisters or sores in the genital area. However, the majority of people with sexually transmitted infections have no symptoms, so consumers should talk to a healthcare professional about STD testing if they are sexually active, have unprotected sex, or have been exposed to a STD.

There are several FDA-approved drugs and vaccines available to treat and prevent many STDs, and these products have met federal standards for safety, effectiveness, and quality and are only available by prescription through a licensed healthcare professional and pharmacy.

For more information on STD symptoms and treatment, visit the Centers for Disease Control and Prevention website at www.cdc.gov/std.

Table 38.1. Fraudulent STD Product Manufacturers

Manufacturer Name	Product Name
Immuneglory (Arenvy Laboratories, Inc)	ImmuneGlory
Viruxo	Viruxo
Masterpeace, Inc.	Disintegrate Formula, Echinacea/Golden Seal, Detox Formula, Burdock Extract,
Int'l Inst of Holistic Health (doctorAJAdams)	Oil of Oregano P73 Physician's Strength, Essaic Tonic Liquid Drops, Colloidal Silver 500ppm (Liquid)
gene-eden/PolyDNA	Gene-Eden
Pacific Naturals	Herpeset, Wartrol
Derma Remedies	H-Stop Dx, H-Guard Dx, Molluscum Dx, Wart Dx
Flor Nutraceuticals	Herpaflör Outbreak Response Topical Liquid, Herpaflör Outbreak Response Tablets, Herpaflör Outbreak Response Combo Pack, Herpaflör Daily Formula Tablets, Herpaflör Complete Package
Medavir	Medavir, ViraBalm, Vyristic Immune Support, Medavir H-Elimination Kit
Never An Outbreak	O2xygen Force (Oxygen Force/OxyForce), DMSO Cream, DMSO Roll-on, DMSO Cream w/Aloe, AlkaLife
EverCLR3	EverCLR3
Chlamydia-Clinic.com	C-Cure

Part Five

STD Risks and Prevention

Chapter 39

Sexual Behaviors That Increase the Likelihood of STD Transmission

Chapter Contents

Section 39.1—Overview of Risky Sexual Behaviors 404

Section 39.2—Choosing High-Risk Partners Increases
STD Risk.. 405

Section 39.3—Oral Sex and HIV Risk 408

Section 39.1

Overview of Risky Sexual Behaviors

"Sexual Risk Behavior: HIV, STD, and Teen Pregnancy Prevention,"
by the Centers for Disease Control and Prevention
(CDC, www.cdc.gov), June 20, 2012.

Many young people engage in sexual risk behaviors that can result in unintended health outcomes. For example, among U.S. high school students surveyed in 2011:

- 47.4% had ever had sexual intercourse;

- 33.7% had had sexual intercourse during the previous three months and of these 39.8% did not use a condom the last time they had sex and 76.7% did not use birth control pills or Depo-Provera to prevent pregnancy the last time they had sex;

- 15.3% had had sex with four or more people during their life.

Sexual risk behaviors place adolescents at risk for HIV [human immunodeficiency virus] infection, other sexually transmitted diseases (STDs), and unintended pregnancy:

- An estimated 8,300 young people aged 13–24 years in the 40 states reporting to CDC had HIV infection in 2009.

- Nearly half of the 19 million new STDs each year are among young people aged 15–24 years.

- More than 400,000 teen girls aged 15–19 years gave birth in 2009.

References

1. CDC. Youth risk behavior surveillance—United States, 2011. *MMWR* 2012;61(SS-4).

2. CDC. Diagnoses of HIV infection and AIDS in the United States and dependent areas, 2009. HIV Surveillance Report, Volume 21.

3. Weinstock H, Berman S, Cates W. Sexually transmitted diseases among American youth: incidence and prevalence estimates, 2000. *Perspectives on Sexual and Reproductive Health* 2004;36(1):6–10.

4. Hamilton BE, Martin JA, Ventura SJ. Births: Preliminary data for 2009. *National Vital Statistics Reports* 2010;59(3).

Section 39.2

Choosing High-Risk Partners Increases STD Risk

Excerpted from "Trends in HIV- and STD-Related Risk Behaviors Among High School Students—United States, 1991–2007," published in the *Morbidity and Mortality Weekly Report* (www.cdc.gov/mmwr), by the Centers for Disease Control and Prevention (CDC), June 1, 2008.

Persons who engage in unprotected sexual intercourse or use injection drugs are at increased risk for human immunodeficiency virus (HIV) infection and sexually transmitted diseases (STDs). Changes in HIV- and STD-related risk behaviors among high school students in the United States during 1991–2005 were reported previously. To update these analyses through 2007, CDC analyzed data from nine biennial national Youth Risk Behavior Surveys (YRBS). This text summarizes the results of that analysis, which indicated that, during 1991–2007, the percentage of U.S. high school students who ever had sexual intercourse decreased 12%, the percentage who had sexual intercourse with four or more persons during their lifetime decreased 20%, and the percentage who were currently sexually active decreased 7%. Among students who were currently sexually active, the prevalence of condom use increased 33%. However, these changes in risk behaviors were not observed in some subgroups. In addition, no changes were detected in the prevalence of sexual risk behaviors from 2005 to 2007, and many students still engaged in behaviors that place them at risk for HIV infection and STDs. Additional efforts to reduce sexual risk behaviors, particularly among black, Hispanic, and male students, must be implemented to meet the Healthy People 2010 national health objective for adolescent sexual behaviors and to decrease rates of HIV infection and STDs.

The biennial national YRBS, a component of CDC's Youth Risk Behavior Surveillance System, used independent, three-stage cluster samples for the 1991–2007 surveys to obtain cross-sectional data representative of public and private school students in grades 9–12 in all 50 states and the District of Columbia. Sample sizes ranged from 10,904 to 16,296. School response rates ranged from 70% to 81%, and student response rates ranged from 83% to 90%; therefore, overall response rates for the surveys ranged from 60% to 70%.

For each cross-sectional national survey, students completed anonymous, self-administered questionnaires that included identically worded questions about sexual intercourse, number of sex partners, condom use, and injection-drug use. Sexual experience was defined as ever having had sexual intercourse. Multiple sex partners was defined as having four or more sex partners during one's lifetime. Current sexual activity was defined as having sexual intercourse during the three months before the survey. Condom use was defined as use of a condom during last sexual intercourse among currently sexually active students. Injection-drug use was defined as ever having used a needle to inject any illegal drug into one's body. Race/ethnicity data are presented only for non-Hispanic black, non-Hispanic white, and Hispanic students (who might be of any race); the numbers of students from other racial/ethnic groups were too small for meaningful analysis.

During 1991–2007, the prevalence of sexual experience decreased 12% overall, from 54.1% to 47.8%. Logistic regression analyses indicated a significant linear decrease overall and among female, male, 9th-grade, 10th-grade, 11th-grade, 12th-grade, black, and white students. Among Hispanic students, no significant change was detected. Among male students, 11th-grade students, and black students, a significant quadratic trend also was detected. Among male students and 11th-grade students, the prevalence of sexual experience declined during 1991–1997 and then leveled off during 1997–2007. Among black students, the prevalence of sexual experience declined during 1991–2001 and then leveled off during 2001–2007. From 2005 to 2007, no significant change was detected in the prevalence of sexual experience overall or among any sex, grade, or racial/ethnic subgroup of students.

During 1991–2007, the prevalence of multiple sex partners decreased 20%, from 18.7% to 14.9%. A significant linear decrease was detected overall and among female, male, 9th-grade, 10th-grade, 11th-grade, 12th-grade, black, and white students. Among Hispanic students, no significant change was detected. A significant quadratic trend also was detected among male students, 11th-grade students, and 12th-grade students. For each group, the prevalence of multiple sex partners declined during 1991–1997 and then leveled off during 1997–2007. From 2005 to 2007, no significant change was detected in the prevalence of multiple sex partners overall or among any sex, grade, or racial/ethnic subgroup of students. During 1991–2007, the prevalence of current sexual activity decreased 7%, from 37.5% to 35.0%. A significant linear decrease was detected overall and among 9th-grade students and black students. Among 9th-grade and 11th-grade students, a significant quadratic trend was detected. For 9th-grade students, the prevalence of current sexual activity remained stable during 1991–1999 and then declined during 1999–2007. For 11th-grade students, the prevalence of current sexual activity declined during 1991–1999 and then remained stable during 1999–2007. From 2005 to 2007, no significant change was detected in the prevalence of current sexual activity overall or among any sex, grade, or racial/ethnic subgroup of students.

During 1991–2007, among students who were currently sexually active, the prevalence of condom use increased 33%, from 46.2% to 61.5%. A significant linear increase in condom use was detected among currently sexually active students overall and among all sex, grade, and racial/ethnic subgroups of students who were currently sexually active. A significant quadratic trend also was detected among currently sexually active students overall and among female students, 10th-grade students, and black students who were currently sexually active. Among currently sexually active students overall, female students, and 10th-grade students, the prevalence of condom use increased during 1991–2003 and then leveled off during 2003–2007. The prevalence of condom use among currently sexually active black students increased during 1991–1999 and then leveled off during 1999–2007. From 2005 to 2007, no significant change was detected in the prevalence of condom use overall or among any sex, grade, or racial/ethnic subgroup of currently sexually active students.

During 1995–2007, the prevalence of injection-drug use remained below 4%. However, a significant linear increase in injection-drug use was detected among black and Hispanic students. From 2005 to 2007, no change was detected in the prevalence of injection-drug use overall or among any subgroup, except for 10th-grade students, whose prevalence decreased from 2.3% to 1.4%.

Section 39.3

Oral Sex and HIV Risk

"Oral Sex and HIV Risk," by the Centers for Disease
Control and Prevention (CDC, www.cdc.gov), June 3, 2009.

Oral Sex Is Not Risk Free

Like all sexual activity, oral sex carries some risk of HIV (human immunodeficiency virus) transmission when one partner is known to be infected with HIV, when either partner's HIV status is not known, and/or when one partner is not monogamous or injects drugs. Even though the risk of transmitting HIV through oral sex is much lower than that of anal or vaginal sex, numerous studies have demonstrated that oral sex can result in the transmission of HIV and other sexually transmitted diseases (STDs). Abstaining from oral, anal, and vaginal sex altogether or having sex only with a mutually monogamous, uninfected partner are the only ways that individuals can be completely protected from the sexual transmission of HIV. However, by using condoms or other barriers between the mouth and genitals, individuals can reduce their risk of contracting HIV or another STD through oral sex.

Oral Sex Is a Common Practice

Oral sex involves giving or receiving oral stimulation (i.e., sucking or licking) to the penis, the vagina, and/or the anus. Fellatio is the technical term used to describe oral contact with the penis. Cunnilingus is the technical term which describes oral contact with the vagina. Anilingus (sometimes called rimming) refers to oral-anal contact. Studies indicate that oral sex is commonly practiced by sexually active male-female and same-gender couples of various ages, including adolescents. Although there are only limited national data about how often adolescents engage in oral sex, some data suggest that many adolescents who engage in oral sex do not consider it to be sex; therefore they may use oral sex as an option to experience sex while still, in their minds, remaining abstinent. Moreover, many consider oral sex to be a safe or no-risk sexual practice. In a national survey of teens conducted for

The Kaiser Family Foundation, 26% of sexually active 15- to 17-year-olds surveyed responded that one "cannot become infected with HIV by having unprotected oral sex," and an additional 15% didn't know whether or not one could become infected in that manner.

Oral Sex and the Risk of HIV Transmission

The risk of HIV transmission from an infected partner through oral sex is much less than the risk of HIV transmission from anal or vaginal sex. Measuring the exact risk of HIV transmission as a result of oral sex is very difficult. Additionally, because most sexually active individuals practice oral sex in addition to other forms of sex, such as vaginal and/or anal sex, when transmission occurs, it is difficult to determine whether or not it occurred as a result of oral sex or other more risky sexual activities. Finally, several co-factors may increase the risk of HIV transmission through oral sex, including: oral ulcers, bleeding gums, genital sores, and the presence of other STDs. What is known is that HIV has been transmitted through fellatio, cunnilingus, and anilingus.

Other STDs Can Also Be Transmitted via Oral Sex

In addition to HIV, other STDs can be transmitted through oral sex with an infected partner. Examples of these STDs include herpes, syphilis, gonorrhea, genital warts (HPV), intestinal parasites (amebiasis), and hepatitis A.

Oral Sex and Reducing the Risk of HIV Transmission

The consequences of HIV infection are life-long. If treatment is not initiated in a timely manner, HIV can be extremely serious and life threatening. However, there are steps you can take to lower the risk of getting HIV from oral sex.

Generally, the use of a physical barrier during oral sex can reduce the risk of transmission of HIV and other STDs. A latex or plastic condom may be used on the penis to reduce the risk of oral-penile transmission. If your partner is a female, a cut-open condom or a dental dam can be used between your mouth and the vagina. Similarly, regardless of the sex of your partner, if your mouth will come in contact with your partner's anus, a cut-open condom or dental dam can be used between your mouth and the anus.

At least one scientific article has suggested that plastic food wrap may be used as a barrier to protect against herpes simplex virus during oral-vaginal or oral-anal sex. However, there are no data regarding the effectiveness of plastic food wrap in decreasing transmission of HIV and other STDs in this manner and it is not manufactured or approved by the FDA (U.S. Food and Drug Administration) for this purpose.

Chapter 40

Sexually Transmitted Diseases and Substance Use

Sexually transmitted diseases (STDs) are infections transmitted mainly through sexual activity, although some STDs can be transmitted by sharing drug injection equipment. In the United States in 2005, there were 976,445 new cases of chlamydia, 339,593 new cases of gonorrhea, 266,000 new cases of herpes, and 8,724 new cases of syphilis. Sexually active adolescents and young adults may be at higher risk of acquiring STDs than older adults.

Recent estimates suggest that persons aged 15 to 24 represent about 25 percent of all persons who were ever sexually active, but nearly half of all new STD cases. In addition, research has documented the association between substance use and STDs.

The National Survey on Drug Use and Health (NSDUH) asks questions to examine health conditions, including STDs. Respondents are provided with a list of health conditions and are asked to indicate whether they have ever been told by a doctor or other medical professional that they had each of these conditions. Individuals who report having ever been told they had any of these conditions then are asked to indicate whether they had been told by a doctor or other medical professional that they had each of the conditions in the past year.

Excerpted from "Sexually Transmitted Diseases and Substance Use," a National Survey on Drug Use and Health (NSDUH) Report, by the Substance Abuse and Mental Health Services Administration (SAMHSA, www.oas.samhsa.gov), March 30, 2007. Reviewed by David A. Cooke, MD, FACP, July 12, 2012.

411

One of the conditions asked about is STDs, such as chlamydia, gonorrhea, herpes, or syphilis. NSDUH also asks persons aged 12 or older to report on their use of alcohol and illicit drugs in the past month.

Those who report having used alcohol are asked about binge and heavy use. Binge alcohol use is defined as drinking five or more drinks on the same occasion (i.e., at the same time or within a couple of hours of each other) on at least 1 day in the past 30 days. Heavy alcohol use is defined as drinking five or more drinks on the same occasion on each of 5 or more days in the past 30 days; all heavy alcohol users are also binge alcohol users. Illicit drugs refer to marijuana/ hashish, cocaine (including crack), inhalants, hallucinogens, heroin, or prescription-type drugs used nonmedically.

This text examines STDs among the civilian, noninstitutionalized U.S. population aged 12 or older, with a focus on young adults aged 18 to 25. In addition, rates of past year STDs are presented by level of past month alcohol use and combination of past month alcohol and illicit drug use among young adults aged 18 to 25. Past month, rather than past year, substance use is presented because most young adults have had at least one drink of alcohol in the past year, thus making past month use a better indicator of recent drinking behavior. All findings presented in this report are based on 2005 NSDUH data.

Prevalence of Sexually Transmitted Diseases, by Demographic Characteristics

In 2005, 0.8 percent of persons aged 12 or older (2.0 million persons) had an STD in the past year (i.e., the year prior to the survey). Persons aged 18 to 25 were more likely to have had an STD than were persons in any other age group. Females aged 12 or older were more likely to have had a past year STD than were their male counterparts (1.2 vs. 0.5 percent). Blacks were more likely to have had a past year STD than were Hispanics, whites, Native Hawaiians, or Other Pacific Islanders, Asians, and persons of two or more races (1.7 vs. 0.9, 0.7, 0.2, 0.2, and 0.3 percent, respectively).

Prevalence of Sexually Transmitted Diseases among Persons Aged 18 to 25

In 2005, 2.1 percent of young adults aged 18 to 25 had a past year STD. Females aged 18 to 25 were 4 times as likely to have had a past year STD as their male counterparts (3.4 vs. 0.8 percent). Black young adults were more likely to have had a past year STD than were white,

Hispanic, and Asian young adults, as well as young adults of two or more races.

Rates of Past Year Sexually Transmitted Diseases, by Past Month Alcohol Use among Persons Aged 18 to 25

The likelihood of having an STD in the past year was related to the frequency of alcohol use during the past month.

Among young adults aged 18 to 25, 1.4 percent of those who did not drink alcohol in the past month had a past year STD compared with 2.5 percent of those who drank but did not binge on alcohol in the past month, 2.4 percent of those who engaged in past month binge alcohol use but not heavy use, and 3.1 percent of past month heavy alcohol users.

Similar patterns were found for males and females.

Rates of Past Year Sexually Transmitted Diseases, by Past Month Alcohol and Illicit Drug Use among Persons Aged 18 to 25

Having an STD in the past year was more common among persons aged 18 to 25 who used both alcohol and an illicit drug in the past month (3.9 percent) than those who used neither alcohol nor an illicit drug (1.3 percent), those who used alcohol but no illicit drugs (2.1 percent), and those who used an illicit drug but not alcohol (2.1 percent).

Similar patterns were found for both males and females.

Chapter 41

Other Behaviors That Increase STD Risk

Chapter Contents

Section 41.1—Douching May Increase Risk of STDs 416

Section 41.2—Body Art Allows Exposure to Bloodborne
Pathogens Such as HIV 419

Section 41.3—Injection Drug Use 421

415

Section 41.1

Douching May Increase Risk of STDs

"Douching," by the Office on Women's Health (www.womenshealth.gov), part of the U.S. Department of Health and Human Services, May 18, 2010.

What is douching?

The word "douche" means to wash or soak in French. Douching is washing or cleaning out the vagina (birth canal) with water or other mixtures of fluids. Most douches are prepackaged mixes of water and vinegar, baking soda, or iodine. You can buy these products at drug and grocery stores. The mixtures usually come in a bottle and can be squirted into the vagina through a tube or nozzle.

Why do women douche?

Women douche because they mistakenly believe it gives many benefits. Women who douche say they do it to:

- clean the vagina;
- rinse away blood after monthly periods;
- get rid of odor;
- avoid sexually transmitted infections (STIs); or
- prevent pregnancy.

How common is douching?

Douching is common among women in the United States. It's estimated that 20 to 40 percent of American women 15 to 44 years old douche regularly. About half of these women douche each week. Higher rates of douching are seen in teens, African-American women, and Hispanic women.

Is douching safe?

Most doctors and the American College of Obstetricians and Gynecologists (ACOG) recommend that women don't douche. Douching can change the delicate balance of vaginal flora (organisms that live in the vagina) and acidity in a healthy vagina. One way to look at it is in a healthy vagina there are both good and bad bacteria. The balance of the good and bad bacteria help maintain an acidic environment. Any changes can cause an overgrowth of bad bacteria, which can lead to a yeast infection or bacterial vaginosis. Plus, if you have a vaginal infection, douching can push the bacteria causing the infection up into the uterus, fallopian tubes, and ovaries.

What are the dangers linked to douching?

Research shows that women who douche regularly have more health problems than women who don't. Doctors are still unsure whether douching causes these problems. Douching may simply be more common in groups of women who tend to have these issues. Health problems linked to douching include the following:

- Vaginal irritation
- Bacterial vaginosis (BV)
- STIs
- Pelvic inflammatory disease (PID)

Some STIs, BV, and PID can all lead to serious problems during pregnancy. These include infection in the baby, problems with labor, and early delivery.

Should I douche to clean inside my vagina?

No. The American College of Obstetricians and Gynecologists suggests women avoid douching completely. In most cases the vagina's acidic environment "cleans" the vagina. If there is a strong odor or irritation it usually means something is wrong. Douching can increase your chances of infection. The only time you should douche is when your doctor tells you to.

What is the best way to clean my vagina?

Most doctors say it's best to let your vagina clean itself. The vagina cleans itself naturally by making mucous. The mucous washes away blood, semen, and vaginal discharge. You should know that even healthy, clean vaginas may have a mild odor.

Keep the outside of your vagina clean and healthy by washing regularly with warm water and mild soap when you bathe. You should also avoid scented tampons, pads, powders, and sprays. These products may increase your chances of getting a vaginal infection.

417

Should I douche to get rid of vaginal odor, discharge, pain, itching, or burning?

No. You should never douche to try to get rid of vaginal odor, discharge, pain, itching, or burning. Douching will only cover up odor and make other problems worse. It's very important to call your doctor right away if you have the following:

- Vaginal discharge that smells bad
- Thick, white, or yellowish-green discharge with or without an odor
- Burning, redness, and swelling in or around the vagina
- Pain when urinating
- Pain or discomfort during sex

These may be signs of an infection, especially one that may be sexually transmitted. Do not douche before seeing your doctor. This can make it hard for the doctor to figure out what's wrong.

Can douching after sex prevent sexually transmitted infections (STIs)?

No. It's a myth that douching after sex can prevent STIs. The only sure way to prevent STIs is to not have sex. If you do have sex, the best way to prevent STIs is to practice safer sex:

- Be faithful. Have sex with only one partner who has been tested for STIs and is not infected.
- Use latex or female condoms every time you have sex.
- Avoid contact with semen, blood, vaginal fluids, and sores on your partner's genitals.

Can douching after sex stop me from getting pregnant?

No. Douching does not prevent pregnancy. It should never be used for birth control.

Can douching hurt my chances of having a healthy pregnancy?

Douching may affect your chances of having a healthy pregnancy. Limited research shows that douching may make it harder for you to

418

get pregnant. In women trying to get pregnant, those who douched more than once a week took the longest to get pregnant.

Studies also show that douching may increase a woman's chance of damaged fallopian tubes and ectopic pregnancy. Ectopic pregnancy is when the fertilized egg attaches to the inside of the fallopian tube instead of the uterus. If left untreated, ectopic pregnancy can be life-threatening. It can also make it hard for a woman to get pregnant in the future.

Section 41.2

Body Art Allows Exposure to Bloodborne Pathogens Such as HIV

"Body Art," by the National Institute of Occupational
Safety and Health (NIOSH), part of the Centers for Disease Control
and Prevention, January 31, 2011.

Body art is popular and growing with an estimated 16,000 body artists working in the United States today. Body art, which typically consists of tattoos and body piercings, is an art form where the artists' canvas is the human body.

When working on this unique medium, artists may come in contact with a client's blood if they are stuck with the needle that they are using on a client (or stuck with a used needle during disposal), or if the client's blood splashes into the eyes, nose, or mouth. Contact with another person's blood may expose workers to bloodborne pathogens such as hepatitis B virus, hepatitis C virus, or human immunodeficiency virus (HIV). These bloodborne pathogens can be dangerous and may cause permanent illness. If an artist gets one of these viruses, he or she may become ill and be unable to support his or her family. Also, since bloodborne pathogens can be spread through contact with blood and other bodily fluids such as semen and vaginal secretions, sexual partners could also be at risk of getting a bloodborne disease.

In the early 1990s as the body art industry grew, professional associations were formed to promote better business practices in the industry and address safety and health issues. Because of concerns voiced by artists in the industry, NIOSH researchers visited several tattooing and piercing studios and found certain practices used in body piercing and tattooing could increase the chance of an artist coming in contact with blood. NIOSH met with many of the tattooing and piercing professional organizations, other government agencies, scientists and the artists themselves to learn more about body art work practices and what could be done to lower artists' chance of exposure to bloodborne diseases.

To lower exposure to blood, NIOSH recommends using safe work practices and staying informed about problems affecting body artists. Recommendations for protecting tattoo artists and body piercers from bloodborne pathogens include the following:

- Seek emergency medical assistance if an artist is exposed to another person's blood. If a tattooist or piercer is exposed to another person's blood, the artist should notify the shop owner and immediately seek medical attention. If treatment is needed, it is more likely to be effective if it begins soon after the exposure happens.

- Use single-use, disposable needles and razors. Disposable piercing needles, tattoo needles, and razors are used on one person and then thrown away. Reusing needles or razors is not safe.

- Safely dispose of needles and razors. Used needles and razors should be thrown away in a sharps disposal container to protect both the client and the person changing or handling the trash bag from getting cut. Sharps disposal containers must be closeable, puncture resistant, leak-proof, and labeled.

- Wash hands before and after putting on disposable gloves. Gloves are always worn while working with equipment and clients, changed when necessary, and are not reused.

- Clean and sterilize reusable tools and equipment. Some tools and equipment can be reused when tattooing or piercing. Reusable tools and equipment should be cleaned and then sterilized to remove viruses and bacteria.

- Frequently clean surfaces and work areas. Chairs, tables, work spaces, and counters should be disinfected between procedures to protect both the health of the client and the artist. Cross-contamination (spreading bacteria and viruses from one surface to another) can occur if surfaces are not disinfected frequently and between clients. Any disinfectant that claims to be able to eliminate the tuberculosis germ can also kill HIV, hepatitis B, and hepatitis C viruses. Use a commercial disinfectant, following the manufacturer's instructions, or a mixture of bleach and water (one part bleach to nine parts water).

Body artists face unique risks for exposure to bloodborne pathogens, but when proper safety and health practices are followed, these risks can be greatly reduced.

Section 41.3

Injection Drug Use

"Drug-Associated HIV Transmission Continues in the United States," by the Centers for Disease Control and Prevention (CDC, www.cdc.gov), March 8, 2007. Reviewed and revised by David A. Cooke, MD, FACP, July 11, 2012.

Sharing syringes and other equipment for drug injection is a well-known route of HIV [human immunodeficiency virus] transmission, yet injection drug use contributes to the epidemic's spread far beyond the circle of those who inject. People who have sex with an injection drug user (IDU) also are at risk for infection through the sexual transmission of HIV. Children born to mothers who contracted HIV through sharing needles or having sex with an IDU may become infected as well.

Since the epidemic began, injection drug use has directly and indirectly accounted for more than one-third (36%) of AIDS [acquired immunodeficiency syndrome] cases in the United States. This disturbing trend appears to be continuing. Of the 42,156 new cases of AIDS reported in 2000, 11,635 (28%) were IDU-associated.

Racial and ethnic minority populations in the United States are most heavily affected by IDU-associated AIDS. In 2000, IDU-associated AIDS accounted for 26% of all AIDS cases among African-American and 31% among Hispanic adults and adolescents, compared with 19% of all cases among white adults/adolescents.

IDU-associated AIDS accounts for a larger proportion of cases among adolescent and adult women than among men. Since the epidemic began, 57% of all AIDS cases among women have been attributed to injection drug use or sex with partners who inject drugs, compared with 31% of cases among men.

Noninjection drugs (such as "crack" cocaine) also contribute to the spread of the epidemic when users trade sex for drugs or money, or when they engage in risky sexual behaviors that they might not engage in when sober. One CDC study of more than 2,000 young adults in three inner-city neighborhoods found that crack smokers were three times more likely to be infected with HIV than non-smokers.

Strategies for IDUs Must Be Comprehensive

Comprehensive HIV prevention interventions for substance abusers must provide education on how to prevent transmission through sex.

Numerous studies have documented that drug users are at risk for HIV through both drug-related and sexual behaviors, which places their partners at risk as well. Comprehensive programs must provide the information, skills, and support necessary to reduce both risks. Researchers have found that many interventions aimed at reducing sexual risk behaviors among drug users have significantly increased the practice of safer sex (e.g., using condoms, avoiding unprotected sex) among participants.

Drug Treatment Slots Are Scarce

In the United States, drug use and dependence are widespread in the general population. Experts generally agree that there are about 1 million active IDUs in this country, as well as many others who use noninjection drugs or abuse alcohol. Clearly, the need for substance abuse treatment vastly exceeds our capacity to provide it. Effective substance abuse treatment that helps people stop using drugs not only eliminates the risk of HIV transmission from sharing contaminated syringes, but, for many, reduces the risk of engaging in risky behaviors that might result in sexual transmission.

For injection drug users who cannot or will not stop injecting drugs, using sterile needles and syringes only once remains the safest, most effective approach for limiting HIV transmission.

To minimize the risk of HIV transmission, IDUs must have access to interventions that can help them protect their health. They must be advised to always use sterile injection equipment; warned never to reuse needles, syringes, and other injection equipment; and told that using syringes that have been cleaned with bleach or other disinfectants is not as safe as using new, sterile syringes.

Access to Sterile Injection Equipment Is Important

Preventing the spread of HIV through injection drug use requires a comprehensive approach that incorporates several basic principles:

- Ensure coordination and collaboration among all providers of services to IDUs, their sex partners, and their children
- Ensure coverage, access to, and quality of interventions
- Recognize and overcome stigma associated with injection drug use
- Tailor services and programs to the diverse populations and characteristics of IDUs

Strategies for prevention should include the following:

- Preventing initiation of drug injection
- Using community outreach programs to reach drug users on the streets
- Improving access to high quality substance abuse treatment programs
- Instituting HIV prevention programs in jails and prisons
- Providing health care for HIV-infected IDUs
- Making HIV risk-reduction counseling and testing available for IDUs and their sex partners

Although they are often politically controversial, multiple studies have shown that needle exchange programs reduce the transmission of disease among IV drug users and do not increase the rates of IV drug use. Making such programs more widespread is an opportunity to further reduce rates of infection spread.

Better Integration of All Prevention and Treatment Services Is Critically Needed

HIV prevention and treatment, substance abuse prevention, and sexually transmitted disease treatment and prevention services must be better integrated to take advantage of the multiple opportunities for intervention—first, to help the uninfected stay that way; second, to help infected people stay healthy; and third, to help infected individuals initiate and sustain behaviors that will keep themselves safe and prevent transmission to others.

Chapter 42

Talking to Sexual Partners Can Reduce STD Risk

Chapter Contents

Section 42.1—Talking to Your Partner about Condoms............ 426

Section 42.2—Telling Your Partner You Have an STD 429

Section 42.3—Sharing Your HIV Status.................................... 432

Section 42.1

Talking to Your Partner about Condoms

It's much smarter to talk about condoms before having sex, but that doesn't make it easy. Some people—even those who are already having sex—are embarrassed by the topic of condoms. But not talking about condoms affects a person's safety. Using condoms properly every time is the best protection against sexually transmitted disease (STDs)—even if you're using another form of birth control like the Pill.

So how can you overcome your embarrassment about talking about condoms? Well, for starters it can help to know what a condom looks like, how it works, and what it's like to handle one. Buy a box of condoms so you can familiarize yourself.

The next thing to get comfortable with is bringing up the topic of condoms with a partner. Practice opening lines. If you think your partner will object, work out your response ahead of time. Here are some possibilities:

Your partner says: "It's uncomfortable."

You might answer this by suggesting a different brand or size. Wearing a condom also may take some getting used to.

Your partner says: "It puts me right out of the mood."

Say that having unsafe sex puts you right out of the mood. Permanently.

Your partner says: "If we really love each other, we should trust each other."

Say that it's because you love each other so much that you want to be sure you're both safe and protect each other.

Your partner says: "Are you nervous about catching something?"

The natural response: "Sometimes people don't even know when they have infections, so it's better to be safe."

Your partner says: "I won't enjoy sex if we use a condom."

Say you can't enjoy sex unless it's safe.

Your partner says: "I don't know how to put it on."

This one's easy: "Here, let me show you."

Timing

After you've familiarized yourself with condoms and practiced your routine, you'll want to pick the right time to bring up the subject with your partner. A good time to do this is long before you're in a situation where you might need a condom. When people are caught up in the heat of the moment, they may find they're more likely to be pressured into doing something they regret later.

Try bringing up the topic in a matter-of-fact way. You might mention that you've bought some condoms and checked them out. Offer to bring the unopened condoms along. Or suggest that your partner buy his or her favorite brand (and then bring some of yours with you, just to be on the safe side). Offer to try different types of condoms to find which works best for both of you.

Make it clear that you won't have sex without a condom. If someone threatens you or says they'd rather break up than wear a condom, it's time for you to say good-bye. Tell the person you won't have sex with someone who doesn't respect you or themselves enough to use protection.

Here are some tips for using condoms:

- Check the expiration date (condoms can dry and crack if they're old). Don't use a condom if it seems brittle or sticky—throw it away and get another one.

427

- Choose condoms made of latex, which is thought to be more effective in preventing STDs. (If one of you has an allergy to latex, use polyurethane condoms instead.)

- If you use lubricants with condoms, always use water-based ones. Shortening, lotion, petroleum jelly, or baby oil can break down the condom.

- Open the condom packet with your hands, not your teeth, and open it carefully so you don't tear the condom.

- Choose a condom with a reservoir tip to catch semen after ejaculation. Lightly pinch the top of the condom and place it at the top of your (or your partner's) penis. This gets rid of trapped air, which can cause a condom to burst.

- Roll the condom down until it's completely rolled out—if it's inside out, throw it away and start over with a new condom.

- Remove the condom immediately after ejaculation, before the penis softens. You or your partner should hold the condom at the base of the penis (the part nearest the guy's body) while he withdraws to prevent the condom from slipping off.

- Slide the condom off the penis, keeping the semen inside. Since condoms can clog the toilet if they are flushed, tie it off or put in a plastic bag (so it's not a health risk for others) and throw it out.

These aren't the only tips on discussing and using condoms. If you want more advice, talk to your friends, siblings, or parents. Yes, parents. Not everyone feels comfortable talking about sex with their parents, but lots of teens do. Parents often have the best tips.

Health professionals are also great sources of advice on sex and sexuality. A doctor or nurse practitioner or someone at a local health or family planning clinic can offer you advice—confidentially if necessary.

Of course, the only way to be 100% protected from pregnancy and STDs is abstinence (not having sex). But if you do decide to have sex, using a condom allows you to protect yourself.

Section 42.2

Telling Your Partner You Have an STD

Megan and Josh have been friends since middle school, and somehow they always knew they'd end up as a couple. But although they shared all kinds of personal secrets over the years, Megan dreaded telling Josh about her STD [sexually transmitted disease]. After she summoned the nerve to talk about it, she was surprised when Josh said he had the same STD—and was wondering how he would tell her.

First, Get Tested

Sexually transmitted diseases—or STDs—affect the body, but living with one can be a strain on a person's emotions as well. If you have an STD, you might feel alone—but you're not. STDs are incredibly common. Luckily, many can be cured. And those that can't (like herpes or HIV/AIDS [human immunodeficiency virus/acquired immunodeficiency syndrome]) can still be treated to help with symptoms, although the infection can still spread to other people.

The trouble happens when people feel perfectly fine and show no signs of having an STD. Since they don't know, they don't get treated. That causes bigger problems because STDs don't just go away on their own. Without treatment, the infection stays in the body and could cause permanent health problems or spread to other people. That's why doctors recommend that people who are having sex (or who have had sex in the past) get tested regularly for STDs.

Why People Need to Tell Their Partners

So what do you do if your test comes back positive? One of the first steps is to tell any sexual partners—past, present, and future. Why?

Their health is at risk, so they need to know what's going on. It's natural to feel apprehensive, even scared, at the thought of discussing your disease. You may worry about rejection and rumors. But to protect your partner (and avoid any future embarrassment or misunderstanding), it's a conversation you need to have.

Need more reasons?

- Not telling a partner about an STD after a confirmed diagnosis may be a criminal offense in some states.

- Some STDs can affect fertility later in life if they're not treated early on.

- Some STDs can cause life-threatening infections, especially if they're not recognized and treated.

- If you're treated for a curable STD but your partner hasn't been, you can get reinfected.

- Telling a future partner allows that person to make an informed decision about his or her own health—such as taking precautions to prevent the spread of disease.

- Telling a past or current partner gives that person the opportunity to get checked out and, if necessary, treated.

Telling a New Partner about an STD

If you have an STD, it's normal to be nervous about telling someone new. Everyone raises the subject differently. Here are some ideas for handling the conversation:

Try imagining that your roles are reversed. What would you expect your partner to do and say if he or she were in your shoes?

Be proud of your intentions. Your willingness to have this difficult conversation shows that you care about the other person and your relationship. We're all more likely to trust and respect people who are honest (and brave!) enough to talk about tough topics like STDs.

It's best to be direct. You could start by saying, "Before we have sex, I want us to talk about STDs and protection. Because I have an STD." Mention the type of STD you have and how you got it. You don't have to share every detail of your past relationships, but showing that you're open to talking and answering questions can help your partner feel more comfortable, too.

It's best to be honest. You may worry about rumors spreading—but isn't it better for your partner to find out because you said something rather than wake up one day with an infection? People are more likely to respect someone's privacy if they feel that person has also respected them.

Allow the conversation to proceed naturally. Listen rather than doing all the talking. Prepare for your partner to be surprised. Each person reacts differently to the news. Some might panic. Some might be full of questions. Others might just need to time to think.

Don't push your partner to make decisions about sex or your relationship right away. It's normal to want acceptance and reassurance after revealing such personal information. But give the other person some space. Making a suggestion like "I know you probably want some time to think about this" shows that you're confident and in control.

Encourage your partner to ask questions. During the conversation, offer information and facts about the STD and its symptoms, such as whether it can be treated or cured. You may want to bring an article or booklet about your STD to give to your partner. If you can't answer all of your partner's questions, that's OK. Say you don't know and then go online together to learn more.

If you and your partner decide not to have sexual intercourse (vaginal, anal, or oral sex), there are other ways you can be intimate or express your feelings for one another. If you do decide to have intercourse, use condoms and practice safe sex techniques.

Telling a Current Partner about an STD

Being diagnosed with an STD while in a relationship can provoke many emotions. You may even begin to question your trust in your partner. Before you blame your partner for infidelity, though, keep in mind that some STDs don't always cause symptoms right away. It is possible that you or your partner contracted the STD in a previous relationship without even knowing it.

These feelings can be hard to confront. But the most important thing to remember is that you and your partner both need to receive medical care as soon as possible.

If you find out that you have an STD while you are in a relationship, talk to your partner as soon as possible. Be honest and straightforward—even if you haven't been in the past. Remember that your partner may be upset and possibly angry, so try to be sensitive.

The most helpful thing you can do is listen to your partner's concerns and fears and offer information about the STD and its symptoms. Give your partner time to absorb this information.

If you and your partner have already had sex, stop until you can both get tested. Talk to a doctor. If you have a curable STD, you will probably need to take medicine as part of your treatment. Take all of your medication exactly as your doctor prescribes and schedule a follow-up exam to make sure the STD is completely gone.

You also might need to take medication if you have an STD, like herpes, that can't be cured. A doctor or a health clinic can give advice on how to avoid passing the infection to your sexual partner.

If you're diagnosed with an STD and you think you've had it for a while, you need to let past sexual partners know. They should get tested, too.

It may be emotionally uncomfortable, but telling partners about STDs is the right thing to do. If you think you have an STD or you have questions about STDs, talk to a doctor, sexual health clinic, or student health center.

Section 42.3

Sharing Your HIV Status

This section includes text from "Do You Have To Tell?," August 23, 2009, and "Sexual Partners," August 24, 2009, by AIDSinfo.gov, part of the U.S. Department of Health and Human Services.

Do You Have to Tell?

After you are diagnosed with HIV (human immunodeficiency virus), you will have to decide whether to share that information with other people, and—if so—whom you should tell.

It is very important that you talk to your current and past sexual partners about your HIV status. If you have shared needles with others to inject drugs, you need to tell them, too. If you are afraid or embarrassed to tell them yourself, the health department in your area can notify your sexual or needle-sharing partners that they may have been exposed to HIV without giving your name.

Disclosure can be a tough process, but you don't have to face it alone. Talk to your healthcare provider and ask for help in finding support groups or other individuals who can help you in the disclosure process.

Sharing your HIV status with those you trust—such as family members, friends, and children—can help with the stresses of having HIV, and can actually improve your overall health. Disclosing your status to your healthcare provider is important to make sure that you receive the best care for your HIV.

In most cases, sharing your HIV status is a personal choice—but it may also be a legal requirement. Many states have laws that require you to tell specific people about your HIV status.

Before you decide to tell people that you are HIV-positive, here are some things to consider:

1. Think about the people you rely on for support, like family, friends, or coworkers.

2. What kind of relationship do you have with these people? What are the pros and cons of telling them you are living with HIV?

3. Are there particular issues a person might have that will affect how much he or she can support you?

4. What is that person's attitude and knowledge about HIV?

5. Why do you want to disclose to this person? What kind of support can this person provide?

6. For each person you want to tell, ask yourself if the person needs to know now—or if it's better to wait.

Sexual Partners

Partner Counseling and Referral Services (PCRS)

Once you have been diagnosed, you will be asked to identify your sexual and needle-sharing partners, so that they can be told that they have been exposed to HIV [human immunodeficiency virus] and need to be tested. Partner notification is one of the most important ways to prevent the spread of HIV. (It's also important, of course, that you use a condom during sex and don't share needles.)

The Partner Counseling and Referral Service (PCRS) can help you with notifying your partner(s). Most state public health departments have a PCRS program. PCRS can also help your partner(s) get counseling, a medical evaluation, treatment, and any other services they may need.

Notifying and Testing Partners

Once you have identified your partners, they should be notified as soon as possible. This gives them an opportunity to protect themselves from infection if they don't have HIV—or, if they are having sex or sharing needles with others—to take steps to protect or notify those partners.

Notification can happen in four ways:

- Provider referral means that your healthcare provider notifies your partner(s) for you.

- Self-referral means that you notify your partner(s) yourself.

- Contract referral means that you make a contract to notify your partner(s) by a particular date. If, by the contract date, your partners have not come in for counseling and testing, the health department will contact them.

- Dual referral means that you and the health department will notify your partner(s) together.

If your partner(s) are notified by your healthcare provider or the health department, they will also be given information about where they can get tested for HIV and where they can find treatment if they need it. Healthcare officials would prefer that people get tested for HIV at the same time they're notified because not everyone follows through on going to the testing sites.

It's possible for your partner(s) to test negative for HIV even when they are already infected if they take the test during the window period. That's the time between when a person is infected with HIV and the time that the body develops antibodies to the virus. Partners are advised to be retested three months after the date of their last known exposure.

Disclosing without Patient Consent

A physician or HIV counselor may disclose a patient's HIV status without his or her consent only under the following conditions:

- The physician or counselor has made a reasonable effort to counsel and encourage the patient to voluntarily provide this information to the spouse or sexual partner.

- The physician or counselor reasonably believes the patient will not provide the information to the spouse or sexual partner.

- Disclosure is necessary to protect the health of the spouse or sexual partner.

Chapter 43

Talking to Your Child or Teen about STDs

Sometimes it's difficult to see your child as anything but that: A child. Yet, in many ways, teens today are growing up faster than ever. They learn about violence and sex through the media and their peers, but they rarely have all the facts. That's why it's so important for you to talk to your kids about sex, particularly sexually transmitted diseases (STDs).

Teens are one of the groups most at risk for contracting STDs. You can help your kids stay safe by talking to them and sharing some important information about STDs and prevention.

Before you tackle this sensitive subject, however, it's important to make sure you not only know what to say, but how and when to say it.

Timing Is Everything

It's never too late to talk to your kids about STDs, even if they're already teens. A late talk is better than no talk at all. But the best time to start having these discussions is some time during the preteen years.

"STDs," August 2011, reprinted with permission from www.kidshealth.org. This information was provided by KidsHealth®, one of the largest resources online for medically reviewed health information written for parents, kids, and teens. For more articles like this, visit www.KidsHealth.org, or www.TeensHealth.org. Copyright © 1995–2012 The Nemours Foundation. All rights reserved.

Of course, the exact age varies from child to child: Some kids are more aware of sex at age 9 than others are at age 11. You'll need to read your child's cues.

No matter how old your child is, if he or she starts having questions about sex, it's a good time to talk about STDs.

Questions are a good starting point for a discussion. When kids are curious, they're often more open to hearing what their parents have to say.

But not all kids ask their parents questions about sex. One way to initiate a discussion is to use a media cue, like a TV program, a movie, or an article in the paper, and ask what your child thinks about it.

Another way is to use the human papillomavirus (HPV) vaccine as a starting point for a conversation. The HPV vaccine is recommended for preteen girls (and also boys), and has the best chance of protecting against infection if the series of shots is given before someone becomes sexually active.

The surest way to have a healthy dialogue is to establish lines of communication early on. If parents aren't open to talking about sex or other personal subjects when their kids are young, kids will be a lot less likely to seek out mom or dad when they're older and have questions.

Spend time talking with your kids from the beginning and it'll be much easier later to broach topics like sex because they'll feel more comfortable sharing thoughts with you.

Tips for Talking

To make talking about STDs a little easier for both you and your kids:

- Be informed. STDs can be a frightening and confusing subject, so it may help if you read up on STD transmission and prevention. You don't want to add any misinformation and being familiar with the topic will make you feel more comfortable. If kids ask for information that you're not sure about, find out the answer from a reliable source and get back to them.

- Ask what your kids already know about STDs and what else they'd like to learn. Remember, though: Kids often already know more than you realize, although much of that information could be incorrect. Parents need to provide accurate information so their kids can make the right decisions and protect themselves.

- Ask what your kids think about sexual scenarios on TV and in movies and use those fictional situations as a way to talk about safe sex and risky behavior.

- Encourage your kids to raise any fears, questions, or concerns they have.

- Make your kids feel that they're in charge of this talk, not you, by getting their opinions on whatever you discuss. If you let their questions lead the way, you'll have a much more productive talk than if you stick to an agenda or give a lecture.

- Explain that the only sure way to remain STD-free is to not have sex or intimate contact with anyone outside of a committed, monogamous relationship, such as marriage. However, those who are having sex should always use condoms to protect against STDs, even when using another method of birth control. Most condoms are made of latex, but both male and female condoms made of polyurethane are available for people with a latex allergy.

Common Questions about STDs

Depending on what your kids have heard from friends and the media, their questions will probably be fairly straightforward, such as:

- **What is an STD?** An STD is a sexually transmitted disease.

- **How does someone catch one?** These infections and diseases are spread from one individual to another during anal, oral, or vaginal sex. They also can be spread by fingers or objects after they have touched genitals or body fluids.

- **What do STDs do to a person's body?** The type of STD determines what kinds of symptoms, if any, someone has. Some STDs cause virtually no symptoms, whereas others can cause the person to have discharge from the vagina or penis, sores, or pain. But even when there are no symptoms, if STDs are untreated, they can lead to damage to the internal organs and may cause long-term health problems, like infertility or cancer. This is why anyone who has had any type of sex (vaginal, oral, or anal) needs to be tested for STDs regularly.

- **Are STDs curable or do you have them forever?** Some STDs like chlamydia and gonorrhea can be cured with antibiotics, but some infections—like herpes or HIV—have no cure.

- **Are people who catch STDs somehow bad?** Getting an STD does not mean that someone is a bad person, just that he or she needs to learn how to prevent future infections.

- **Can you tell that someone has an STD just by looking at him or her?** People often may not even know that they're infected themselves. Although there may be visible signs around the genitals with certain kinds of STDs, like genital warts and herpes, most of the time, there is no way to look at someone and know that he or she has an STD.

Answering any of these questions or others as openly as possible is the best approach. It's up to you to gently correct any misinformation your kids may have learned. And always answer questions honestly without being overly dramatic.

It can be tough, but try not to be too emotional or preachy. You want your kids to know that you're there to support and help, not condemn.

Finding Reliable Information

Communicating with your kids may not be simple, but it's necessary. If you're always available to talk, discussions will come easier. Literature from your doctor's office or organizations like Planned Parenthood can provide answers.

And websites like TeensHealth.org discuss STDs and sex in teen-friendly language. Viewing them together can help you and your kids start talking.

Your child's school can be an information resource. Find out when sexuality will be covered in health or science class and read the texts that will be taught. The PTA (Parent Teacher Association) may even offer sessions about talking to teens where you can share tips and experiences with other parents.

And don't shy away from discussing STDs or sex out of fear that talking will make kids want to have sex. Informed teens are not more likely to have sex; but when they do become sexually active they are more likely to practice safe sex.

If you try these tactics and still don't feel comfortable talking about STDs, make sure your kids can talk to someone who will have accurate information: A doctor, counselor, school nurse, teacher, or another family member.

Kids and teens need to know about STDs, and it's better that they get the facts from someone trustworthy instead of discovering them on their own.

Chapter 44

Sex Education and STD Prevention

Chapter Contents

Section 44.1—Overview of Sex Education 440

Section 44.2—What Programs Effectively Prevent STDs
in Youth? 448

Section 44.3—Are Abstinence Only Sexual Education
Programs Effective? 450

Section 44.4—Behavioral Intervention May Reduce
STD Rates 460

Section 44.1

Overview of
Sex Education

What Is Sex Education?

Sex education, which is sometimes called sexuality education or sex and relationships education, is the process of acquiring information and forming attitudes and beliefs about sex, sexual identity, relationships, and intimacy. Sex education is also about developing young people's skills so that they make informed choices about their behavior, and feel confident and competent about acting on these choices. It is widely accepted that young people have a right to sex education. This is because it is a means by which they are helped to protect themselves against abuse, exploitation, unintended pregnancies, sexually transmitted diseases, and HIV [human immunodeficiency virus] and AIDS [acquired immunodeficiency syndrome]. It is also argued that providing sex education helps to meet young people's rights to information about matters that affect them, their right to have their needs met, and to help them enjoy their sexuality and the relationships that they form.

What Are the Aims of Sex Education?

Sex education aims to reduce the risks of potentially negative outcomes from sexual behavior, such as unwanted or unplanned pregnancies and infection with sexually transmitted diseases including HIV. It also aims to contribute to young people's positive experience of their sexuality by enhancing the quality of their relationships and their ability to make informed decisions over their lifetime. Sex education that works, by which we mean that it is effective, is sex education that contributes to both these aims thus helping young people to be safe and enjoy their sexuality.

What Skills Should Sex Education Develop?

If sex education is going to be effective it needs to include opportunities for young people to develop skills, as it can be hard for them to act on the basis of only having information.

The skills young people develop as part of sex education are linked to more general life-skills. Being able to communicate, listen, negotiate with others, ask for and identify sources of help and advice, are useful life-skills which can be applied to sexual relationships. Effective sex education develops young people's skills in negotiation, decision-making, assertion, and listening. Other important skills include being able to recognize pressures from other people and to resist them, dealing with and challenging prejudice, and being able to seek help from adults—including parents, carers, and professionals—through the family, community, and health and welfare services.

Sex education that works also helps equip young people with the skills to be able to differentiate between accurate and inaccurate information, and to discuss a range of moral and social issues and perspectives on sex and sexuality, including different cultural attitudes and sensitive issues like sexuality, abortion, and contraception.

Forming Attitudes and Beliefs

Young people can be exposed to a wide range of attitudes and beliefs in relation to sex and sexuality. These sometimes appear contradictory and confusing. For example, some health messages emphasize the risks and dangers associated with sexual activity and some media coverage promotes the idea that being sexually active makes a person more attractive and mature. Because sex and sexuality are sensitive subjects, young people and sex educators can have strong views on what attitudes people should hold, and what moral framework should govern people's behavior—these too can sometimes seem to be at odds. Young people can be very interested in the moral and cultural frameworks that bind sex and sexuality. They often welcome opportunities to talk about issues where people have strong views, like abortion, sex before marriage, lesbian and gay issues, and contraception and birth control. It is important to remember that talking in a balanced way about differences in opinion does not promote one set of views over another, or mean that one agrees with a particular view. Part of exploring and understanding cultural, religious, and moral views is finding out that you can agree to disagree.

441

People providing sex education have attitudes and beliefs of their own about sex and sexuality and it is important not to let these influence negatively the sex education that they provide. For example, even if a person believes that young people should not have sex until they are married, this does not imply withholding important information about safer sex and contraception. Attempts to impose narrow moralistic views about sex and sexuality on young people through sex education have failed. Rather than trying to deter or frighten young people away from having sex, effective sex education includes work on attitudes and beliefs, coupled with skills development, that enables young people to choose whether or not to have a sexual relationship taking into account the potential risks of any sexual activity.

Effective sex education also provides young people with an opportunity to explore the reasons why people have sex, and to think about how it involves emotions, respect for one self and other people and their feelings, decisions, and bodies. Young people should have the chance to explore gender differences and how ethnicity and sexuality can influence people's feelings and options. They should be able to decide for themselves what the positive qualities of relationships are. It is important that they understand how bullying, stereotyping, abuse, and exploitation can negatively influence relationships.

So What Information Should Be Given to Young People?

Young people get information about sex and sexuality from a wide range of sources including each other, through the media including advertising, television, and magazines, as well as leaflets, books, and websites (such as www.avert.org) which are intended to be sources of information about sex and sexuality. Some of this will be accurate and some inaccurate. Providing information through sex education is therefore about finding out what young people already know and adding to their existing knowledge and correcting any misinformation they may have. For example, young people may have heard that condoms are not effective against HIV or that there is a cure for AIDS. It is important to provide information which corrects mistaken beliefs. Without correct information young people can put themselves at greater risk.

Information is also important as the basis on which young people can develop well-informed attitudes and views about sex and sexuality. Young people need to have information on all the following topics:

- Sexual development and reproduction: The physical and emotional changes associated with puberty and sexual reproduction, including fertilization and conception, as well as sexually transmitted diseases and HIV.

- Contraception and birth control: What contraceptives there are, how they work, how people use them, how they decide what to use or not, and how they can be obtained.

- Relationships: What kinds of relationships there are, love and commitment, marriage and partnership, and the law relating to sexual behavior and relationships as well as the range of religious and cultural views on sex and sexuality and sexual diversity.

In addition, young people should be provided with information about abortion, sexuality, and confidentiality, as well as about the range of sources of advice and support that is available in the community and nationally.

When Should Sex Education Start?

Sex education that works starts early, before young people reach puberty, and before they have developed established patterns of behavior. The precise age at which information should be provided depends on the physical, emotional, and intellectual development of the young people as well as their level of understanding. What is covered and also how, depends on who is providing the sex education, when they are providing it, and in what context, as well as what the individual young person wants to know about.

It is important for sex education to begin at a young age and also that it is sustained. Giving young people basic information from an early age provides the foundation on which more complex knowledge is built up over time. For example, when they are very young, children can be informed about how people grow and change over time, and how babies become children and then adults, and this provides the basis on which they understand more detailed information about puberty provided in the pre-teenage years. They can also when they are young, be provided with information about viruses and germs that attack the body. This provides the basis for talking to them later about infections that can be caught through sexual contact.

Does Sex Education at an Early Age Encourage Young People to Have Sex?

Some people are concerned that providing information about sex and sexuality arouses curiosity and can lead to sexual experimentation.

However, in a review of 48 studies of comprehensive sex and STD/HIV education programmes in U.S. schools, there was found to be strong evidence that such programmes did not increase sexual activity. Some of them reduced sexual activity, or increased rates of condom use or other contraceptives, or both. It is important to remember that young people can store up information provided at any time, for a time when they need it later on.

When Should Parents Start Talking to Young People about Sex?

Sometimes it can be difficult for adults to know when to raise issues, but the important thing is to maintain an open relationship with children which provides them with opportunities to ask questions when they have them. Parents and carers can also be proactive and engage young people in discussions about sex, sexuality, and relationships. Naturally, many parents and their children feel embarrassed about talking about some aspects of sex and sexuality. Viewing sex education as an on-going conversation about values, attitudes, and issues as well as providing facts can be helpful. The best basis to proceed on is a sound relationship in which a young person feels able to ask a question or raise an issue if they feel they need to. It has been shown that in countries like The Netherlands, where many families regard it as an important responsibility to talk openly with children about sex and sexuality, this contributes to greater cultural openness about sex and sexuality and improved sexual health among young people.

The role of many parents and carers as sex educators changes as young people get older and are provided with more opportunities to receive formal sex education through schools and community settings. However, it doesn't get any less important. Because sex education in school tends to take place in blocks of time, it can't always address issues relevant to young people at a particular time, and parents can fulfill a particularly important role in providing information and opportunities to discuss things as they arise.

Who Should Provide Sex Education?

Sex education can take place in a variety of settings, both in and out of school. In these different contexts, different people have the opportunity and responsibility to provide sex education for young people.

Parents/Carers

At home, young people can easily have one-to-one discussions with parents or carers which focus on specific issues, questions, or concerns. They can have a dialogue about their attitudes and views. Sex education at home also tends to take place over a long time, and involve lots of short interactions between parents and children. There may be times when young people seem reluctant to talk, but it is important not to interpret any diffidence as meaning that there is nothing left to talk about. As young people get older advantage can be taken of opportunities provided by things seen on television for example, as an opportunity to initiate conversation. It is also important not to defer dealing with a question or issue for too long as it can suggest that you are unwilling to talk about it. There is evidence that positive parent-child communication about sexual matters can lead to greater condom use among young men and a lower rate of teenage conception among young women.

Teachers

In school the interaction between the teacher and young people takes a different form and is often provided in organized blocks of lessons. It is not as well suited to advising the individual as it is to providing information from an impartial point of view. The most effective sex education acknowledges the different contributions each setting can make. School programmes which involve parents, notifying them what is being taught and when, can support the initiation of dialogue at home. Parents and schools both need to engage with young people about the messages that they get from the media, and give them opportunities for discussion.

Young People

In some countries, the involvement of young people themselves in developing and providing sex education has increased as a means of ensuring the relevance and accessibility of provision. Consultation with young people at the point when programmes are designed, helps ensure that they are relevant and the involvement of young people in delivering programmes may reinforce messages as they model attitudes and behavior to their peers. As part of their school-based Sex and Relationship Education programme, the UK-based organization Apause involves peer-educators to achieve positive behavior change among students aged 13 and 14, with an aim to reduce the rates of first intercourse before the age of 16.

Effective School-Based Sex Education

School-based sex education can be an important and effective way of enhancing young people's knowledge, attitudes, and behavior. There is widespread agreement that formal education should include sex education and what works has been well-researched. Evidence suggests that effective school programmes will include the following elements:

- A focus on reducing specific risky behaviors

- A basis in theories which explain what influences people's sexual choices and behavior

- A clear and continuously reinforced message about sexual behavior and risk reduction

- Providing accurate information about, the risks associated with sexual activity, about contraception and birth control, and about methods of avoiding or deferring intercourse

- Dealing with peer and other social pressures on young people; providing opportunities to practice communication, negotiation, and assertion skills

- Uses a variety of approaches to teaching and learning that involve and engage young people and help them to personalize the information

- Uses approaches to teaching and learning which are appropriate to young people's age, experience, and cultural background

- Is provided by people who believe in what they are saying and have access to support in the form of training or consultation with other sex educators

Formal programs with all these elements have been shown to increase young people's levels of knowledge about sex and sexuality, put back the average age at which they first have sexual intercourse, and decrease risk when they do have sex.

In addition to this, effective sex education is supported by links to sexual health services and takes into account the messages about sexual values and behavior young people get from other sources (such as friends and the media). It is also responsive to the needs of the young people themselves—whether they are girls or boys, on their own or in a single sex or mixed sex group, and what they know already, their age, and experiences.

In 2010 the UK [United Kingdom] missed an important opportunity to introduce structured, compulsory sex and relationship education in all English state schools. The measure, seen by many as controversial, had been designed by government to ensure all 15-year-olds would receive sex education. The Labour Secretary of State for Children, Schools and Families, Ed Balls MP, described his disappointment that political opponents "could not agree to make personal, social, and health education statutory."

Taking Sex Education Forward

Providing effective sex education can seem daunting because it means tackling potentially sensitive issues and involving a variety of people—parents, schools, community groups, and health service providers. However, because sex education comprises many individual activities, which take place across a wide range of settings and periods of time, there are lots of opportunities to contribute.

The nature of a person's contribution depends on their relationship, role, and expertise in relation to young people. For example, parents are best placed in relation to young people to provide continuity of individual support and education starting from early in their lives. School-based education programs are particularly good at providing information and opportunities for skills development and attitude clarification in more formal ways, through lessons within a curriculum. Community-based projects provide opportunities for young people to access advice and information in less formal ways. Sexual health and other health and welfare services can provide access to specific information, support, and advice. Sex education through the mass media, often supported by local, regional, or national government and non-governmental agencies and departments, can help to raise public awareness of sex health issues.

Further development of sex education partly depends on joining up these elements in a coherent way to meet the needs of young people. There is also a need to pay more attention to the needs of specific groups of young people like young parents, young lesbian, gay, and bisexual people, as well as those who may be out of touch with services and schools and socially vulnerable, like young refugees and asylum-seekers, young people in care, young people in prisons, and also those living on the street.

The circumstances and context available to parents and other sex educators are different from place to place. Practical or political realities in a particular country may limit people's ability to provide young people with comprehensive sex education combining all the elements in the best way possible. But the basic principles outlined here apply everywhere. By making our own contribution and valuing that made by others, and by being guided by these principles, we can provide more sex education that works and improve the support we offer to young people.

Section 44.2

What Programs Effectively Prevent STDs in Youth?

Excerpted from "Effective HIV and STD Prevention
Programs for Youth," by the Centers for Disease Control and
Prevention (CDC, www.cdc.gov), July 12, 2011.

Just as schools are critical settings for preparing students academically, they are also vital partners in helping young people take responsibility for their own health. School health programs can help youth adopt lifelong attitudes and behaviors that support overall health and well-being—including behaviors that can reduce their risk for HIV [human immunodeficiency virus] and other sexually transmitted diseases (STDs).

HIV/STD prevention programs implemented by schools include prevention education programs designed specifically to reduce sexual risk behaviors and youth asset-development programs, which provide adolescents with more general skills that help them engage in healthy behaviors and solve problems.

Effective HIV/STD Prevention Education Programs

Research shows that well-designed and well-implemented HIV/STD prevention programs can decrease sexual risk behaviors among students, including the following:

- Delaying first sexual intercourse
- Reducing the number of sex partners

- Decreasing the number of times students have unprotected sex

- Increasing condom use

A review of 48 research studies found that about two-thirds of the HIV/STD prevention programs studied had a significant impact on reducing sexual risk behaviors, including a delay in first sexual intercourse, a decline in the number of sex partners, and an increase in condom or contraceptive use. Notably, the HIV prevention programs were not shown to hasten initiation of sexual intercourse among adolescents, even when those curricula encouraged sexually active young people to use condoms.

In addition to determining programs that are most effective in reducing sexual health risk behaviors among youth, scientists also have identified key common attributes among these programs. Effective HIV/STD prevention programs tend to be those that have the following characteristics:

- Are delivered by trained instructors

- Are age-appropriate

- Include components on skill-building, support of healthy behaviors in school environments, and involvement of parents, youth-serving organizations, and health organizations

Traits common among effective programs should guide the development of curricula and the integration of program activities for HIV/STD prevention in schools and communities.

Youth Asset-Development Programs: A Promising Approach

A second approach to HIV prevention seeks to increase the skills of children and adolescents to avoid health risks, including sexual risk behaviors. Youth asset-development programs, including those conducted in schools, teach youth how to solve problems, communicate with others, and plan for the future. They also help youth develop positive connections with their parents, schools, and communities.

Youth asset-development programs typically address multiple health risk behaviors and are commonly provided to children and adolescents over a number of years. Evidence indicates that these programs can be associated with long-term reductions in sexual risk behaviors.

449

Section 44.3

Are Abstinence Only Sexual Education Programs Effective?

In recent years there has been discussion about what form sex education should take, and the advantages and disadvantages of adopting an abstinence based approach as an alternative to a more comprehensive approach. Despite recent changes in public policy within the United States which has seen a cessation of federal funding for abstinence only programs of sex education, programs of this kind continue in both the United States, other parts of the developed world, and are even expanding in some of the countries most affected by HIV [human immunodeficiency virus] and AIDS [acquired immunodeficiency syndrome] because of funding made available through the PEPFAR (President's Emergency Plan For AIDS Relief) program.

What Is an Abstinence Based Approach to Sex Education?

An abstinence based approach to sex education focuses on teaching young people that abstaining from sex until marriage is the best means of ensuring that they avoid infection with HIV, other sexually transmitted infections, and unintended pregnancy. As well as seeing abstinence from sex as the best option for maintaining sexual health, many supporters of abstinence based approaches to sex education also believe that it is morally wrong for people to have sex before they are married. Abstinence approaches are represented in programs such as Aspire and True Love Waits (both developed in the United States), which aim to teach young people that they should commit to abstaining from sex until marriage.

Although not all abstinence education programs are the same, they share the fundamental purpose of teaching the social, psychological, and health gains to be realized by abstaining from sexual activity. As such, abstinence education tends to include the following teaching objectives, which are derived from a definition given in Federal Law in the United States:

- abstinence from sexual activity outside marriage is the expected standard for all school age children;

- abstinence from sexual activity is the only certain way to avoid out of wedlock pregnancy, sexually transmitted diseases, and other associated health problems;

- a mutually faithful, monogamous relationship in the context of marriage is the expected standard of sexual activity;

- sexual activity outside the context of marriage is likely to have harmful psychological and physical effects;

- bearing children out of wedlock is likely to have harmful consequences for the child, the child's parents, and society;

- how to reject sexual advances and that alcohol and drug use increases vulnerability to sexual advances;

- the importance of attaining self-sufficiency before engaging in sexual activity.

How Does This Differ from Comprehensive Sex Education?

The main difference between abstinence based and comprehensive approaches to sex education is that comprehensive approaches do not focus either solely or so closely on teaching young people that they should abstain from sex until they are married. Although comprehensive approaches do explain to young people the potential benefits of delaying having sex until they are emotionally and physically ready, they also make sure that they are taught how to protect themselves from infections and pregnancy when they do decide to have sex. In the United Kingdom, this approach has been taken by the organization Apause, which includes the postponement of first intercourse as part of their wider school-based Sex and Relationships Education program.

Descriptions of what programs of comprehensive sex education comprise are contained in guidelines produced by SIECUS (Sexuality Information and Education Council of the United States) and UNESCO [United Nations Educational, Scientific, and Cultural Organization].

Can Abstinence Based and Comprehensive Approaches to Sex Education Be Combined?

Some people have argued that is it possible to combine the main elements of both comprehensive and abstinence based approaches to sex education in one approach. These people point out that supporters of both abstinence based and comprehensive approaches share the view that sex education plays an important role in HIV prevention and both approaches emphasize the potential benefits of delaying having sexual intercourse in terms of helping young people avoid HIV, other STIs, and unintended pregnancies. On the basis of this it has been argued that abstinence based and comprehensive approaches can be reconciled into one inclusive approach which is sometimes called abstinence plus.

In abstinence plus sex education, although the main emphasis is on abstaining from sex as the preferred choice of protection, young people are also provided with information about contraception and disease prevention so that they can protect themselves when they do become sexually active. One example of an abstinence plus approach is the United States developed Reducing the Risk. The RISK approach comprises of a school based curricula which explicitly emphasize that students should avoid unprotected intercourse, either by not having sex or (for students who choose to have sex) by using contraceptives.

So Why Is There So Much Disagreement?

Despite the similarities in some of the things that supporters of abstinence based and comprehensive approaches believe about sex education and what it can achieve in terms of young people's sexual health, it is probably overly optimistic to think that it is possible to build consensus on a single approach. This is because these superficial similarities mask profound differences in the values and attitudes which inform the views of supporters of abstinence based and comprehensive sex education.

Moral and religious views: Many supporters of abstinence based sex education have a background in or connection to Christian organizations that have strong views about sex and sexuality. Not only do they often believe that sex should only take place in the context of marriage, but some are also opposed to same sex relationships and abortion. As a result of the strong faith basis for their beliefs about sex, supporters of abstinence education see the main objective as being to equip (and encourage) young people to refuse or avoid sex altogether, and they may exclude from their programs any other information that they believe conflicts with this view. This may result in an abstinence only course failing to include basic information about what activities transmit HIV and how such transmission can be avoided.

Even where supporters of abstinence based sex education disavow a strong religious basis for their beliefs about what young people should be taught, they often highlight issues about fidelity to one partner, and reject provision of information about steps young people can take to protect themselves against disease and unintended pregnancy because they argue that to do so sends a mixed message.

In contrast, most supporters of comprehensive sex education regard having sex and issues to do with sexuality as matters of personal choice that should not be dictated by religious or political dogmas. Working from an understanding of human rights, which means that people are entitled to access information about matters that affect them and the decisions that they make, they see sex education as being about providing young people with the means by which they can protect themselves against abuse and exploitation as well as unintended pregnancies, sexually transmitted diseases, and HIV/AIDS. They argue that without access to information about all aspects of sex and sexuality making these decisions freely is impossible. While they think that it is important that sex education is sensitive to faith issues, they assert that sex education should not be based on any set of specific religious values.

Different problem, different solution: These fundamentally different views about sex and sexuality mean that supporters of abstinence based and comprehensive approaches to sex education see the problem of what to do about young people and sex quite differently and therefore reach quite different conclusions about the solution. If, as supporters of comprehensive sex education tend to believe, the underlying premise of sexual health interventions is to meet social and utilitarian ideals then the solutions that are proposed are more likely to include earlier and more comprehensive sex education, more liberal abortion laws, and freely available contraception. By contrast if, as supporters of abstinence based approaches feel, the underlying motive has a strong religious dimension then the solutions are more likely to revolve around abstinence campaigns and be characterized by reluctance to promote contraception.

But Which Method of Sex Education Is Best?

One of the ways in which the debate between supporters of abstinence and comprehensive approaches to sex education has been framed is in terms of which is the most effective.

Although at first glance the evidence can seem confusing, with claims coming from both groups about the proven effectiveness of programs embodying their values, when only the most reliable studies are taken into account the position is clear. There is good evidence, from reviews of studies and studies of programs implemented in the United States, United Kingdom, and other European countries and countries in Africa and Asia, that comprehensive sex education can reduce behaviors that put young people at risk of HIV, STIs, and unintended pregnancy. Studies have repeatedly shown too that this kind of sex education does not lead to the earlier onset of sexual activity among young people and, in some cases, will even lead to it happening later.

In contrast, there is no such robust evidence for the effectiveness of abstinence education. Almost all the studies that have claimed to show any positive outcomes are not well enough designed to sustain these claims so it is not possible to infer whether they work or not from the research reports. Several academic reviews suggest that abstinence only programs generally have no effects on young people's sexual behavior. In just a few cases abstinence only programs may encourage young people to delay first sexual intercourse in the short-term. Worryingly, some of these studies also suggest that compared to other young people those who do receive abstinence only programs may be less knowledgeable about STDs and less likely to believe that condoms provide effective protection against them.

What Does Research Show about the Effects of Abstinence Based Approaches?

The research that is available currently shows at best mixed outcomes for abstinence based approaches to sex education, benefiting some young people in the short term but placing them at greater risks later.

Two studies suggest that for some young people making pledges to abstain from sexual intercourse until marriage does lead to delay in the timing of their first sexual intercourse. But these young people tend to hold strong religious beliefs and enjoy being an exclusive group among peers who do not take abstinence pledges. This means that pledging abstinence is not appropriate for young people who do not hold strong religious views and, moreover, if lots of young people are involved in making pledges (as using abstinence education as a method of sex education requires) the sense of being special will be dissipated. In addition, the majority of young people who take abstinence pledges still have sex before they are married and when they do they report using condoms less often than non-pledgers and are more likely to substitute anal or oral sex for vaginal sexual intercourse.

In April 2007 the results were published of a Congressionally mandated evaluation of federally funded abstinence based programs in American schools. The investigation, which looked at four programs offering a range of settings and strategies, found that rates of abstinence and unprotected sex in students who took part in the programs were virtually identical to rates among students who had been randomly assigned to not take part. The ages at first sexual intercourse were also nearly identical, as were the numbers of sexual partners. It appears that the programs had no impact on how the students behaved.

With regards to HIV prevention, a systematic review of all relevant studies concluded, "Evidence does not indicate that abstinence only interventions effectively decrease or exacerbate HIV risk among participants in high-income countries; trials suggest that the programs are ineffective." Nevertheless the authors stressed the lack of robust data and the need for more rigorous trials. They noted that most studies have been conducted among American youth, which may limit the generalizability of their findings.

Assessing the effectiveness of abstinence plus sex education programs, in comparison to abstinence only programs, is hampered by the lack of academic reviews. However, one recent and very robust review suggests that neither are very effective and that there are good grounds for believing that failure to provide young people with information about contraception prevents them from knowing about facts which have the greatest potential to protect them against pregnancy and STDs.

What Is the Difference in the Content of Abstinence Based and Comprehensive Programs of Sex Education?

Another way in which the debate gets framed is in relation to differences in beliefs about what the real facts are that young people should be presented with in the context of sex education. Many supporters of abstinence based sex education say that comprehensive programs are too positive about the protective potential of contraceptives and understate their failure rate and the risks of contracting HIV or another STI. In addition, they criticize programs of comprehensive sex education for placing too little emphasis on abstinence and sending young people a mixed message by referring both to abstaining from or delaying when they first have sexual intercourse, and the benefits of using contraception.

For their part critics of abstinence based programs have said that they are too negative about the effectiveness of contraception and sometimes include inaccurate information about failure rates. Proponents of abstinence based approaches have been accused of overstating condom failure rates, exaggerating the risks of infection with HIV and other STIs, reinforcing gender and sexuality stereotypes, and presenting sex and sexuality in an overly negative way.

The criticisms leveled against comprehensive programs of sex education are difficult to sustain because research suggests that in practice many sex educators are very concerned not to present sex in too positive a light and tend to avoid coverage of sensitive and potentially embarrassing subjects like homosexuality and abortion. Young people consistently report that the underlying message is that they should not have sex. Moreover, much of the evidence for the ineffectiveness of condoms and other contraceptives cited by critics of comprehensive programs is highly suspect, being based on poor quality research or the outcome of a partial reading of its results.

In contrast, those criticisms leveled at abstinence based approaches do seem to have a firmer foundation. Some reviews of program materials suggest factual inaccuracies—such as massively overestimating the prevalence of HIV and STIs and the failure rates of condoms when properly used—are common. These reviews have also shown that these programs tend to project stereotypes about gender, repress information about positive aspects of sexual relationships, and overstate the emotional risks and dangers associated with sex.

Is It Realistic to Encourage Abstinence until Marriage?

The premise on which abstinence based sex education is founded—that it is reasonable to wait until marriage before having sex for the first time and then be faithful to that one partner for life—may well be unrealistic for many young people because it fails to reflect the nature of modern, industrial societies in which people marry later in life, if at all. And with the high frequency of breakdown in marriage, people are very likely to have several sexual partners over their lifetime.

Across the United States, the United Kingdom, and the rest of Europe data on sexual lifestyles consistently show that the age at which people first marry has risen to around 30 years old and that about a fifth of marriages end in divorce or separation within five years. Yet while the age at which people marry has risen, the age at which they first have sexual intercourse has been falling to around 16 years old, and a diminishing minority of people report that their first sexual partner was also their marriage partner. Data on young people's sexual lifestyles and behavior from countries in the developing world where HIV is most prevalent also suggest that advice to abstain from sex until marriage may be wildly out of step with accepted cultural norms.

So Can We Decide Whether One Approach Is Better Than the Other?

It is very important to note that debates about research into the effectiveness of different types of sex education, and criticisms of the extent to which programs contain factual inaccuracies and are guilty of stereotyping, do not always represent objective attempts to weigh the evidence that these studies have produced. While the debate between supporters of both approaches has populated these areas of difference it is not in pursuit of a resolution of their differences but rather a definitive answer that suits their moral agenda. There is no doubt that, whatever evidence is assembled, people who hold particular strong moral views are unlikely to give up supporting their preferred approach regardless of whether it works or whether someone else thinks it presents a distorted picture of the facts.

Which View Is in the Ascendancy?

There is no doubt that abstinence based approaches gathered political and financial support in the United States during the early 2000s when they were strongly associated with the moral and religious inclinations of the Republican Party and the Presidency of George W. Bush. Indeed, more than 80% of the $1.5 billion spent on abstinence education since 1982 was spent under the Bush administration, with the 2007 budget granting approximately $204 million to abstinence only education programs.

However, the Obama administration has withdrawn Federal support for abstinence only programs within the United States. The budget plans for 2010 have proposed that over $100 million will be directed to teenage pregnancy programs which have been shown to be evidentially effective.

The effect that the change in policy in the United States will have on sex education in countries severely affected by HIV and AIDS which receive funding via PEPFAR is not yet clear. When PEPFAR was reauthorized in 2008, the requirement that a third of funds allocated to HIV prevention be spent on abstinence only programs was replaced with the requirement of a written report to Congress if less than a half of HIV prevention funds are spent on abstinence only sex education. Although the effects of this change in legislation remain to be seen, HIV and AIDS organizations have argued that it sustains a bias towards abstinence only programs in countries which receive PEPFAR funding.

In the United Kingdom, abstinence education has no support in public policy and receives no funding from government, although there is an expectation that sex educators in schools will emphasize the potential benefits of delaying or abstaining from sexual activity alongside providing information about contraception, sexual health services, sexuality, and gender issues.

What Is the Current Situation with Abstinence Based Sex Education in the United States?

The impact of the radical shift in public policy in the United States away from abstinence based sex education is yet to be determined. However, the current position seems to be one in which abstinence education has become somewhat entrenched in some states.

A survey in 2009 found that while 21 states and the District of Columbia mandate that public schools teach sex education, many more spell out requirements on how the topics of abstinence and contraception should be dealt with in the context of any teaching. The survey found that in general there was a greater tendency to require that abstinence be stressed than programs that cover contraception.

In contrast to this trend, some states seem to have been actively engaged in consolidating comprehensive provision and an increasing number have chosen not to receive federal funding for abstinence based sex education.

Is Abstinence Education Supported by Young People, Parents, and Schools?

Surveys of teachers, parents, and young people consistently show that abstinence based sex education has little widespread public support. State based studies, such as a survey of parents in North Carolina and another in Minnesota conducted in 2005 and 2006–2007 respectively, show an overwhelming majority supporting the provision of sex education via schools and that it be comprehensive. These results support evidence gleaned in previous studies which have found overwhelming support for sex education in school and little local controversy about its provision and organization within schools.

In the United Kingdom an even greater proportion of parents and young people support comprehensive approaches to sex education. Young people want AIDS education in school and want to be informed of the facts that will enable them to make their own informed decisions.

Why Is the Debate about Abstinence Education Important in Terms of HIV/AIDS Prevention?

Globally, the greatest HIV and AIDS burden falls on young people. Sex education is recognized as a major component of HIV prevention targeting young people; what form it takes and whether or not it works impacts directly on the HIV risk to which they are exposed. AIDS education for young people is a crucial factor in determining the extent to which they are at risk of HIV infection.

With considerable amounts of money continuing to be dedicated to abstinence only programs under the President's Emergency Plan For AIDS Relief, abstinence education is being promoted in some of the countries worst affected by HIV and AIDS. This raises a number of concerns about whether this is an appropriate approach in contexts where HIV is very prevalent and sexual intercourse before marriage is widespread, and, particularly, whether such programs will withhold accurate information about condoms.

All the evidence clearly shows that the best way to progress HIV prevention through sex education is through comprehensive programs. Despite generating considerable debate and political support, particularly in the United States, abstinence education represents, primarily, a minority moral movement rather than an effective response to the sexual health needs and behavior of young people.

As the experiences around the world demonstrate—a good example of which can be found in Uganda—what works in terms of sex education for HIV prevention is a comprehensive approach that is sensitive to the needs and experiences of particular groups. For unmarried, sexually active young people abstinence messages are not effective, whereas promoting faithfulness to one partner, condom use, and abstinence is effective. Abstinence messages work to some extent for younger sexually inactive people, but they need to have information about contraception and risk-reduction behavior for when they do decide to have sex. Everyone has the right to the information that can enable them to protect themselves against HIV infection—it is neither Christian nor moral to refuse them.

Section 44.4

Behavioral Intervention May Reduce STD Rates

"SAFE Studies Show Behavioral Intervention Reduces STIs in San Antonio, Texas," by the National Institute for Allergy and Infectious Diseases (NIAID, www.niaid.nih.gov), part of the National Institutes of Health, November 10, 2010.

For more than 20 years, NIAID has funded the Sexual Awareness for Everyone (SAFE) study at The University of Texas Health Science Center, San Antonio, targeting risky sexual behaviors in African- and Mexican-American communities that often lead to sexually transmitted infections (STIs). The behavioral intervention fine-tuned by the research team has been extremely effective at reducing STIs in these minority groups. In fact, SAFE is recognized by the Centers for Disease Control and Prevention as a best evidence program to reduce chlamydia and gonorrhea infections and risky sex behaviors.

SAFE researchers have conducted three randomized trials using a unique behavioral intervention to reduce the prevalence of chlamydia and gonorrhea. But before the trials began, researchers spent 18 months collecting qualitative information from the target groups to better understand the needs, beliefs, and practices that would have to be addressed in the intervention as well as cultural strengths that could be used to motivate change.

"We believed that STIs could be prevented through a culture- and gender-specific behavioral-cognitive intervention," explained anthropologist Rochelle Shain, PhD, who led the study. The intervention had three goals: 1) to make individuals aware that their (and their partners') behaviors can place them at high risk of contracting STIs, 2) to increase their motivation to change risky behavior, and 3) to provide them with the skills and support to do so. This reasoning was based on an adaptation of the AIDS Risk Reduction model.

Trials Taught Risk Recognition, Risk Reduction, and Communication, Then Measured Infections

In SAFE 1, the first of the three trials, 617 female study volunteers were randomized to control and intervention groups. The latter participated in three weekly interactive sessions that focused on risk recognition, commitment to reduce risk, and communication skill-building. Each small group was matched by a facilitator of the same ethnicity. The sessions aimed to empower individuals and cultivate self-confidence, raise their consciousness with regard to relationship needs with male partners, dispel myths associated with STI transmission, negotiate condom use, and educate about consequences of STIs.

At one-year follow-up, the researchers reported a 38 percent reduction of gonorrhea and/or chlamydia among women assigned to intervention. The intervention worked equally well for African- and Mexican-Americans, the depressed and non-depressed, and adolescents and adults. Behaviors responsible for this reduction included reducing number of partners and rate of partner turnover, practicing mutual monogamy, not having sex with a man before he was fully treated for STIs, avoiding unsafe sex, and not douching after sex.

Subsequent studies tested the addition of support groups (SAFE 2) and the inclusion of male partners (SAFE 3). In SAFE 2, women were assigned to intervention with and without the option of monthly support groups; one year later, both groups of women were more than 40 percent less likely to have chlamydia and/or gonorrhea. After five years, these trends persisted. A third trial, SAFE 3, included male partners and produced even greater STI reductions for women and men.

Results: Variety Is the Spice of Life

Dr. Shain attributes the success of SAFE to its multifaceted approach. "Individuals can choose different paths to avoid STIs," she explains. "SAFE is not limited to encouraging condom use, but includes a mix of options." These options include practicing abstinence or limited periods of abstinence, engaging in mutual monogamy, reducing number of partners and concurrency, not settling for an unsatisfactory relationship, taking time between partners to be selective, using condoms consistently and correctly, learning how to eroticize condom use, not douching after sex, and increasing health-seeking behavior.

Since STI infection is associated with poverty, low educational levels, and low self-esteem, SAFE stresses empowerment and treats the whole person. For example, program materials include a detailed self-help booklet to help participants obtain a GED, find employment, seek housing assistance, and more. Participants are put in touch with their community's cultural strengths, such as love of family and avoidance of infertility.

Chapter 45

Preventing STDs with Safer Sex

Chapter Contents

Section 45.1—What Is "Safer" Sex?... 464

Section 45.2—Condoms: Do They Work to Prevent STDs?....... 470

Section 45.3—Tips for Using Condoms and Dental Dams
to Prevent STDs.. 475

Section 45.4—Spermicides Alone Do Not Protect
against STDs 479

Section 45.1

What Is "Safer" Sex?

Safer Sex ("Safe Sex") at a Glance

- [It] reduces our risk of getting a sexually transmitted disease (STD).

- Using condoms makes vaginal or anal intercourse safer sex.

- Using condoms or other barriers makes oral sex safer sex.

- Having sex play without intercourse can be even safer sex.

- Safer sex can be very pleasurable and exciting.

- Want to get tested for STDs? Find a health center.

We all care about protecting ourselves and the ones we love. For sexually active people that means practicing safer sex. We can use it to reduce our risk of getting sexually transmitted diseases (STDs). It lets us protect ourselves—and our partners—while we enjoy sex play with them. Safer sex is for responsible people who care about their and their partners' pleasure and health.

How Can I Lower My Risk Using Safer Sex?

One way to have safer sex is to only have one partner who has no sexually transmitted infections and no other partners than you.

But, this isn't always the safest kind of safer sex. That's because most people don't know when they have infections. They are very likely to pass them on without knowing it.

Another other reason is that some people aren't as honest as they should be. In fact, about one out of three people will say they don't have an infection when they know they do, just to have sex. So most of us have to find other ways to practice safer sex.

Another way to practice safer sex is to only have sex play that has no risk—or a lower risk—of passing STDs. This means no vaginal or anal intercourse. Many of us find that great sex is about a lot more than a penis going in a vagina or anus. It is about exploring the many other ways you and your partner can turn each other on. Not only is it a way to discover new sexual pleasures, it's also safer.

No-risk safer sex play includes:

- masturbation;
- mutual masturbation;
- cybersex;
- phone sex;
- sharing fantasies.

Low-risk safer sex play includes:

- kissing;
- fondling—manual stimulation of one another;
- body-to-body rubbing—frottage, "grinding," or "dry humping";
- oral sex (even safer with a condom or other barrier);
- playing with sex toys—alone or with a partner.

The highest risk kinds of sex play are:

- vaginal intercourse;
- anal intercourse.

How Different Sexually Transmitted Infections Get Passed Along

Infections are passed in different ways. Here are the basics:

Vaginal or Anal Intercourse without a Condom—High Risk for Passing

- Chancroid
- Chlamydia
- Cytomegalovirus (CMV)
- Genital warts

- Gonorrhea
- Hepatitis B
- Herpes
- Human immunodeficiency virus (HIV)
- Human papilloma virus (HPV)
- Pelvic inflammatory disease (PID)
- Pubic lice
- Scabies
- Syphilis
- Trichomoniasis

Oral Sex without a Condom—High Risk for Passing

- CMV
- Gonorrhea
- Hepatitis B
- Herpes
- Syphilis

Skin-to-Skin Sex Play without Sexual Intercourse—Risky for Passing

- CMV
- Herpes
- HPV
- Pubic lice
- Scabies

Lots of other infections, from the flu to mononucleosis, can also be passed during sex play.

Luckily, we can use condoms during vaginal and anal intercourse to make them safer.

Is Oral Sex Safer Sex?

When it comes to HIV, oral sex is safer sex than vaginal or anal intercourse. But other infections, like herpes, syphilis, and hepatitis

B, can be passed by oral sex. Condoms or other barriers can also be used to make oral sex even safer.

How Can I Use Sheer Glyde or Dental Dams to Make Oral Sex Safer?

Dental dams are small, thin, square pieces of latex used to protect the throat during certain kinds of dental work. They can also be placed on the vulva or the anus when the mouth, lips, or tongue are used to sexually arouse a partner. Like the condom, dams keep partners' body fluids out of each other's bodies. They also prevent skin-to-skin contact. A special kind of dam, the Sheer Glyde dam, has been approved by the FDA [U.S. Food and Drug Administration] especially for safer sex. Like dental dams, Sheer Glyde dams are available online, in some drugstores, and at many Planned Parenthood health centers.

If Sheer Glyde dams or dental dams aren't handy, you can use plastic wrap or a cut-open condom.

How Can I Have Safer Sex with My Sex Toys?

Many people like to spice up sex play with sex toys—dildos, vibrators, strap-ons, butt plugs, and more. These toys need special care, too, when used alone or with partners. Unless they are kept clean between uses, they can build up bacteria, which can cause an infection. And if they are shared between partners, they can pass along sexually transmitted diseases.

The best way to keep sex toys clean and safe is to protect them with a latex condom. The condom should be changed whenever the toy is passed from partner to partner or from one body opening to another—mouth, anus, or vagina.

If you don't use condoms to keep a sex toy clean, it's important to clean it before and after every use. Sex toys are made of many different materials—silicone, jelly rubber, vinyl, stainless steel, acrylic, etc. They all may have to be cleaned different ways. Some toys can be soaked in water—and some cannot. Please read the instructions on the package carefully. Never use breakable household objects, like glass bottles, as sex toys.

Keeping your sex toys clean will help them last longer, and they'll give you pleasure instead of infections.

How Can I Use Lubricant for Safer Sex?

A good lubricant can go a long way in making sure that safer sex is pleasurable and fun. Lubricant is important in safer sex because it also makes condoms and dams slippery and less likely to break. Lubricants make safer sex feel better by cutting down on the dry kind of friction that a lot of people find irritating.

When buying lube, it's important to find the right kind—one that works for you and for your condom. Never use oil-based lube with a latex or non-latex rubber condom. Use only water or silicone-based lube with latex and non-latex rubber condoms. Read the package insert if you have any questions about what you can use.

What about Safer Sex and Drugs and Alcohol?

Alcohol and other drugs can make you forget you promised yourself to have safer sex. The use of too much alcohol or any amount of drugs often leads to high-risk sex.

How Does Safer Sex Make Sex Feel Better?

Worrying about sexually transmitted infections can make sex less satisfying. Safer sex can reduce that worry. Practicing safer sex can also help you and your partner:

- add variety to sexual pleasure;
- make sex play last longer by postponing orgasms;
- increase intimacy and trust;
- strengthen relationships;
- improve communication—verbal and nonverbal.

The bottom line is that safer sex can be fun. It is a great way to explore who we are sexually, express our feelings, bond with others, and have a good time. Practicing safer sex can enhance our pleasure—and who doesn't want more pleasure?

Am I Ready for Safer Sex?

Which of the following statements are true for you?

- I am ready to let my partner know where and how I like to be touched.
- I am ready to buy condoms, even if it's embarrassing.
- If I decide I want to use sex toys, I'm ready to keep them clean.

- I am ready to let my partner know my limits when it comes to taking risks.

- I am ready to say no to sex when I don't want to have it.

- I am ready to have regular physical exams and tests for sexually transmitted infections.

- I am ready to talk with my health care provider about my sex life.

- I am ready to enjoy sex without having to get high.

If you answered "True" to more than half of these questions, you are well on your way to being ready for safer sex. Congratulations!

How Do Condoms Make Sex Safer?

Condoms work by forming a barrier between the penis and anus, vagina, or mouth. The barrier keeps one partner's fluids from getting into or on the other. And condoms reduce the amount of skin-to-skin contact. There are two main kinds of condoms—latex condoms and female condoms.

Latex condoms are great safer sex tools for anal or vaginal intercourse. They are easy to get at a pharmacy, grocery store, or at a Planned Parenthood health center. They are cheap. And they come in a variety of shapes, sizes, and textures.

People with latex allergies can use condoms made of non-latex rubber or plastic. They also make sex safer, but they are not as widely available as latex condoms.

Female condoms reduce your risk of infection, too. Female condoms aren't quite as easy to find as latex condoms, but they are available in some drugstores and many Planned Parenthood health centers. You can also order them online if you can't find them in your neighborhood. Follow the instructions on the package for using female condoms correctly.

Section 45.2

Condoms: Do They Work to Prevent STDs?

Excerpted from "Condoms and STDs: Fact Sheet for Public
Health Personnel," by the Centers for Disease Control and Prevention
(CDC, www.cdc.gov), September 13, 2011.

Consistent and correct use of male latex condoms can reduce (though not eliminate) the risk of STD [sexually transmitted disease] transmission. To achieve the maximum protective effect, condoms must be used both consistently and correctly. Inconsistent use can lead to STD acquisition because transmission can occur with a single act of intercourse with an infected partner. Similarly, if condoms are not used correctly, the protective effect may be diminished even when they are used consistently. The most reliable ways to avoid transmission of sexually transmitted diseases (STDs), including human immunodeficiency virus (HIV), are to abstain from sexual activity or to be in a long-term mutually monogamous relationship with an uninfected partner. However, many infected persons may be unaware of their infections because STDs are often asymptomatic or unrecognized.

This text presents evidence concerning the male latex condom and the prevention of STDs, including HIV [human immunodeficiency virus], based on information about how different STDs are transmitted, the physical properties of condoms, the anatomic coverage or protection that condoms provide, and epidemiologic studies assessing condom use and STD risk.

Are Condoms Effective in Preventing STDs?

Latex condoms, when used consistently and correctly, are highly effective in preventing the sexual transmission of HIV, the virus that causes AIDS. In addition, consistent and correct use of latex condoms reduces the risk of other sexually transmitted diseases (STDs), including diseases transmitted by genital secretions, and to a lesser degree, genital ulcer diseases. Condom use may reduce the risk for genital human papillomavirus (HPV) infection and HPV-associated diseases, e.g., genital warts and cervical cancer.

There are two primary ways that STDs are transmitted. Some diseases, such as HIV infection, gonorrhea, chlamydia, and trichomoniasis, are transmitted when infected urethral or vaginal secretions contact mucosal surfaces (such as the male urethra, the vagina, or cervix). In contrast, genital ulcer diseases (such as genital herpes, syphilis, and chancroid) and human papillomavirus (HPV) infection are primarily transmitted through contact with infected skin or mucosal surfaces.

Laboratory studies have demonstrated that latex condoms provide an essentially impermeable barrier to particles the size of STD pathogens.

Condoms can be expected to provide different levels of protection for various STDs, depending on differences in how the diseases are transmitted. Condoms block transmission and acquisition of STDs by preventing contact between the condom wearer's penis and a sex partner's skin, mucosa, and genital secretions. A greater level of protection is provided for the diseases transmitted by genital secretions. A lesser degree of protection is provided for genital ulcer diseases or HPV because these infections also may be transmitted by exposure to areas (e.g., infected skin or mucosal surfaces) that are not covered or protected by the condom.

Epidemiologic studies seek to measure the protective effect of condoms by comparing risk of STD transmission among condom users with nonusers who are engaging in sexual intercourse. Accurately estimating the effectiveness of condoms for prevention of STDs, however, is methodologically challenging. Well-designed studies address key factors such as the extent to which condom use has been consistent and correct and whether infection identified is incident (i.e., new) or prevalent (i.e., pre-existing). Of particular importance, the study design should assure that the population being evaluated has documented exposure to the STD of interest during the period that condom use is being assessed. Although consistent and correct use of condoms is inherently difficult to measure, because such studies would involve observations of private behaviors, several published studies have demonstrated that failure to measure these factors properly tends to result in underestimation of condom effectiveness.

Epidemiologic studies provide useful information regarding the magnitude of STD risk reduction associated with condom use. Extensive literature review confirms that the best epidemiologic studies of condom effectiveness address HIV infection. Numerous studies of discordant couples (where only one partner is infected) have shown consistent use of latex condoms to be highly effective for preventing sexually acquired HIV infection. Similarly, studies have shown that condom use reduces the risk of other STDs. However, the overall strength of the evidence regarding the effectiveness of condoms in reducing the risk of other STDs is not at the level of that for HIV, primarily because fewer methodologically sound and well-designed studies have been completed that address other STDs. Critical reviews of all studies, with both positive and negative findings point to the limitations in study design in some studies which result in underestimation of condom effectiveness; therefore, the true protective effect is likely to be greater than the effect observed.

Overall, the preponderance of available epidemiologic studies have found that when used consistently and correctly, condoms are highly effective in preventing the sexual transmission of HIV infection and reduce the risk of other STDs.

The following includes specific information for HIV infection, diseases transmitted by genital secretions, genital ulcer diseases, and HPV infection.

HIV: The Virus That Causes AIDS

Latex condoms, when used consistently and correctly, are highly effective in preventing the sexual transmission of HIV, the virus that causes AIDS [acquired immunodeficiency syndrome].

HIV infection is, by far, the most deadly STD, and considerably more scientific evidence exists regarding condom effectiveness for prevention of HIV infection than for other STDs. The body of research on the effectiveness of latex condoms in preventing sexual transmission of HIV is both comprehensive and conclusive. The ability of latex condoms to prevent transmission of HIV has been scientifically established in "real-life" studies of sexually active couples as well as in laboratory studies.

Laboratory studies have demonstrated that latex condoms provide an essentially impermeable barrier to particles the size of HIV.

Latex condoms cover the penis and provide an effective barrier to exposure to secretions such as urethral and vaginal secretions, blocking the pathway of sexual transmission of HIV infection.

Epidemiologic studies that are conducted in real-life settings, where one partner is infected with HIV and the other partner is not, demonstrate that the consistent use of latex condoms provides a high degree of protection.

472

Other Diseases Transmitted by Genital Secretions

Latex condoms, when used consistently and correctly, reduce the risk of transmission of STDs such as gonorrhea, chlamydia, and trichomoniasis.

STDs such as gonorrhea, chlamydia, and trichomoniasis are sexually transmitted by genital secretions, such as urethral or vaginal secretions.

Laboratory studies have demonstrated that latex condoms provide an essentially impermeable barrier to particles the size of STD pathogens. The physical properties of latex condoms protect against diseases such as gonorrhea, chlamydia, and trichomoniasis by providing a barrier to the genital secretions that transmit STD-causing organisms.

Epidemiologic studies that compare infection rates among condom users and nonusers provide evidence that latex condoms can protect against the transmission of STDs such as chlamydia, gonorrhea, and trichomoniasis.

Genital Ulcer Diseases and HPV Infections

Genital ulcer diseases and HPV infections can occur in both male and female genital areas that are covered or protected by a latex condom, as well as in areas that are not covered. Consistent and correct use of latex condoms reduces the risk of genital herpes, syphilis, and chancroid only when the infected area or site of potential exposure is protected. Condom use may reduce the risk for HPV infection and HPV-associated diseases (e.g., genital warts and cervical cancer).

Genital ulcer diseases include genital herpes, syphilis, and chancroid. These diseases are transmitted primarily through "skin-to-skin" contact from sores/ulcers or infected skin that looks normal. HPV infections are transmitted through contact with infected genital skin or mucosal surfaces/secretions. Genital ulcer diseases and HPV infection can occur in male or female genital areas that are covered (protected by the condom) as well as those areas that are not.

Laboratory studies have demonstrated that latex condoms provide an essentially impermeable barrier to particles the size of STD pathogens.

Protection against genital ulcer diseases and HPV depends on the site of the sore/ulcer or infection. Latex condoms can only protect against transmission when the ulcers or infections are in genital areas that are covered or protected by the condom. Thus, consistent and correct use of latex condoms would be expected to protect against transmission of genital ulcer diseases and HPV in some, but not all, instances.

Epidemiologic studies that compare infection rates among condom users and nonusers provide evidence that latex condoms provide limited protection against syphilis and herpes simplex virus-2 transmission. No conclusive studies have specifically addressed the transmission of chancroid and condom use, although several studies have documented a reduced risk of genital ulcers associated with increased condom use in settings where chancroid is a leading cause of genital ulcers.

Condom use may reduce the risk for HPV-associated diseases (e.g., genital warts and cervical cancer) and may mitigate the other adverse consequences of infection with HPV; condom use has been associated with higher rates of regression of cervical intraepithelial neoplasia (CIN) and clearance of HPV infection in women, and with regression of HPV-associated penile lesions in men. A limited number of prospective studies have demonstrated a protective effect of condoms on the acquisition of genital HPV.

Although condom use has been associated with a lower risk of cervical cancer, the use of condoms should not be a substitute for routine screening with Pap smears to detect and prevent cervical cancer, nor should it be a substitute for HPV vaccination among those eligible for the vaccine.

Section 45.3

Tips for Using Condoms and Dental Dams to Prevent STDs

"Tips for Using Condoms and Dental Dams," by the U.S. Department of Veterans Affairs (VA, www.va.gov), October 3, 2011.

Some people think that using a condom makes sex less fun. Other people have become creative and find condoms sexy. Not having to worry about infecting someone will definitely make sex much more enjoyable.

If you are not used to using condoms, practice, practice, practice.

Condom Dos and Don'ts

- Use lubricated latex condoms. Always use latex, because lamb-skin condoms don't block HIV (human immunodeficiency virus) and STDs (sexually transmitted diseases), and polyurethane condoms break more often than latex. Shop around and find your favorite brand. Try different sizes and shapes (yes, they come in different sizes and shapes!). There are a lot of choices—one will work for you.

- Store condoms loosely in a cool, dry place (not your wallet). Make sure your condoms are fresh—check the expiration date. Throw away condoms that have expired, been very hot, or been washed in the washer. If you think the condom might not be good, get a new one. You and your partner are worth it.

- Open the package carefully, so that you don't rip the condom. Be careful if you use your teeth. Make sure that the condom package has not been punctured (there should be a pocket of air). Check the condom for damaged packaging and signs of aging such as brittleness, stickiness, and discoloration.

- Put on the condom after the penis is erect and before it touches any part of a partner's body. If a penis is uncircumcised (uncut), the foreskin must be pulled back before putting on the condom.

- Make sure the condom is right-side out. It's like a sock—there's a right side and a wrong side. Before you put it on the penis, unroll the condom about half an inch to see which direction it is unrolling. Then put it on the head of the penis and hold the tip of the condom between your fingers as you roll it all the way down the shaft of the penis from head to base. This keeps out air bubbles that can cause the condom to break. It also leaves a space for semen to collect after ejaculation.

- If you use a lubricant (lube), it should be a water-soluble lubricant (for example, ID Glide, K-Y Jelly, Slippery Stuff, Foreplay, Wet, Astroglide) in order to prevent breakdown of the condom. Products such as petroleum jelly, massage oils, butter, Crisco, Vaseline, and hand creams are not considered water-soluble lubricants and should not be used.

- Put lubricant on after you put on the condom, not before—it could slip off. Add more lube often. Dry condoms break more easily.

- Withdraw the penis immediately after ejaculation, while the penis is still erect; grasp the rim of the condom between your fingers and slowly withdraw the penis (with the condom still on) so that no semen is spilled.

- Throw out the used condom right away. Tie it off to prevent spillage or wrap it in bathroom tissue and put it in the garbage. Condoms can clog toilets. Use a condom only once. Never use the same condom for vaginal and anal intercourse. Never use a condom that has been used by someone else.

Do You Have to Use a Condom for Oral Sex?

It is possible for oral sex to transmit HIV, whether the infected partner is performing or receiving oral sex. But the risk is low compared with unprotected vaginal or anal sex.

If you choose to perform oral sex, and your partner is male, use a latex condom on the penis, or if you or your partner is allergic to latex, plastic (polyurethane) condoms can be used.

If you choose to have oral sex, and your partner is female, use a latex barrier (such as a natural rubber latex sheet, a dental dam, or a cut-open condom that makes a square) between your mouth and the vagina. A latex barrier such as a dental dam reduces the risk of blood or vaginal fluids entering your mouth. Plastic food wrap also can be used as a barrier.

If you choose to perform oral sex with either a male or female partner and this sex includes oral contact with your partner's anus (anilingus or rimming), use a latex barrier (such as a natural rubber latex sheet, a dental dam, or a cut-open condom that makes a square) between your mouth and the anus. Plastic food wrap also can be used as a barrier. This barrier is to prevent getting another sexually transmitted disease or parasites, not HIV.

If you choose to share sex toys, such as dildos or vibrators, with your partner, each partner should use a new condom on the sex toy; and be sure to clean sex toys between each use.

Female Condom

Most people have never heard of these, but they may be helpful for you. The female condom is a large condom made of polyurethane fitted with larger and smaller rings at each end that help keep it inside the vagina. They may seem a little awkward at first, but can be an alternative to the male condom. They are made of polyurethane, so any lubricant can be used without damaging them. Female condoms generally cost more than male condoms, and if you aren't used to them, you'll definitely need to practice.

- Store the condom in a cool dry place, not in direct heat or sunlight.

- Throw away any condoms that have expired—the date is printed on individual condom wrappers.

- Check the package for damage and check the condom for signs of aging such as brittleness, stickiness, and discoloration. The female condom is lubricated, so it will be somewhat wet.

- Before inserting the condom, you can squeeze lubricant into the condom pouch and rub the sides together to spread it around.

- Put the condom in before sex play because pre-ejaculatory fluid, which comes from the penis, may contain HIV. The condom can be inserted up to eight hours before sex.

- The female condom has a firm ring at each end of it. To insert the condom, squeeze the ring at the closed end between the fingers (like a diaphragm), and push it up into the back of the vagina. The open ring must stay outside the vagina at all times, and it will partly cover the lip area.

- Do not use a male condom with the female condom.

- Do not use a female condom with a diaphragm.

- If the penis is inserted outside the condom pouch or if the outer ring (open ring) slips into the vagina, stop and take the condom out. Use a new condom before you start sex again.

- Don't tear the condom with fingernails or jewelry.

- Use a female condom only once and properly dispose of it in the trash (not the toilet).

Dental Dams and Plastic Wrap

Even though oral sex is a low-risk sexual practice, you may want to use protection when performing oral sex on someone who has HIV.

Dental dams are small squares of latex that were made originally for use in dental procedures. They are now commonly used as barriers when performing oral sex on women, to keep in vaginal fluids or menstrual blood that could transmit HIV or other STDs.

Some people use plastic wrap instead of a dental dam. It's thinner. Here are some things to remember:

- Before using a dental dam, first check it visually for any holes.

- If the dental dam has cornstarch on it, rinse that off with water (starch in the vagina can lead to an infection).

- Cover the woman's genital area with the dental dam.

- For oral-anal sex, cover the opening of the anus with a new dental dam.

- A new dental dam should be used for each act of oral sex; it should never be reused.

Section 45.4

Spermicides Alone Do Not Protect against STDs

Spermicides are a type of vaginal barrier method. They prevent pregnancy by acting as a barrier to sperm so they can't reach and fertilize one of the eggs that your ovaries produce each month. If you decide to use a spermicide, you need to use it every time you have sexual intercourse. Make sure you wash your hands before you put any of these contraceptives into your vagina. Also, women who are allergic to nonoxynol-9 should not use any method that contains spermicide or works with spermicide. Women who are having frequent daily intercourse may increase their risk of getting HIV [human immunodeficiency virus] if they use spermicides because of vaginal irritation. Condoms are more effective than spermicide.

What Are Spermicides?

There are different forms of spermicides, including vaginal creams, foams, films, suppositories, and sponges. Spermicides work by forming a chemical barrier that either kills sperm or paralyzes them. So the sperm can't pass through your cervix to fertilize the egg.

Spermicides can be used alone as a form of contraception, but they are much more effective when used with another type.

Where Can I Get Spermicide?

You can get spermicide over-the-counter at drug stores. No prescription is needed. It costs between $0.50–$1.50 per use.

How Effective Is Spermicide against Pregnancy?

Spermicide alone is one of the less effective forms of contraception against pregnancy.

If women use spermicide every time they have sexual intercourse and follow instructions perfectly every time, it is 82% effective. This means that if 100 women use spermicide all the time and always use it correctly, 18 women will become pregnant in a year.

If women use spermicide, but not perfectly, it is 72% effective. This means that if 100 women use spermicide, 28 women or more will become pregnant in a year.

Does Spermicide Protect against STIs?

No. It is much better to use condoms for STI [sexually transmitted infection] and HIV protection.

What Kinds of Spermicide Are There and How Do I Use Them?

Contraceptive foam, which is a spermicide in an aerosol form, is inserted deep into your vagina using a small applicator. Contraceptive cream or jelly can also be inserted deep into the vagina with a small applicator. Contraceptive creams or jellies are good to use with diaphragms. Follow the directions on the package. You should insert foams, creams, or jellies no more than 30–60 minutes before you have intercourse. You should wait several minutes after you insert them before you have intercourse.

The small, oval-shaped vaginal suppositories are placed deep in the vagina and release a contraceptive foam 10–15 minutes after you insert one. Because of this, you should not have intercourse until 15 minutes after insertion, so there is time for the foaming to occur.

A vaginal contraceptive film (VCF) is a two-inch by two-inch flat package with wax paper-like tissues, each containing the spermicide nonoxynol-9. You should put the film on a dry fingertip and insert it up into the vagina at least 15 minutes before you have intercourse.

The effectiveness of the spermicides usually lasts only for about an hour, so you will need to insert more if you are having sexual intercourse for more than an hour. Each time you have sexual intercourse, you should insert more spermicide into your vagina.

What about Douching after Intercourse?

Douching is not recommended after intercourse. There are no benefits and it is not safe because it can cause an increased risk in pelvic inflammatory disease, bacterial vaginosis (an infection of the vagina), and ectopic pregnancy (implantation of the fertilized egg outside of the uterus). Your body makes everything it needs to keep it clean. All you should be using to clean the outside of your vagina is water and soap. However, if you decide to douche in spite of this warning, you should wait at least six hours after intercourse so that the spermicide does not get washed away.

Are There Any Problems with Spermicides?

Some women are allergic to spermicides, while others have some irritation in or around their vagina. You are more likely to get urinary tract infections. If you are having frequent daily intercourse, you may be more likely to get HIV.

What If I Have Problems with Spermicides?

You should call your health care provider if you have any of the following:

- Soreness in your vagina
- Rash in or around your vagina
- Discharge that smells bad or that comes in a larger amount than normal

Chapter 46

Preventing STDs after Possible or Certain Exposure

Chapter Contents

Section 46.1—Expedited Partner Therapy 484

Section 46.2—Preventing STDs after a Sexual Assault 488

Section 46.3—Post-Exposure Prophylaxis: Taking HIV
              Drugs If You've Been Exposed to the Virus
              through Blood or Sexual Contact 492

Section 46.1

Expedited Partner Therapy

Excerpted from the Executive Summary of "Expedited Partner Therapy in the Management of Sexually Transmitted Diseases," a report by the Centers for Disease Control and Prevention (CDC, www.cdc.gov), 2006. Reviewed by David A. Cooke, MD, FACP, July 10, 2012.

Expedited partner therapy (EPT) is the practice of treating the sex partners of persons with sexually transmitted diseases (STD) without an intervening medical evaluation or professional prevention counseling. The usual implementation of EPT is through patient-delivered partner therapy (PDPT), although other methods may be employed.

Evidence

For STDs [sexually transmitted diseases] other than syphilis, partner management based on patient referral or provider referral has had only modest success in assuring partner treatment, largely attributable to limitations of available financial and personnel resources. EPT is believed to have been widely employed in women with trichomoniasis. Recent surveys document occasional use by many primary care providers in the management of patients with gonorrhea and chlamydial infection, and consistent use by a few. A retrospective case control study and two process-oriented analyses suggested that EPT holds promise as a partner management option. These studies contributed to CDC decisions to fund four randomized controlled trials (RCTs) designed to compare EPT with standard partner management approaches in men and women with gonorrhea, chlamydial infection, or trichomoniasis; and to assess behavioral predictors of treatment and reinfection.

Persistent or Recurrent Infection

The first RCT of EPT followed 1,787 women in 6 cities after treatment for chlamydial infection. Recurrent infection was documented at follow-up visits 1 month and 4 months later in 12% of women randomized to EPT and 15% of those managed by patient referral. The second RCT enrolled 2,751 men and women with gonorrhea or chlamydial infection from both public and private care settings in a single metropolitan area. Persistent or recurrent infection with either disease was found in 9.9% of subjects randomized to EPT and 13.0% of those who had standard patient-referral or provider-referral of their partners. EPT was more effective in preventing gonorrhea at follow-up than chlamydial infection. Chlamydial infection was present at follow-up in 7.6% of women who denied all sex since treatment, suggesting that a higher than expected rate of treatment failure accounted for some infections at follow-up. In the third available RCT, 977 men with symptomatic urethritis (principally gonorrhea and chlamydial infection) were randomized to EPT, patient referral, or patient referral enhanced by written education materials. Follow-up testing for gonorrhea and chlamydial infection 4–8 weeks later was accomplished in 37.5% of patients. Persistent or recurrent infection was found in 43% of subjects in the patient referral group (referent), 14% of men randomized to enhanced patient referral, and 23% of men randomized to EPT. For trichomoniasis, in an as yet unpublished RCT of 463 women randomized to the same interventions as the male urethritis trial, with 80% follow-up, the prevalences of infection 3–7 weeks later were not significantly different for patient referral (6%), enhanced patient referral (9%), or EPT (9%).

Behavioral Outcomes

The four available RCTs evaluated the association of EPT with index cases' reports of success in partner notification, confidence that their partners were treated, and sexual behaviors likely to predict reinfection. In two trials that enrolled male index cases, men randomized to EPT were equally or more likely to notify their partners than those randomized to the control strategies. Female index cases with chlamydial infection or gonorrhea who were randomized to EPT had either equivalent success or enhanced success in notifying partners compared with women randomized to standard partner management. In all three trials of gonorrhea or chlamydial infection, EPT was associated with at least equivalent and typically increased confidence by both male and female index cases that their partners had received treatment, including direct observation that their partners took medication. Two trials that addressed both gonorrhea and chlamydial infection found EPT to be associated with significantly reduced rates of sex with untreated partners at follow-up. The trichomoniasis trial showed general equivalence of EPT with desirable behavioral outcomes compared with standard patient referral.

Cost Effectiveness

Preliminary economic analyses suggest that EPT is a cost-saving and cost effective partner management strategy.

Limitations

The data available to support EPT for chlamydial infection were derived in larger and geographically more diverse samples of patients than those for gonorrhea. Nevertheless, the evidence in favor of EPT, as measured by the rate of persistent or recurrent infection at follow-up, is stronger for gonorrhea than for chlamydial infection, perhaps due to a higher than expected rate of persistent chlamydial infection in women. This finding confounds the assessment of EPT in women with chlamydial infection. Assuring the treatment of infected men's female partners is a high priority to prevent ongoing transmission and community spread.

As for all RCTs, the extent to which the results of the available trials can be safely generalized to other populations and settings is not certain. Owing to modest sample sizes in some disease-specific patient groups, and varying effect sizes, not all outcomes of interest have been shown to be statistically significant. For example, further data are desirable on the use of EPT in male index cases. The available data do not support the routine use of EPT in the management of trichomoniasis, and no published data support the use of EPT for chlamydial infection or gonorrhea in men who have sex with men (MSM). Although substantial numbers of adolescents were included in the available trials, there is little experience in patients younger than 18 years old.

Issues in Implementation of EPT

Among several pragmatic issues that will influence implementation of EPT as an STD prevention strategy, a dominant one is the possibility of undetected STD in partners. The potential for undiagnosed pelvic inflammatory disease (PID) is of concern when EPT is used to treat the female partners of men with gonorrhea or chlamydial infection. Therefore, EPT intended for female partners should be accompanied by warnings about the symptoms of PID and advice that women seek medical attention in addition to accepting treatment. Undiagnosed gonorrhea and chlamydial infection are common in the partners of women with trichomoniasis, and undiagnosed HIV infection and other morbidities have been found in many partners of STD-infected MSM.

The legality of EPT is uncertain in some states and overt statutory impediments exist in others; the practice is clearly legal only in a few states. The medicolegal ramifications may be uncertain in the event of adverse outcomes in the recipients of EPT. Other barriers include direct and indirect costs, including limitations on third-party insurance coverage; missed opportunities for prevention counseling of partners; risks of allergic reactions and other adverse drug effects; administrative barriers; privacy issues; and the attitudes and beliefs of health care providers and agencies about the practice.

Conclusions

Both clinical and behavioral outcomes of the available studies indicate that EPT is a useful option to facilitate partner management among heterosexual men and women with chlamydial infection or gonorrhea. The evidence indicates that EPT should be available to clinicians as an option for partner management, although ongoing evaluation will be needed to define when and how EPT can be best utilized. EPT represents an additional strategy for partner management that does not replace other strategies, such as standard patient referral or provider-assisted referral, when available. Along with medication, EPT should be accompanied by information that advises recipients to seek personal health care in addition to EPT. This is particularly important when EPT is provided to male patients for their female partners, and for male partners with symptoms. Existing data suggest that EPT has a limited role in partner management for trichomoniasis. No data support its use in the routine management of syphilis, and there is no experience with EPT for gonorrhea or chlamydial infection among MSM.

Section 46.2

Preventing STDs after a Sexual Assault

Excerpted from "For People Who Have Been Sexually Assaulted... What You Need to Know about STDs and Emergency Contraception," by the New Jersey Department of Health and Senior Services (www.state.nj.us), February 2009.

People who have been sexually assaulted often are worried about their risk of becoming pregnant or contracting a sexually transmitted disease (STD) and have a lot of questions about many subjects. This text is intended to give you information about STDs, including HIV [human immunodeficiency virus], and emergency contraception. If you have questions about this information or would like further information, please ask your health care provider to assist you.

Sexually Transmitted Diseases (STDs) and Sexual Assault

STDs (also called sexually transmitted infections or STIs) are infections that are spread through oral, vaginal, or anal sex. If left untreated, STDs can cause serious damage to the reproductive organs, lead to infertility, or lead to other serious health problems. Most STDs are curable if diagnosed and treated early. Even if an STD is not curable, treatment can minimize the effects on your body.

Risk of Getting an STD from Sexual Assault

The risk of getting an STD from sexual assault is low. Gonorrhea and chlamydia are the STDs most commonly diagnosed after sexual assault. Both of these are curable if diagnosed early. The risk of being infected with HIV from an assault is extremely low.

If an STD is diagnosed after a sexual assault, it does not always mean that the infection occurred during the assault. That is, it is possible that a person had an STD without knowing it before being assaulted.

Signs and Symptoms of STDs

Most of the time, people with an STD will not have any symptoms. However, some signs that a person might have an STD include:

- itching or burning in the genital or anal area;
- painful urination;
- lower abdominal pain;
- bumps or sores in the genital or anal area;
- unusual bleeding or discharge.

Sometimes even if a person has symptoms of an STD, these will go away on their own, but the person will still have an STD. Other times symptoms are very mild and a person might not think anything of them. Even if symptoms are mild or not present, an untreated STD can still cause serious damage to a person's body. Therefore, it is very important to see a health care provider for an examination that includes STD tests to find out if you have been infected after a sexual assault, even if you do not have any symptoms.

STD Testing and Treatment after Assault

After being assaulted, it is important to have an exam as soon as possible to test for possible infection. You also have the option of having a sexual assault forensic medical examination. During this type of exam, a specially trained nurse, called a sexual assault nurse examiner or SANE, will provide a medical assessment and collect evidence.

If you seek medical care after an assault, your health care provider or SANE may give you medications for certain STDs in case you were exposed to these during the assault. These medications, however, are not 100% effective so it is important to look for any symptoms and to follow up with your health care provider in two to three weeks for additional evaluation and to ensure you have been effectively treated. Also, keep in mind that your health care provider may decide to wait for STD test results to determine appropriate treatment before giving you medication.

Could I Infect Someone with an STD?

It is possible to infect someone with whom you are having oral, anal, or vaginal sex with an STD if you were infected during an assault. It is a good idea to wait to have sex until you have had the appropriate follow-up tests two to three weeks after your initial health care visit and you have received the results of any STD follow-up tests. If you do have oral, anal, or vaginal sex, it is important to use a latex barrier, such as a condom.

HIV/AIDS and Sexual Assault

Risk of Getting HIV from Sexual Assault

The risk of being infected with HIV (the virus that causes AIDS [acquired immunodeficiency syndrome]) through a sexual assault is low. Penetration of the vagina or anus by a penis, or contact with blood is the most likely way HIV would be transmitted during a sexual assault. There is a lower risk of being infected through oral sex.

If there is a reason to believe you may have been exposed to HIV, there is medicine that might help prevent HIV/AIDS if taken within 72 hours. The SANE, or other health care provider you see, will know if this is an option for you.

Signs and Symptoms of HIV/AIDS

HIV infection is a long-term illness. A person can look and feel healthy with no symptoms of HIV for years with the virus in their body. Sometimes a person will have flu-like symptoms within a few weeks of being infected with HIV but often there are no symptoms. Symptoms may become more severe later.

HIV Testing and Treatment after Assault

It is important to have an HIV test as soon as possible after an assault. HIV is usually detected through a simple blood test. Sometimes cells taken from the mouth or a urine sample will be used instead. Rapid HIV testing, using blood or oral fluid, may be available at the initial examination and/or follow- up testing. Results with this type of test are available within 20–40 minutes. However, these preliminary results need to be confirmed with a test sent to a laboratory. Also, if a person has been infected with HIV, it can take up to six months for a test to detect HIV. Therefore, even if your test results are negative (do not show HIV), it is important to have follow-up tests periodically up to six months after the assault. The timeframe for follow-up tests that is often suggested is four to six weeks, three months, and six months after a suspected exposure to HIV.

Pregnancy and Emergency Contraception

Women who have been sexually assaulted are often worried about becoming pregnant from the assault. It is possible to prevent pregnancy even after an assault with emergency contraception (also called EC) if taken within 120 hours, or five days. If EC is not an option for you for medical reasons, your regular or emergency health care provider or SANE will explain this to you as well as answer any questions you might have about EC.

EC (emergency contraception) is a way to prevent pregnancy even after unprotected vaginal intercourse. Many women who have been raped choose this option to prevent pregnancy. The most common method of EC is in pill form (also called ECPs, or morning after pills).

Emergency contraception pills should be taken within 120 hours or five days of unprotected vaginal intercourse. Therefore, it is important to seek health care as soon as possible if there is any chance you may have gotten pregnant from an assault.

EC prevents pregnancy in one or more ways: By temporarily stopping eggs from being released, stopping fertilization, or stopping a fertilized egg from attaching to the womb. EC will not work if you are already pregnant and will not cause an abortion.

EC can cause some women to feel nauseous. Other side effects might be sore breasts, headaches, or abdominal cramping. These side effects usually last for one day. EC can also cause a woman's next period to come early.

If you are confused about your risk for pregnancy or if you have any questions or concerns, your regular or emergency health care provider or SANE should be able to help you figure out what health care procedures are best for you.

Section 46.3

Post-Exposure Prophylaxis: Taking HIV Drugs If You've Been Exposed to the Virus through Blood or Sexual Contact

"Post-Exposure Prophylaxis," AIDSinfo.gov, part of the U.S. Department of Health and Human Services, May 19, 2011.

What is post-exposure prophylaxis (PEP)?

PEP involves taking anti-HIV [human immunodeficiency virus] drugs as soon as possible after you may have been exposed to HIV to try to reduce the chance of becoming HIV positive. There are two types of PEP: (1) Occupational PEP (sometimes called oPEP), and (2) non-occupational PEP, (sometimes called nPEP). Workplace exposure (oPEP) is when someone working in a health-care setting is potentially exposed to material infected with HIV. nPEP is when someone is potentially exposed to HIV outside the workplace (e.g., condom breakage, sexual assault, etc.)

To be effective, PEP must begin within 72 hours of exposure, before the virus has time to rapidly replicate in your body. PEP consists of two to three antiretroviral medications and should be taken for 28 days. Your doctor will determine what treatment is right for you based on how you were exposed to HIV. The medications have serious side effects that can make it difficult to finish the program. PEP is not 100% effective; it does not guarantee that someone exposed to HIV will not become infected with HIV.

Who needs PEP?

PEP is usually used for anyone who may have been exposed to HIV.

Healthcare workers have the greatest risk. They can be exposed to HIV by the following:

- Needle sticks or cuts

- Getting blood or other body fluids in their eyes or mouth

- Getting blood or other body fluids on their skin when it is chapped, scraped, or affected by dermatitis

The risk of HIV transmission in these ways is extremely low—less than 1% for all exposures.

PEP can also be used to treat people who may have been exposed to HIV by accident (e.g., condom breakage) or sexual assault.

When should I take PEP if I've been exposed?

PEP is most effective if you take it within 72 hours of possible HIV exposure. The longer you wait to start PEP, the greater the risk of becoming HIV positive.

Your healthcare provider will consider whether PEP is right for you based on how you might have been exposed and whether you know for sure that the individual who might have exposed you is HIV positive. You may be asked to return for more HIV testing at four to six weeks, three months, and six months to determine your HIV status.

Where can I get PEP?

Some of the places you can go to seek treatment include your doctor's office, emergency rooms, urgent care clinics, or a local HIV clinic.

Chapter 47

Preventing Mother-to-Child HIV Transmission

HIV Testing and Pregnancy

HIV [human immunodeficiency virus] testing is recommended for all pregnant women. HIV testing is provided to pregnant women in two ways: Opt-in or opt-out testing. In areas with opt-in testing, women may be offered HIV testing. Women who accept testing will need to sign an HIV testing consent form. In areas with opt-out testing, HIV testing is automatically included as part of routine prenatal care. With opt-out testing, women must specifically ask not to be tested and sign a form refusing HIV testing. The Centers for Disease Control and Prevention (CDC) recommends that opt-out testing be provided to all pregnant women.

Ask your health care provider about HIV testing in your area. If HIV opt-out testing is not available, ask to be tested for HIV.

What are the benefits of HIV testing for pregnant women?

A mother who knows early in her pregnancy that she is HIV infected has more time to make important decisions. She and her health care provider will have more time to decide on effective ways to protect her health and prevent mother-to-child transmission of HIV. She can also take steps to prevent passing HIV to her partner.

Excerpted from "HIV and Pregnancy," by AIDSinfo (www.aidsinfo.nih.gov), part of the National Institutes of Health, updated February 2012.

495

How will I be tested for HIV?

The most common HIV test is the HIV antibody test. HIV antibodies are a type of protein the body produces in response to HIV infection. An HIV antibody test looks for HIV antibodies in a person's blood, urine, or fluids from the mouth. When a person has a positive result from an HIV antibody test, a second and different type of antibody test is done to confirm that the person is indeed infected with HIV. The second test is called a confirmatory HIV test. To be diagnosed with HIV, a person's confirmatory HIV test must also be positive.

Getting results from an HIV antibody blood test generally takes only a few days. (Results from some tests that use fluids from the mouth are ready within an hour.) Getting results from a confirmatory HIV test can take longer—from a few days to a few weeks after the test. People generally receive their results during a follow-up visit with a health care provider. It is important to keep your appointment for your HIV test results.

Pregnant women who test positive for HIV have many options to stay healthy and protect their babies from becoming HIV infected. Health care providers recommend that women infected with HIV take anti-HIV medications to prevent mother-to-child transmission of HIV and, if needed, for their own health.

If you are diagnosed with HIV, your health care provider will answer your questions about HIV and discuss ways to help you and your baby stay healthy. Together you can make decisions about HIV care during your pregnancy.

What happens if I ask not to be tested for HIV?

You will not be tested for HIV. However, your health care provider will likely re-emphasize the importance of HIV testing. You may be offered counseling on how HIV is spread and ways to prevent HIV transmission. Throughout your pregnancy, your health care provider may encourage you to reconsider your decision not to be tested.

Where can I find information on HIV testing in my state?

The U.S. Department of Health and Human Services (HHS) offers information on HIV testing for each state. Contact HHS at 877-696-6775 or 202-619-0257. You can also find information on your state health department website.

Mother-to-Child Transmission of HIV

HIV is transmitted (passed) from one person to another through specific body fluids—blood, semen, genital fluids, and breast milk. Having unprotected sex or sharing needles with a person infected with HIV are the most common ways HIV is transmitted.

Mother-to-child transmission of HIV is when a woman infected with HIV transmits HIV to her baby during pregnancy, during labor and delivery, or by breastfeeding. Because HIV can be transmitted through breast milk, women infected with HIV should not breastfeed their babies. In the United States, baby formula is a safe and healthy alternative to breast milk.

Although the risk is very low, HIV can also be transmitted to a baby through food that was previously chewed (prechewed) by a mother or caretaker infected with HIV. To be safe, babies should not be fed prechewed food.

HIV cannot be transmitted through casual contact, such as hugging and closed-mouth kissing. HIV also cannot be transmitted by items such as toilet seats, door knobs, or dishes used by a person infected with HIV.

When are anti-HIV medications used to prevent mother-to-child transmission of HIV?

Anti-HIV medications are used at the following times to reduce the risk of mother-to-child transmission of HIV:

- During pregnancy, pregnant women infected with HIV receive a regimen (combination) of at least three different anti-HIV medications.

- During labor and delivery, pregnant women infected with HIV receive intravenous (IV) AZT [azidothymidine] and continue to take the medications in their regimens by mouth.

- After birth, babies born to women infected with HIV receive liquid AZT for six weeks. (Babies of mothers who did not receive anti-HIV medications during pregnancy may be given other anti-HIV medications in addition to AZT.)

In addition to taking anti-HIV medications to reduce the risk of mother-to-child transmission of HIV, a pregnant woman infected with HIV may also need anti-HIV medications for her own health. Some women may already be on a regimen before becoming pregnant.

However, because during pregnancy some anti-HIV medications may not be safe to use or may be absorbed differently by the body, the medications in a woman's regimen may change.

How do anti-HIV medications help prevent mother-to-child transmission of HIV?

Taking anti-HIV medications during pregnancy reduces the amount of HIV in an infected mother's body. Having less HIV in the body reduces the risk of mother-to-child transmission of HIV.

Some anti-HIV medications also pass from the pregnant mother to her unborn baby through the placenta (also called the afterbirth). The anti-HIV medication in the baby's body helps protect the baby from HIV infection. This is especially important during delivery when the baby may be exposed to HIV in the mother's genital fluids or blood.

After birth, babies born to women infected with HIV receive anti-HIV medication. The medication reduces the risk of infection from HIV that may have entered the babies' bodies during delivery.

Anti-HIV Medications for Use in Pregnancy

I am HIV infected and pregnant. When should I start taking anti-HIV medications?

When to start taking anti-HIV medications depends on your health, how much HIV has affected your body, and how far along you are in your pregnancy. In general, people infected with HIV who are not pregnant begin taking anti-HIV medications when their CD4 [cluster of differentiation 4] counts fall below 500 cells/mm^3 or if they develop certain other infections. Pregnant women infected with HIV must also consider whether they need anti-HIV medications for their own health or only to prevent mother-to-child transmission of HIV.

Women who need anti-HIV medications for their own health:

- may be taking anti-HIV medications before becoming pregnant; or

- may start taking anti-HIV medications when they become pregnant.

Women who need anti-HIV medications only to prevent mother-to-child transmission of HIV can consider waiting until after the first trimester of pregnancy to take anti-HIV medications. However, starting medications earlier may be more effective at reducing the risk of mother-to-child transmission of HIV.

All pregnant women infected with HIV should be taking anti-HIV medications by the second trimester of pregnancy. Women diagnosed with HIV later in pregnancy should start taking anti-HIV medications as soon as possible.

What anti-HIV medications should I use during my pregnancy?

All pregnant women infected with HIV should take a regimen (combination) of at least three anti-HIV medications. However, the specific medications in your regimen will depend on your individual needs. To select a regimen, your health care provider will review your medical history and order blood tests to assess your health and the stage of your HIV infection. Your health care provider will also consider:

- why you need anti-HIV medications—for your own health or only to prevent transmitting HIV to your baby;

- changes in how your body may absorb medications during pregnancy; and

- the potential of anti-HIV medications to harm your baby or cause birth defects.

I am currently taking anti-HIV medications and just learned I'm pregnant. What should I do?

Continue taking your anti-HIV medications until you talk to your health care provider. Stopping treatment could harm both you and your baby.

If you are in the first trimester of pregnancy, tell your health care provider right away if you are taking Sustiva (or Atripla, an anti-HIV medication that contains Sustiva). Sustiva alone or in Atripla may cause birth defects that develop during the first few months of pregnancy. Your health care provider may recommend safe alternatives for these medications. After the first trimester, Sustiva or Atripla can be used safely.

Talk to your health care provider about the anti-HIV medications in your regimen. Because pregnancy can affect how the body absorbs medications, the doses of some medications you take may change later in pregnancy.

If you are taking anti-HIV medications and your viral load is more than 500 copies/mL, your current regimen may not be effective at suppressing HIV. Your health care provider will recommend a test to see if the medications are still working against HIV (drug-resistance testing) and use the test results to find more effective anti-HIV medications.

I used to take anti-HIV medications, but I don't anymore. What should I do?

Talk to your health care provider about all anti-HIV medications you have used, the results of past drug-resistance testing, and why you no longer take anti-HIV medications. Your medical history, past drug-resistance test results, and additional drug-resistance testing will help you and your health care provider select a new regimen that is safe for use during pregnancy.

Whether you were on anti-HIV medications before becoming pregnant or are just starting a regimen, your health care provider will:

- explain the risks and benefits of using anti-HIV medications during pregnancy;

- stress the importance of taking anti-HIV medications exactly as directed; and

- arrange for additional medical or social support you may need to help you have a healthy pregnancy.

Safety of Anti-HIV Medications during Pregnancy

I am HIV infected and pregnant. Is it safe to use anti-HIV medications during my pregnancy?

Women infected with HIV can safely use many anti-HIV medications during pregnancy to protect their health and to prevent transmitting HIV to their babies. However, some anti-HIV medications can cause problems when used during pregnancy. Knowing more about the safety of anti-HIV medications and pregnancy will help you and your health care provider decide what medications are right for you.

Is my baby at risk from anti-HIV medications I take during pregnancy?

It's not known if babies will have any long-term effects from the anti-HIV medications their mothers use during pregnancy. However, the risk of mother-to-child transmission of HIV is known. And the illness that results when HIV infection is passed from a mother to her child is very real. Because anti-HIV medications can greatly reduce the risk of passing HIV infection from a mother to her child during pregnancy, all pregnant women infected with HIV should take anti-HIV medications.

Information on the use of anti-HIV medications during pregnancy is limited. But enough information is known to make recommendations about the safety of the most commonly used medications from the three most commonly used classes of anti-HIV medications—protease inhibitors (PIs), non-nucleoside reverse transcriptase inhibitors (NNRTIs), and nucleoside reverse transcriptase inhibitors (NRTIs). (Not enough information is known to make recommendations about use during pregnancy of entry inhibitors and integrase inhibitors, two additional classes of anti-HIV medications.)

What should I know about protease inhibitors (PIs)?

There may be a link between the use of some PIs and high blood sugar (hyperglycemia) or diabetes. For some women, the risk of hyperglycemia increases in pregnancy. It is unclear if taking PIs adds to this risk. Talk to your health care provider about the use of PIs during pregnancy and about when to have blood tests to check for hyperglycemia or diabetes.

What should I know about non-nucleoside reverse transcriptase inhibitors (NNRTIs)?

Two NNRTIs, Sustiva and Viramune, should be used in first few months of pregnancy.

- Sustiva may cause birth defects that develop during the first few months of pregnancy. Therefore, if possible, use of Sustiva should be avoided in the first trimester of pregnancy. Atripla, a combination pill that contains Sustiva, should also be avoided in the first trimester of pregnancy. After the first trimester, Sustiva or Atripla can be used safely.

- Viramune increases the risk of very serious liver damage in women with CD4 counts greater than 250 cells/mm^3. Viramune should only be started in pregnant women with CD4 counts higher than 250 cells/mm^3 if the benefits very clearly outweigh the risks. Women who begin using Viramune during pregnancy are carefully monitored for early signs of liver damage. Women taking Viramune without problems before they become pregnant can safely continue to take the medication. Liver damage from Viramune use in pregnancy has not been seen in women already taking the medication without side effects.

501

What should I know about nucleoside reverse transcriptase inhibitors (NRTIs)?

Using NRTIs can sometimes lead to lactic acidosis, a condition caused by the buildup of a specific acid in the blood. Women should not take the combination of Zerit and Videx during pregnancy because the combination has caused deaths from lactic acidosis and liver failure. Women taking NRTIs during pregnancy are watched carefully for signs of lactic acidosis.

Talk to your health care provider about the safety of anti-HIV medications during pregnancy. There are many anti-HIV medications to choose from that will keep you and your baby healthy.

Preventing Transmission of HIV during Labor and Delivery

I am HIV infected and pregnant. Will I need anti-HIV medications during labor and delivery?

Women infected with HIV take anti-HIV medications during labor and delivery to reduce the risk of mother-to-child transmission of HIV. During labor and delivery, women continue to take the anti-HIV medications they took throughout their pregnancies. They also receive an anti-HIV medication called AZT intravenously to protect their babies from HIV in the mother's genital fluids or blood during labor and delivery.

Talk to your health care provider about the use of anti-HIV medications during labor and delivery well before your due date.

Will I have a vaginal or a cesarean delivery?

The risk of mother-to-child transmission of HIV is low for women who take anti-HIV medications during pregnancy and have a viral load less than 1,000 copies/mL near the time of delivery.

For some HIV-infected mothers, a scheduled cesarean delivery (also called a C-section) at 38 weeks of pregnancy (two weeks before the due date) can reduce the risk of mother-to-child transmission of HIV. A scheduled cesarean delivery is recommended for HIV-infected women who:

- have not received anti-HIV medications during pregnancy;

- have a viral load greater than 1,000 copies/mL or an unknown viral load near the time of delivery.

If, before her scheduled cesarean delivery, a woman's water breaks (also called rupture of membranes) or she goes into labor, a cesarean delivery may not reduce the risk of mother-to-child transmission of HIV. If there is not another pregnancy-related reason to have a cesarean delivery, the risks of going ahead with the scheduled cesarean delivery may be greater than the benefits. Depending on an individual woman's situation, a vaginal delivery may be the best alternative to a planned cesarean delivery.

What are the risks of delivery?

All deliveries have risks—even for mothers without HIV infection. In general, a cesarean delivery has greater risks than a vaginal delivery.

For the mother, the risk of infection or a blood clot in the legs or lungs is greater with a cesarean delivery than with a vaginal delivery. All women who have a cesarean delivery, including women infected with HIV, should receive antibiotics to prevent infection. For the infant, the risk of temporary breathing difficulties may be greater with a cesarean delivery.

Talk to your health care provider about the risks and benefits of each type of delivery early in your pregnancy.

Women Infected with HIV and Their Babies after Birth

I am HIV infected and pregnant. What are the chances my baby will be born with HIV?

In the United States and Europe, fewer than two babies in 100 born to mothers infected with HIV are infected with the virus. This is because most women infected with HIV and their babies receive anti-HIV medications to prevent mother-to-child transmission of HIV and do not breastfeed. If you take anti-HIV medications during pregnancy and labor and delivery, if your baby receives anti-HIV medications after birth, and if you do not breastfeed your baby, the risk of passing HIV to your baby is very low.

Will my newborn baby receive anti-HIV medications?

Yes. Within 6 to 12 hours after delivery, babies born to women infected with HIV receive an anti-HIV medication called AZT. AZT helps prevent mother-to-child transmission of HIV. The babies receive AZT for six weeks. (In certain situations, some babies may receive other anti-HIV medications in addition to AZT.)

When will my baby be tested for HIV?

HIV testing for babies born to women with known HIV infection is recommended at 14 to 21 days, at one to two months, and again at four to six months. Testing for babies is done using a virologic HIV test. Virologic HIV tests look directly for the presence of HIV in the blood.

- To be diagnosed with HIV, a baby must have positive results from two virologic HIV tests.

- To know for certain that a baby is not infected with HIV, the baby must have two negative virologic HIV tests, the first at one month of age or older, and the second at least one month later.

Babies who are HIV-infected receive a combination of anti-HIV medications to treat HIV. At four to six weeks of age, babies infected with HIV also start a medication called Bactrim. (Bactrim is also given as a precaution when it's not known if a baby is HIV infected or not.) Bactrim helps prevent *Pneumocystis jiroveci* pneumonia (PCP), a type of pneumonia that can develop in people with advanced HIV.

What is the best way to feed my baby?

Because HIV can be transmitted through breast milk, women infected with HIV who live in the United States should not breastfeed. In the United States, infant formula is a safe and healthy alternative to breast milk. Although the risk is very low, HIV can be transmitted to a baby through food that was previously chewed (prechewed) by a mother or caretaker infected with HIV. To be safe, babies should not be fed prechewed food.

Will my anti-HIV medications change after I give birth?

After your baby is born, you and your health care provider may decide to stop or change your anti-HIV regimen. The decision to continue, change, or stop your anti-HIV medications will depend on several factors, including the following:

- current expert recommendations on the use of anti-HIV medications;

- your CD4 count and viral load;

- issues that make it hard to take medications exactly as directed;

- whether or not your partner is infected with HIV;

- the preferences of you and your health care provider.

Don't stop taking any of your anti-HIV medications without first talking to your health care provider. Stopping your medications may limit the number of anti-HIV medications that will work for you and may cause your HIV infection to worsen.

Having a new baby is exciting! However, caring for a new baby while dealing with the physical and emotional changes that follow childbirth can be stressful. It may be difficult to take your anti-HIV medications exactly as directed. If you feel sad or overwhelmed or have concerns about taking your medications, talk to your health care provider. Together you can make a plan to keep you and your baby healthy.

Chapter 48

Needle Exchange Programs: Preventing STDs in Injection Drug Users

Needle exchange programs are one of the main harm reduction measures that aim to curb the spread of blood-borne viruses such as HIV [human immunodeficiency virus] and Hepatitis C among injecting drug users (IDUs). With an estimated one in five injecting drug users worldwide infected with HIV and 30 percent of HIV infections outside sub-Saharan Africa resulting from injecting drug use, such programs are key to bringing the global epidemic under control.

Harm reduction programs aim to reduce the negative consequences of drug use, by reducing the harm self-inflicted by the user through unsafe practices and the harm inflicted upon society. The provision of needle exchanges and other harm reduction measures, however, is generally poor, and opposition to them is impairing the fight against HIV.

Needle Exchange and HIV

Advocates of harm reduction argue that HIV transmission through blood can be effectively averted through needle exchanges as they empower IDUs to protect themselves and others from HIV. Studies have found that through offering an accessible alternative to needle sharing, HIV transmission within IDU communities can be brought under control. However, this form of harm reduction can be controversial and the scale of implementation varies between countries.

How Does a Needle Exchange Operate?

Needle exchange schemes provide access to sterile syringes and other injecting equipment such as swabs and sterile water to reduce the risk of IDUs coming into contact with other users' blood. Needle exchange programs that offer safe syringe access may be run by NGOs, hospitals or medical facilities, and local or national governments. Needles may be provided at drop-in centers, outreach points, or from vans that service different points within a city or area. In some places, vending machines are used to distribute needles, functioning as a 24-hour service when other sites are shut.

Sometimes a needle exchange may only distribute the same number of syringes that they receive from a user, whereas others may require a lower return rate or not require any return at all. Some needle exchange programs may provide a high number of sterile syringes to a single user so they in turn can distribute them among IDU populations not accessing such programs.

As well as providing clean needles, a needle exchange scheme can also act as a gateway through which users learn about safe injection practices and equipment disposal, safer sex education, access to other prevention services such as substitution therapy, and referral to treatment. The World Health Organization says that without such complementary measures, needle exchange programs will not control HIV infection among injecting drug users.

The U.K.'s [United Kingdom's] medical advisory body recommends that needles are provided in different sizes, and are distributed in a quantity that meets need rather than being limited arbitrarily.

Where Do Needle Exchanges Exist?

Many countries that report injecting drug use and HIV among their injecting populations do not have needle/syringe exchanges. Globally, only 82 countries have needle exchange programs. Moreover, it is evident that although countries report having NSP sites, injecting drug users are still not accessing enough needles/syringes. For example, in Germany there are 250 needle/syringe exchanges, yet injecting drug users only receive an average of two needles/syringes each, per year. It is recommended that in order for needle exchanges to prevent HIV transmission and to make an impact on the HIV epidemic a distribution rate of 200 needle/syringes per IDU, per year is needed. So far this target has only been met by three low- and middle-income countries—Bangladesh, India, and Slovakia.

Low numbers of NSP sites and low distribution rates can be due to a variety of reasons; for example, the lack of resources, public and/or political opposition to harm reduction, as well as laws which criminalize harm reduction.

Overall, Western European countries and Australia are the leaders in harm reduction, and some of the highest distribution levels in the world are among these countries. In 2009, Australia distributed an average of 213 needles/syringes per IDU, per year. However, many countries are failing to deliver an adequate harm reduction service.

As of March 2009, only 184 needle exchange programs existed in 36 U.S. states, plus Washington, DC, and Puerto Rico. For over two decades, the U.S. government forbade funding for such services, but in 2009 the federal funding ban was lifted. This should lead to needle exchange services becoming far more widespread throughout the United States. Currently, the needle/syringe rate is 22 per IDU, per year—far below the recommended rate and one of the lowest in the world.

Throughout Eastern Europe and Central Asia, a promising scale up of harm reduction services has occurred in recent years in many countries, notably Ukraine (which increased the number of NSPs by nearly a thousand to 1,323 between 2008 and 2010). A study focusing on 14 European countries, including Estonia, Slovakia, and Belgium, found a 33 percent increase in the number of syringes distributed by needle and syringe programs between 2003 and 2007. However, distribution levels remain low across this region.

Despite an average of one in six IDUs in Asia living with HIV, most Asian countries have a long way to go before the needle exchange services which exist make an impact on their HIV epidemics. Whilst some countries have many NSPs, in several cases they are only reaching a very low percentage of the country's injecting drug users, who receive very few clean needles/syringes per year. Despite increasing the number of NSPs from 92 in 2006 to 901 in 2010, syringe distribution in China remains very low, at an average of 32 needles/ syringes per IDU, per year.

Apart from a few notable exceptions needle exchanges across Latin America and the Caribbean, Africa, and the Middle East are largely non-existent or where they exist inadequate. Brazil, Mauritius, and Iran are some of the countries which have the most advanced NSPs throughout these regions, although the number of syringes they distribute is low.

Evidence of the Effectiveness of Needle Exchanges

There is clear evidence that needle exchange programs have reduced HIV transmission rates among injecting drug users in areas where they have been established. One of the most definitive studies of needle exchange programs was carried out in 1997, focusing on 81 cities worldwide. It found that HIV infection rates increased by 5.9 percent per year in the 52 cities without needle exchange programs, and decreased by 5.8 percent per year in the 29 cities that did provide them.

A study of HIV among IDUs in New York between 1990 and 2001, found that HIV prevalence fell from 54 percent to 13 percent following the introduction of needle exchange programs.

According to an Australian government study, investment in needle exchange programs from 1991 to 2000 averted 25,000 HIV infections and 21,000 hepatitis C infections. A later Australian study examining the impact of needle exchanges in the following decade revealed they had prevented 32,000 HIV infections and almost 100,000 hepatitis C infections. Furthermore, it is believed the needle exchanges led to healthcare cost savings of over AU$1 billon, equating to a five-fold return on investment for every dollar spent.

The effectiveness of needle exchanges in preventing needle reuse and the potential transmission of HIV has been reflected in a Canadian report. The study found that between 2008 and 2009, needle sharing increased from 10 to 23 percent following the closure of Victoria's only fixed needle exchange. On the other hand, needle sharing among those studied in Vancouver, which has a number of needle exchanges, remained at less than 11 percent.

The World Health Organization (WHO) released a report in 2004 that reviewed the effectiveness of needle exchange programs in many countries, and examined whether they promoted or prolonged illicit drug use. The results produced convincing evidence that needle exchange programs significantly reduce HIV infection, and no evidence that they encourage drug use.

A Case Study: Needle Exchanges in the United States

There has been a long-standing opposition to needle exchanges in the United States, with a ban on federal funding for them being in place for more than twenty years. This funding ban was overturned in 2009 but while in place denied needle exchanges a crucial source of funding. Needle exchange coverage is therefore very poor compared to many other countries of similar economic development.

When the ban was lifted in December 2009, House Speaker Nancy Pelosi labeled it "a big victory for science and for public health." One needle exchange advocate claimed:

"Hundreds of thousands of Americans will not get HIV/AIDS [acquired immunodeficiency syndrome] or hepatitis C, thanks to Congress repealing the federal syringe funding ban."

However, the repeal was not lifted without a fight, in an indication of how strong the opposition is to needle exchanges.

At one stage, the repeal contained a clause restricting federally-funded needle exchanges to locations at least 1,000 feet away from schools, parks, playgrounds, youth centers, and similar areas where children congregate. This clause would have severely limited the areas where needle exchanges could operate, and underlined conservative opposition to them. Some needle exchange advocates used a map of Chicago to highlight the fact that the amendment would make nearly all parts of the city off limits, and that a city cemetery would be one of the few areas where a federally-funded needle exchange could operate.

A similar restriction would have applied to all needle exchanges in the capital, Washington, DC, whose spending is authorized separately from the rest of the country. The author of the DC amendment, Representative Jack Kingston, believed the mere presence of a needle exchange within proximity of a school would in some way encourage drug use:

"There's a mixed signal when we're telling kids stay off drugs, but in some cases 200 feet away, we're allowing people to exchange needles."

In response to Representative Kingston's amendment, Dr. Anthony Fauci, director of the National Institute of Allergy and Infectious Diseases at the National Institutes of Health, said:

"It does not result in an increase in drug abuse, and it does decrease the incidence of HIV. The idea that kids are going to walk out of school and start using drugs because clean needles are available is ridiculous."

A *Washington Post* editorial was scathing of the Congressman's attempt to hamper needle exchange operations in the U.S. capital: "In a city that is in the grips of a harrowing AIDS epidemic, Mr. Kingston's move was unconscionable."

Now the ban on federally-funded needle exchanges has been lifted, without unnecessarily strict restrictions on where they operate, the United States can perhaps make inroads into its HIV epidemic among injecting drug users.

Other Examples of Harm Reduction

Like needle exchanges, other harm reduction measures exist to minimize the harmful consequences associated with drug use. The provision of these programs is often hindered by laws which prohibit carrying drug paraphernalia and the fear of discrimination brought by the association with such programs.

Maintenance therapy: Maintenance therapy, or opioid substitution treatment, involves the provision of drugs such as methadone or buprenorphine, in pill or liquid form, to drug users as a way of minimizing risks associated with injecting. These programs aim to curb needle sharing, the use of contaminated street drugs, overdoses, and crimes associated with funding drug addiction. Methadone or buprenorphine substitution therapy exists in just over 70 countries worldwide.

Drug substitution treatment has proven effective in rehabilitating and stabilizing IDUs, and in reducing HIV infection rates. For example, researchers from the University of Philadelphia monitored 152 injecting users receiving methadone maintenance treatment and 103 injecting users on no treatment over a period of 18 months, all of whom were HIV negative at the beginning of the study. The results showed that over the 18 months, only 3.5 percent of those receiving methadone became infected with HIV, in contrast to 22 percent not on treatment.

A report by WHO [World Health Organization] in March 2005 reviewed many global studies and concluded that substitution treatment is a critical component of HIV prevention policy, significantly reducing opioid dependency and HIV infection rates. In addition, studies have also found a decline in crime rates and commercial sex work when IDUs no longer have to find ways to fund their expensive addictions.

Several studies have shown that prescribing injectable opiates—including heroin—can help heroin addicts who have failed on traditional maintenance therapy. The Randomized Injectable Opioid Treatment Trial (RIOTT), which took place in three U.K. cities, targeted the 5 percent of addicts who were not benefiting from existing treatments and were continuing to inject street heroin despite receiving oral methadone. Individuals in all three groups—those receiving injectable heroin, injectable methadone, or oral methadone—decreased their consumption of street heroin, with the biggest decrease among those receiving injectable heroin. Programs such as these would be beneficial for HIV prevention among problem drug users as reducing their use of street heroin also reduces the likelihood of using contaminated needles. This was in addition to a substantial reduction in crime.

The risk of HIV infection through the use of methamphetamine (crystal meth) is high, yet substitution treatment for meth addiction does not currently exist. As well as the HIV risk associated with injecting meth, one effect of the drug is a high sex drive, which can lead to an increase in sexual partners and riskier sexual behavior. In the United States the use of meth by men who have sex with men (MSM) is 20 times higher than in the general population and is believed to be a major cause of new HIV infections among MSM. If substitution treatment was made available to meth users the risks associated with this drug could be substantially reduced.

Despite evidence of the effectiveness and need for opioid substitution therapy 88 countries and territories which report injecting drug use do not have opioid substitution therapy in place, including 50 countries which also report HIV among injecting drug users.

Safer injection facilities (SIFs): These provide an environment where drug users can inject in a safer manner and under medical supervision. Like needle exchange programs they may offer drug education and referral for treatment. They also aim to reduce public disorder issues and risks associated with injection drug use such as large congregations of injectors in public places and litter, particularly syringes. Such facilities exist in only eight countries including Germany, Switzerland, the Netherlands, Spain, Australia, and Canada.

After Frankfurt introduced SIFs in the early 1990s, cases of HIV among IDUs declined, as did overdose cases in the city which dropped dramatically from 147 in 1991 to 22 in 1997. This decline can be attributed to the city's overall harm reduction approach, though overdose cases dropped steeply in the year following the introduction of SIFs. Furthermore, IDUs who overdose in safer injection facilities are 10 times less likely to require hospitalization. Research of Vancouver's Insite, North America's first SIF, found that there was no association between the facility and the rate of drug trafficking or other crimes linked to drug use. Moreover, in the two-year period following the opening of Insite, the fatal overdose rate declined by 35 percent in the surrounding area.

The Insite facility had faced pressure by Canada's Conservative government, and was threatened with closure under drug trafficking and possession laws. However, a 2008 ruling allowed it to remain open. In the judge's opinion, Canada's Controlled Drugs and Substances Act violated individuals' constitutional rights:

"It denies the addict access to a health care facility where the risk of morbidity associated with infectious disease is diminished, if not eliminated . . . While there is nothing to be said in favor of the injection of controlled substances that leads to addiction, there is much to be said against denying addicts health care services that will ameliorate the effects of their condition."

Safer crack smoking resources: Like needle exchange programs they distribute clean crack-smoking implements in order to curb the risks associated with sharing of equipment.

These have not been implemented on as wide a scale as needle exchange programs but have shown to be effective in cutting behaviors associated with HIV transmission. An Ottowan needle exchange that also began providing sterile crack-smoking equipment, such as glass stems and rubber mouthpieces, found the proportion of participants sharing implements every time decreased from 37 percent six months prior to implementation, to 12 percent 6 months after.

Pharmacy sale of syringes: Non-prescription over-the-counter sale of syringes is another way to allow drug users access to sterile needles. In the United States, some states have amended drug paraphernalia laws to exclude syringes. Pharmacies that provide clean injecting equipment may also offer similar secondary services as needle exchanges such as providing information and referrals. In Australia, pharmacy-based needle and syringe programs account for 15% of all syringes used for injecting drugs.

An examination of the 96 largest metropolitan areas in the United States found both the proportion of IDUs living with, and becoming infected with, HIV, was lower in the 60 areas that permitted the purchase of syringes without prescription compared to the 36 metropolitan areas that did not allow this.

Supplying tin foil to deter injecting: One method of helping habitual drug users avoid the harms of injecting is supplying tin foil to encourage smoking of drugs instead. Heroin can be boiled on a piece of foil and then its vapors inhaled. Some countries such as Holland and Spain supply foil through their needle exchanges. In England, however, it is illegal to do so, though it is believed that around 100 of the known 1300 needle exchanges break the law and supply foil. An Early Day Motion in the British Parliament aims to overturn section 9A of the Misuse of Drugs Act which restricts the supply of tin foil.

Again, while no one would claim that smoking heroin is a healthy activity, for people who are addicted to the drug and normally inject, smoking can be a preferable option: "Smoking drugs is by no means safe, but is a great deal safer than injecting drugs—which is particularly associated with overdose, blood-borne viruses, drug-related litter, greater dependency, abscesses, and vein damage," Jamie Bridge, International Harm Reduction Association.

Safe needle disposal: Various disposal methods exist so contaminated needles are unable to injure another person. These include drop-off points located in buildings such as police departments, clinics, community organizations or medical waste facilities; mail-back programs where used needles are sent in a special container to a collection site; residential pick-up services; and in-home disposal services that safely destroy the needle. Programs that offer safer syringe disposal may well be part of a general needle exchange service.

Community-based outreach programs: These work with injecting drug users to distribute clean equipment, promote condom use, and provide information about prevention and rehabilitation. Injecting communities are often secretive and distrustful of authorities. Outreach programs focus on accessing these hidden groups, opening an important route to providing support. In some cases, former IDUs are recruited and trained as peer-outreach workers. Some IDUs are likely to be involved in sex work to fund their expensive addiction, so provision of sexual health information and condom promotion play key roles in preventing HIV transmission through other routes. Involving communities in the development of harm reduction programs can help to ensure that policies around harm reduction are suitable for local context and meet the needs of IDUs.

A report from the WHO reviewed data from over 40 studies on outreach prevention methods and concluded that these significantly reduce high-risk behavior in IDUs and are successful in directing them to rehabilitation services.

In 2006, UNAIDS [Joint United Nations Programme on HIV/AIDS] published a report that reviewed several high coverage prevention programs (50 percent of local IDU population accessing more than one prevention initiative) in transitional and developing countries. The inclusion of harm reduction measures was one of the key factors in achieving high coverage.

A Case Study: Harm Reduction in Russia

Given that the Russian AIDS epidemic is being driven by injecting drug use, harm reduction measures like needle exchanges and substitution therapy are crucial. However, HIV prevention for drug users is largely inaccessible with opioid substitution therapy being illegal and needle exchange coverage hugely inadequate. It is estimated that in 2008 just 7 percent of Russian injecting drug users were accessing needle exchanges. This is reflected across the wider Eastern Europe and Central Asia region, which Russia dominates, and it is no coincidence that this is the only large part of the world where HIV prevalence is increasing.

Russia's leading figures in psychiatry and addiction have rejected opioid substitution as an effective way of dealing with the harms of drug use. In an official memorandum they wrote:

"The effective way to solve the problem of drug addiction treatment is an intensive search for and introduction of new methods and means that focus on complete cessation of drugs use by patients with addiction, their socialization into a new life style free from drugs, but not on exchanging from one drug to another."

In 2009, Global Fund prevention programs were almost cut after the organization, under its strict guidelines, deemed the country too wealthy to continue to receive funding. The Russian government chose not to step in, instead saying it would focus on broader health promotion. Given Russia's stance, the Global Fund felt it had no option but to extend funding for prevention efforts directed at vulnerable groups until 2011. An editorial in *The Lancet* outlined the difficulties of providing prevention services for drug users and stressed the need for harm reduction initiatives in the country:

"In Russia, the opposition to harm reduction programs has meant that needle exchange is mostly run by non-governmental organizations (NGOs). The government has repeatedly refused to allow methadone substitution to be offered to people who inject drug, despite many international calls to support this evidence-based intervention . . . We urge the Russian Government to continue to fund effective and science-driven harm reduction programs, in addition to its general health promotion efforts."

The Controversy of Harm Reduction

Harm reduction measures are supported and implemented by NGOs, health authorities, governments, and multilateral organizations worldwide. However, such methods for dealing with the harms of drugs have been surrounded by controversy since the mid-1980s when needle exchanges and substitution treatments were first introduced in Western Europe. Drugs policy is often discussed in a very moralistic way, with many politicians adopting stances that do not take into account scientific evidence. Because of the impact of drug abuse on society, and perhaps the mind-altering nature of drugs, legislators want to show they are "tough on drugs," even if their policies contribute to the damage they claim to be against.

Some countries have strategies that involve forcing drug users to abstain or have treatment. Currently there are up to several hundred thousand people who use drugs who are detained in order to undergo treatment, of whom very few have access to maintenance therapy. The WHO maintains that drug detention centers are not effective at preventing drug use and that they can undermine effective harm reduction programs and increase HIV risk.

Advocates of needle exchanges and other harm reduction measures point to the evidence that such programs reduce the incidence of HIV infection and do not encourage drug use. Furthermore, they say having abstinence as the only goal worth pursuing is unrealistic, and as long as people continue to take drugs, they should be encouraged to do so in the least harmful way possible. It is argued that the benefits of harm reduction transcend beyond the drug user into society, not only by reducing death, crime, and HIV infection but through supporting education. This is recognized by the England and Wales National Institute for Health and Clinical Excellence who state that "While NSPs (needle and syringe programs) can help reduce the harm caused to people who inject drugs, the consequent reduction in the prevalence of blood-borne viruses benefits wider society". Moreover, studies show that harm reduction measures can also result in financial savings, for example for every $1 spent on methadone treatment, at least $5 is saved through alleviating public spending in sectors such as healthcare or prisons.

"Harm reduction recognizes that containment and reduction of drug-related harms is a more feasible option than efforts to eliminate drug use entirely . . . [it] does not focus on abstinence: Although harm reduction supports those who seek to moderate or reduce their drug use, it neither excludes nor presumes a treatment goal of abstinence," U.K. Harm Reduction Alliance.

The arguments against harm reduction range from moderate to extreme. Some believe that needle exchange services are a waste of money and only promote injecting drug use, when the message should be abstinence from drugs. Opioid substitution treatment is a difficult concept for many to accept; critics argue that this prolongs drug addiction or provides users with drugs to sell on the street to fund further drug use. Although outreach work is the most accepted form of harm reduction, some believe its activities, such as teaching safer injecting methods, is a waste of resources. There is also strong opposition to safe injection rooms and heroin prescription for problem IDUs, often the most contentious forms of harm reduction.

In 2004, Republican Congressman, Mark Souder, then chairman of the U.S. Subcommittee on Criminal Justice, Drug Policy, and Human Resources, criticized harm reduction supporters:

"Advocates of this position hold that dangerous behaviors, such as drug abuse, should be accepted by society and those who choose such lifestyles—or become trapped in them—should be enabled to continue these behaviors in a less harmful manner."

In response the president of the International Harm Reduction Association summarized the debate over needle exchange programs and other harm reduction measures as one which "divides participants into those who base their judgments on data from those who base their judgments on other considerations than data."

The controversy surrounding harm reduction exists at the highest levels of global decision making. Harm reduction is supported by many United Nations bodies including the General Assembly, UNAIDS, the UN Office on Drugs and Crime, and the World Health Organization. However, the 2009 Political Declaration of the UN Commission on Narcotics Drugs, which outlines international cooperation on drug strategy for the next 10 years, does not refer to it at all. This omission was encouraged by several states including the United States and Russia as well as Sweden, Italy, and Japan. Even the Vatican weighed into the debate, criticizing harm reduction, to which one group in favor responded:

"By making a statement against harm reduction, the Vatican has indicated that its moral objection to drug use is more important than its commitment to the sanctity of life."

The Future of Needle Exchanges and Harm Reduction

It is also argued that countries must significantly scale up harm reduction services for IDUs if benefits are to be population-wide. However, despite notable progress by some countries to improve their harm reduction services, barriers remain, and the future of HIV prevention for injecting drug users in many countries remains uncertain.

Even in countries that have increased access to sterile needles and other harm reduction methods, progress is often insufficient, and in many parts of the world authorities refuse to implement or sufficiently support such programs for political or moralistic reasons.

In 2010 a report claimed that in low and middle income countries prevention of the HIV epidemic among injecting drug users is failing due to funding shortfalls for HIV-related harm reduction programs. The report found spending in 2007 totaled $12.80 per injector, far less than the estimated average need of $256 per injector per year in 2010.

While this situation exists, it seems inevitable that the spread of HIV among drug users will continue to outpace attempts to control it. As Michel Sidibé, Executive Director of UNAIDS identified:

"The vicious cycle of secrecy, social exclusion, drug use, criminalization, and HIV spread must be broken."

Chapter 49

STD Vaccines and Microbicides

Chapter Contents

Section 49.1—Anti-HIV Drug Acts to Block Herpes Virus 520

Section 49.2—Herpevac Trial 522

Section 49.3—Shutting Down the Genital
Herpes Virus with Microbicides 526

Section 49.4—Preventive HIV Vaccines 528

Section 49.5—Therapeutic HIV Vaccines 531

Section 49.6—Understanding the HPV Vaccine 533

Section 49.7—HPV Vaccine Information
for Preteens and Teens 538

Section 49.8—HPV Vaccine Soon to Be Recommended
for Preteen Boys as Well as Girls 541

Section 49.1

Anti-HIV Drug Acts to Block Herpes Virus

"NIH Researchers Show How Anti-HIV Drug Acts
to Block Herpes Virus," by the National Institutes of Health
(NIH, www.nih.gov), October 20, 2011.

An anti-HIV [human immunodeficiency virus] drug also discovered to stop the spread of the genital herpes virus does so by disabling a key DNA [deoxyribonucleic acid] enzyme of the herpes virus, according to findings by researchers at the National Institutes of Health and other institutions.

The study was published online in [the October 20, 2011 issue of] *Cell Host and Microbe* and was conducted by researchers at the Catholic University of Leuven, Belgium; the University of Rome; Gilead Sciences, Inc., Foster City, California; and the NIH's Eunice Kennedy Shriver National Institute of Child Health and Human Development (NICHD).

The findings explain the results of a recent clinical trial showing that the anti-HIV drug tenofovir, when it is formulated as a vaginal gel, could reduce the risk of herpes simplex virus (HSV) infections—as well as HIV infections—in women.

Tenofovir taken orally had been demonstrated to inhibit reproduction of HIV, but had not been known to block the genital herpes virus.

"HIV infection is closely associated with herpes viral infection. When people with genital herpes are exposed to HIV, they are more likely to become infected than are people who do not carry the herpes virus," said Leonid Margolis, PhD, head of the Section on Intercellular Interactions at NICHD and one of the authors of the study. "Human tissues convert tenofovir to a form that suppresses HIV. We found that this form of tenofovir also suppresses HSV [herpes simplex virus]. This discovery may help to identify drugs to treat the two viruses even more effectively."

Discoveries leading to new uses for previously approved drugs have the potential to save millions of dollars, Dr. Margolis said. New drugs typically undergo years of testing for safety and effectiveness before they are approved for patients. Finding new uses for an approved drug increases the value of the initial investment in testing, because most of the testing has previously been completed.

The researchers examined individual cells and groups of cells infected with HSV and found that high concentrations of tenofovir prevent the ability of this virus to reproduce. They also confirmed that tenofovir itself did not damage the cells. These tests included the type of cells that line the vagina, which are targets for infection with HSV and HIV.

Tenofovir is converted by cellular enzymes to another chemical form. The researchers found that this form of tenofovir suppresses not only HIV, but HSV as well. Specifically, the researchers showed that this active form of tenofovir can disable an enzyme that the virus needs to reproduce.

The researchers also examined the effects of tenofovir in tissues samples. They injected HSV into tonsil tissue and cervix tissue, and then applied tenofovir. They found that after 12 days, levels of the virus were only 1 to 13 percent of viral levels in untreated tissue. Tenofovir also blocked viral reproduction in tissue infected with both HIV and HSV simultaneously.

Using tenofovir to treat lab mice infected with the herpes virus also prevented symptoms of the disease and prolonged the animals' survival, the researchers found.

The vaginal gel showed activity against HSV apparently because of the high concentration of tenofovir that it contains. In contrast, when tenofovir is taken orally, tissue levels do not reach sufficient levels to significantly affect HSV.

"When using the gel, the amount of tenofovir on the affected tissues is about 100 times the amount in the body when taking tenofovir in pill form," said Dr. Margolis. "That explains why its anti-herpes activity wasn't noticed before. Thus, under proper conditions, an anti-HIV drug becomes an anti-HSV drug."

In previous research, Dr. Margolis' team showed that an anti-HSV drug, acyclovir, is converted inside the infected cells into an anti-HIV drug. They now believe the next step will be to find the form in which such drugs are most potent against both viruses at the same time.

Section 49.2

Herpevac Trial

"Questions and Answers: The Herpevac Trial for Women," by the National Institute of Allergy and Infectious Diseases (NIAID, www.niaid.nih.gov), part of the National Institutes of Health, January 5, 2012.

What is the Herpevac trial for women?

The Herpevac trial for women is a clinical study investigating a vaccine to protect women against genital herpes disease. The trial, which began in 2002 and concluded in 2010, was conducted at 50 sites in the United States and Canada and was sponsored by GlaxoSmithKline (GSK) Biologicals in cooperation with the National Institute of Allergy and Infectious Diseases (NIAID), part of the NIH. The study chair is Robert Belshe, MD, director of the Center for Vaccine Development at the Saint Louis University School of Medicine in Missouri.

How many participants were involved in the study?

The Herpevac Trial for Women involved 8,323 women ages 18–30. At the time of their enrollment, the study participants were free of the two common types of herpes simplex viruses (HSV): HSV-1, the primary cause of cold sores and an increasing cause of genital herpes, and HSV-2, the common cause of genital herpes. Approximately 31,000 women were screened in order to identify eligible participants.

What was the study's design?

The study was a randomized, double-blind, controlled Phase III clinical trial. Participants were randomly assigned to receive either the investigational herpes vaccine or a version of Havrix, an FDA [U.S. Food and Drug Administration]-approved, licensed vaccine to protect against hepatitis A. This was done to give all participants an opportunity to be protected against either genital herpes or hepatitis A. GSK developed the candidate herpes vaccine and is also the manufacturer of Havrix.

The investigational herpes vaccine is a subunit vaccine containing a glycoprotein from HSV along with an adjuvant to boost immune response. The Havrix vaccine administered to study participants was provided at a lower dose and smaller volume than it is routinely provided in medical practice. This was done to ensure that the vaccine could be administered in the same number of doses as the candidate herpes vaccine. Each volunteer was vaccinated at the beginning of the study and again after one month and six months following the first injection. The participants were followed for 20 months after the initial injection and evaluated for HSV infection and genital herpes disease. Throughout the study, participants were regularly counseled on how to reduce their risk of acquiring HSV.

What were the results of the trial?

The trial was successfully conducted according to protocol and met statistical targets in terms of enrollment and participant follow up. The vaccine proved to be well-tolerated and its safety profile was similar to that observed in previous trials. According to the initial data analysis publicly announced in September 2010, the trial produced a point estimate of overall vaccine effectiveness of 20 percent with a confidence interval that included zero. In other words, the vaccine was not effective at preventing genital herpes disease among the study population of women. At that time, study collaborators stated that evaluation of the trial data would continue and that a more detailed analysis would be provided at a later time.

A subsequent, more detailed analysis published in the *New England Journal of Medicine* on Jan. 5, 2012, found that the investigational vaccine provided some protection against HSV-1, although it did not protect against HSV-2. Specifically, there were 58 percent fewer cases of genital herpes caused by HSV-1 and 35 percent fewer HSV-1 infections among women who received the investigational vaccine, compared to those who received the control vaccine. The recent analysis also found that among women enrolled in the control group, HSV-1 caused more cases of genital herpes than HSV-2. [Reference: RB Belshe et al. Efficacy results of a trial of a herpes simplex vaccine. *New England Journal of Medicine* 366(1):26–35 (2012).]

Why was the trial important?

The Herpevac Trial for Women produced important scientific information to guide future research toward a vaccine to prevent genital herpes. It also provided emerging data about genital herpes and the changing role of HSV-1 in infection.

An estimated one in four women in the United States has genital herpes, making it one of the most common infectious diseases. HSV, the cause of genital herpes disease, may be transmitted through sexual or other skin-to-skin contact, and can be spread even when the infected individual shows no symptoms. Once in the body, HSV migrates to nerve cells and remains there permanently where it can reactivate to cause painful outbreaks in the infected individual. HSV can cause severe illness in infants born to HSV-infected women, and the virus has been identified as a risk factor for HIV transmission in adults. There is no cure for herpes infection, and there is no vaccine to prevent it.

When the investigational vaccine was tested in two earlier studies involving fewer men and women who did not have genital herpes but whose sexual partners were known to be infected, the candidate vaccine prevented genital herpes disease in more than 70 percent of the female volunteers but had no clear effect in men. Further, the candidate vaccine reduced by roughly 40 percent the risk of developing antibodies to herpes, which are used as an indicator that a person has been infected with HSV. These studies formed the basis for conducting the larger Herpevac study. Results of these two earlier studies were published in November 2002 in the *New England Journal of Medicine*. [Reference: LR Stanberry et al. Glycoprotein-D-adjuvant vaccine to prevent genital herpes. *New England Journal of Medicine* 347(21):1652–1661 (2002).]

Though it failed to reach its primary goal, the Herpevac Trial for Women produced important scientific information to guide future research toward a vaccine to prevent genital herpes. The researchers suspect that the differences between the 2002 studies and the Herpevac Trial were due to immunologic and behavioral differences in the populations studied, which may have affected participants' protection from HSV-1 and HSV-2.

The trial results also provided emerging data about genital herpes and the changing role of HSV-1 in infection. Although HSV-1 is typically associated with cold sores and HSV-2 with genital lesions, HSV-1 has become a growing cause of genital disease, an observation echoed in this analysis. Among women enrolled in the control group of the Herpevac trial, HSV-1 was found to cause more cases of genital herpes than HSV-2.

How was participant safety monitored during the trial?

Participant safety was closely monitored throughout the trial, both by the study investigators and by a data and safety monitoring board

(DSMB). The DSMB is an independent committee composed of clinical research experts, herpes virus experts, and statisticians that provides additional oversight of a clinical study. The DSMB regularly reviews data while a clinical trial is in progress to ensure the safety of participants and that any benefits shown in the study are quickly made available to all participants.

The investigational herpes vaccine used in the trial had been previously tested in more than 7,000 volunteers; results from these studies suggested that it was well-tolerated and safe.

Was there any risk to participants that the vaccine could cause herpes infection?

No. The herpes vaccine formulation used in the study did not contain live virus and was incapable of infecting participants with herpes virus. The candidate vaccine contained only a specific fragment of a herpes virus protein to stimulate immune responses.

Will researchers continue to analyze the data from the Herpevac Trial to better understand the results?

Yes. Researchers will continue to examine serum samples from the Herpevac study to better understand why the vaccine protected women from genital disease caused by HSV-1, but not HSV-2.

Section 49.3

Shutting Down the Genital Herpes Virus with Microbicides

"Shutting Down the Genital Herpes Virus," by the National Institutes of Allergy and Infectious Diseases (NIAID, www .niaid.nih.gov), part of the National Institutes of Health, January 5, 2011.

Once acquired, herpes simplex virus (HSV) 2—a common, sexually transmitted infection (STI) that can cause painful, recurring sores around the genitals—never goes away. Although genital herpes symptoms can be controlled with antiviral drugs, preventing HSV-2 infection altogether is an important public health goal because HSV-2 infection increases a person's risk of acquiring HIV [human immunodeficiency virus], the virus that causes AIDS [acquired immunodeficiency syndrome].

NIAID grantee Judy Lieberman, MD, PhD, and her colleagues at Harvard Medical School in Boston made headway toward this goal by creating a fatty liquid that effectively silenced the expression of HSV-2 genes and protected mice from an otherwise lethal dose of the virus. Significantly, the liquid's power seemed long-lasting. In one experiment, the scientists found that their product continued to have the desired effect in mouse vaginas for at least nine days.

The liquid the Boston group is developing is one of a class of experimental substances called microbicides. Several dozen microbicides are being tested in labs, animal studies, and human clinical trials. Whether formulated as a gel, cream, or foam, microbicides would be applied to the vagina prior to intercourse, giving women a discreet way to protect themselves from STIs. An ideal microbicide would not only be safe, easy to use, and inexpensive but also it would be effective even if applied many hours or days before intercourse.

Microbicides can work in different ways. Some create an impenetrable barrier and act like a chemical condom, while others maintain the acidity of the vaginal fluid, boosting its ability to destroy germs. The substance being tested in Dr. Lieberman's lab incorporates short strips of genetic material, called small interfering RNA (siRNA), which specifically target and "silence" the genes HSV-2 needs to reproduce and spread. Dr. Lieberman and colleagues including Deborah Palliser, PhD, and David Knipe, PhD, were the first to show an siRNA-based microbicide worked in an animal model of HSV-2 infection.

RNA Interference

Since its discovery—first in plants and insects and later in higher animals—the naturally occurring viral defense process called RNA interference (RNAi) has generated great excitement throughout the scientific world. Researchers hope to harness the gene-silencing effects of RNAi with lab-created siRNAs that can target the genetic machinery of viruses while sparing host tissue. Significant challenges remain, however. For example, investigators must devise a way to incorporate virus-specific siRNAs into an inert carrier and then deliver them to the appropriate body cells so that the siRNAs can do their silencing work.

Dr. Lieberman and her co-workers have shown that there are ways to work around and potentially overcome these hurdles. They mixed siRNAs targeting two HSV-2 genes with fat molecules called lipids. The siRNA-containing lipid complex was effectively taken up by both surface and deeper layers of mouse vaginal cells and almost completely extinguished the HSV-2 genes' activity. Importantly, the siRNA liquid did not appear to cause inflammation, suggesting that it might be a good candidate for further study as a microbicide. For clinical use, however, it would need to be formulated in a gel that could be retained in a woman's vagina.

Aside from work on microbicide candidates, Dr. Lieberman's lab is also trying to find ways to induce immune cells to take up siRNAs targeted against HIV genes. Unlike vaginal mucosal cells, lymphocytes do not readily take up siRNA-containing lipids. Recently, Dr. Lieberman and her colleagues reported success in overcoming this problem. They combined an siRNA with a protein fragment that enabled siRNAs to be delivered to all types of human white blood cells, including lymphocytes, macrophages, and dendritic cells, all prime targets of HIV. Dr. Lieberman and her co-workers next intend to test these siRNAs in immunodeficient mice transplanted with human blood cells that are susceptible to HIV infection.

References

Palliser D et al. An siRNA-based microbicide protects mice from lethal herpes simplex virus 2 infection. *Nature* DOI: 10.1038/ nature04263 (2006).

Peer D et al. Selective gene silencing in activated leukocytes by targeting siRNAs to the integrin lymphocyte function-associated antigen-1. *Proc Natl Acad Sci* DOI: 10.1073/pnas.0608491104 (2007).

Section 49.4

Preventive HIV Vaccines

Excerpted from "Preventive HIV Vaccines," by AIDSinfo (www.aidsinfo .nih.gov), part of the National Institutes of Health, May 2006. Reviewed and revised by David A. Cooke, MD, FACP, July 10, 2012.

What is a vaccine?

A vaccine is a medical product designed to stimulate your body's immune system in order to prevent or control an infection. An effective preventive vaccine trains your immune system to fight off a particular microorganism so that it can't establish a serious infection or make you sick.

What is the difference between a preventive HIV (human immunodeficiency virus) vaccine and a therapeutic HIV vaccine?

Therapeutic HIV vaccines are designed to control HIV infection in people who are already HIV positive. Preventive HIV vaccines are designed to protect HIV negative people from becoming infected or getting sick. This text focuses on preventive HIV vaccines.

Although there is currently no vaccine to prevent HIV, researchers are developing and testing potential HIV vaccines. The goal is to develop a vaccine that can protect people from HIV infection, or at least lessen the chance of getting HIV or AIDS [acquired immunodeficiency syndrome] should a person be exposed to the virus.

To date, no HIV vaccine has been shown to be sufficiently effective for preventing infection to be approved for general use. However, encouraging results have been seen with some experimental vaccines.

A large study in 2009 performed in Thailand using a combination of the ALVAC and AIDSVAX vaccines showed modest protection against HIV infection in humans. Additional studies are underway to determine whether the effectiveness of this combination can be improved.

In January 2012, an experimental vaccine against SIV (simian immunodeficiency virus, a close relative of HIV) showed substantial protection against infection in monkeys. Trials of a human-adapted version of the vaccine are planned in the near future.

How does a preventive vaccine work?

When your body encounters a microorganism, your immune system mounts an attack on the invader. After the microorganism is defeated, your immune system continues to "remember" how to quickly beat the invader should it try to infect you again.

A vaccine is designed to resemble a real microorganism. The vaccine trains your immune system to recognize and attack the real microorganism should you ever encounter it. If you've received an effective vaccine, your immune system will "remember" how to quickly attack and defeat a particular microorganism for many years.

Can an HIV vaccine give me HIV or AIDS?

The experimental HIV vaccines currently being studied in clinical trials do not contain any real HIV, and therefore cannot cause HIV or AIDS. However, some HIV vaccines in trials could prompt your body to produce antibodies against HIV. These HIV antibodies could cause you to test positive on a standard HIV test, even if you don't actually have HIV.

Other tests are available that can distinguish between vaccinated and infected people.

What are the different types of vaccine?

There are three main types of vaccines that are being studied for the prevention of HIV infection and AIDS:

- Subunit vaccines, also known as component or protein vaccines, contain only individual parts of HIV, rather than the whole virus. Instead of collecting these parts from the virus itself, the HIV subunits are made in the laboratory using genetic engineering techniques. These man-made subunits alone—without the rest of the virus—can prompt the body to produce an anti-HIV immune response, although that response may be too weak to actually protect against future HIV infection.

- Recombinant vector vaccines take advantage of non-HIV viruses that either don't cause disease in humans or have been deliberately weakened so that they can't cause disease. These weakened (attenuated) viruses are used as vectors, or carriers, to deliver copies of HIV genes into the cells of the body. Once inside cells, the body uses the instructions carried in the copies of HIV genes to produce HIV proteins. As with subunit vaccines, these HIV proteins can stimulate an anti-HIV immune response. Most of the recombinant vector vaccines for HIV deliver several HIV genes (but not the complete set) and may therefore create a stronger immune response. Some of the virus vectors being studied for HIV vaccines include ALVAC (a canarypox virus), MVA (modified vaccinia virus Ankara, a type of cowpox virus), VEE (Venezuelan equine encephalitis, a virus that normally infects horses), and adenovirus-5 (a human virus that doesn't usually cause serious disease) based vectors.

- DNA (deoxyribonucleic acid) vaccines also introduce HIV genes into the body. Unlike recombinant vector vaccines, DNA vaccines do not rely on a virus vector. Instead, "naked" DNA containing HIV genes is injected directly into the body. Cells take up this DNA and use it to produce HIV proteins. As with subunit and recombinant vector vaccines, the HIV proteins trigger the body to produce an immune response against HIV.

Again, none of these vaccines contain real HIV or anything else that could cause HIV infection or AIDS.

What is a prime-boost vaccination strategy?

A single type of HIV vaccine may be used alone, or it may be used in combination with another type of HIV vaccine. One approach to combined HIV vaccination is called the prime-boost strategy. In this approach, administration of one type of HIV vaccine (such as a DNA vaccine) is followed by later administration of a second type of HIV vaccine (such as a recombinant vector vaccine). The goal of this approach is to stimulate different parts of the immune system and enhance the body's overall immune response to HIV.

Section 49.5

Therapeutic HIV Vaccines

Excerpted from "Therapeutic HIV Vaccines," by AIDSinfo
(www.aidsinfo.nih.gov), part of the National Institutes of
Health, May 2006. Reviewed by David A. Cooke, MD, FACP,
July 10, 2012.

What is a vaccine?

A vaccine is a medical product designed to stimulate your body's
immune system in order to prevent or control an infection. An effective
vaccine trains your immune system to fight a particular microorganism
so that it can't make you sick.

Although there are currently no vaccines to prevent or treat HIV
[human immunodeficiency virus], researchers are developing and testing potential HIV vaccines. HIV vaccines designed to prevent HIV
infection in HIV negative people are called preventive vaccines. HIV
vaccines designed to help control HIV infection in people who are already HIV positive are called therapeutic vaccines. This text focuses
on therapeutic HIV vaccines.

What is a therapeutic HIV vaccine?

A therapeutic HIV vaccine (also known as a treatment vaccine) is a
vaccine used in the treatment of an HIV infected person. Therapeutic
HIV vaccines are designed to boost the body's immune response to HIV
in order to better control the infection.

Currently, there are no therapeutic HIV vaccines approved by the
Food and Drug Administration (FDA). However, therapeutic HIV vaccines are being tested in clinical trials to find out if they are safe and
effective in treating people with HIV.

Researchers hope that if therapeutic vaccines are able to strengthen
the body's natural anti-HIV immune response, people with HIV will
not have to rely exclusively on the antiretroviral drugs now used to
treat HIV infection. Currently, antiretroviral drugs must be taken for
life, and some cause serious side effects.

531

All experimental therapeutic HIV vaccines are in very early stages of research, and no therapeutic vaccine is anticipated to be available to the general public for many years, if at all.

Will a therapeutic HIV vaccine be able to cure HIV?

Probably not. If therapeutic vaccines are effective, they may be able to help keep HIV infection under control. However, most researchers do not think therapeutic HIV vaccines will be able to completely eliminate HIV infection, because the virus hides in certain cells of the body where it can last for decades.

Will a therapeutic vaccine rule out the need for antiretroviral drugs?

Even an effective therapeutic HIV vaccine probably won't be able to replace antiretroviral drugs entirely. At best, a therapeutic HIV vaccine may help control HIV infection and keep people healthy while minimizing the need for antiretroviral drugs.

Who is eligible to receive a therapeutic vaccine?

Therapeutic vaccines are designed specifically for HIV positive people who have healthy immune systems.

Therapeutic vaccine recipients must have strong immune systems for the vaccine to generate an effective anti-HIV immune response. Clinical trials of therapeutic vaccines are recruiting volunteers with CD4 counts greater than 250 cells/mm^3, and most studies require a CD4 count greater than 350 cells/mm^3. People with weaker immune systems may be unable to produce a good immune response to a therapeutic HIV vaccine, and are therefore not eligible for these trials. Most trials require that therapeutic vaccine recipients continue taking antiretroviral drugs during the study.

What are the side effects of therapeutic vaccines?

Because testing is ongoing, not all of the side effects of therapeutic vaccines are known. However, side effects observed so far in clinical trials have been similar to the side effects that occur with FDA-approved vaccines.

These side effects include the following:

- Soreness, swelling, redness, or pain at the site of injection

- Mild flu-like symptoms (fever, chills, muscle pain or weakness, nausea, headache, and dizziness)

Section 49.6

Understanding the HPV Vaccine

"HPV Vaccine Information for Young Women—Fact Sheet,"
by the Centers for Disease Control and Prevention
(CDC, www.cdc.gov), September 15, 2011.

Two vaccines are available to prevent the human papillomavirus (HPV) types that cause most cervical cancers. These vaccines are Cervarix (GlaxoSmithKline) and Gardasil (Merck). One of the HPV vaccines, Gardasil, also prevents genital warts as well as anal, vulvar, and vaginal cancers. Both vaccines are given in three shots over six months.

Why the HPV Vaccine Is Important

Genital HPV is a common virus that is passed from one person to another through direct skin-to-skin contact during sexual activity. Most sexually active people will get HPV at some time in their lives, though most will never even know it. HPV infection is most common in people in their late teens and early 20s. There are about 40 types of HPV that can infect the genital areas of men and women. Most HPV types cause no symptoms and go away on their own. But some types can cause cervical cancer in women and other less common cancers— like cancers of the anus, penis, vagina, and vulva (area around the opening of the vagina) and oropharynx (back of throat including base of tongue and tonsils). Other types of HPV can cause warts in the genital areas of men and women, called genital warts. Genital warts are not a life-threatening disease. But they can cause emotional stress and their treatment can be very uncomfortable. Every year, about 12,000 women are diagnosed with cervical cancer and 4,000 women die from this disease in the United States. About 1% of sexually active adults in the United States have visible genital warts at any point in time.

Which girls/women should receive HPV vaccination?

HPV vaccination is recommended with either vaccine for 11- and 12-year-old girls. It is also recommended for girls and women age 13 through 26 years of age who have not yet been vaccinated or completed the vaccine series; HPV vaccine can also be given to girls beginning at age 9 years.

Will sexually active females benefit from the vaccine?

Ideally females should get the vaccine before they become sexually active and exposed to HPV. Females who are sexually active may also benefit from the vaccine, but they may get less benefit from it. This is because they may have already gotten one or more of HPV types targeted by the vaccines. However, few sexually active young women are infected with all HPV types prevented by the vaccines, so most young women could still get protection by getting vaccinated.

Can pregnant women get the vaccine?

The vaccines are not recommended for administration to pregnant women. Although studies show that HPV vaccines do not cause problems for babies born to women who received HPV vaccination when pregnant, more research is still needed. A pregnant woman should not get any doses of either HPV vaccine until her pregnancy is completed.

Getting the HPV vaccine when pregnant is not a reason to consider ending a pregnancy. If a woman realizes that she got one or more shots of an HPV vaccine while pregnant, she should do two things:

- Wait until after her pregnancy to finish the remaining HPV vaccine doses.

- Call the pregnancy registry [800-986-8999 for Gardasil or 888-452-9622 for Cervarix]. These pregnancy registries help us learn more about how pregnant women respond to each of the vaccines.

Should girls and women be screened for cervical cancer before getting vaccinated?

Girls and women do not need to get an HPV test or Pap test to find out if they should get the vaccine. However, it is important that women continue to be screened for cervical cancer, even after getting all three shots of either HPV vaccine.

Effectiveness of the HPV Vaccines

The vaccines target the HPV types that most commonly cause cervical cancer. One of the vaccines also protects against the HPV types that cause most genital warts. Both vaccines are highly effective in preventing specific HPV types and the most common health problems from HPV.

The vaccines are less effective in preventing HPV-related disease in young women who have already been exposed to one or more HPV types. That is because the vaccines can only prevent HPV before a person it is exposed to it. HPV vaccines do not treat existing HPV infections or HPV-associated diseases.

How long does vaccine protection last?

Research suggests that vaccine protection is long-lasting. Current studies (with up to about six years of follow-up data) indicate that the vaccines are effective, with no evidence of decreasing immunity.

What does the vaccine not protect against?

The vaccines do not protect against all HPV types—so they will not prevent all cases of cervical cancer. About 30% of cervical cancers will not be prevented by the vaccines, so it will be important for women to continue getting screened for cervical cancer (regular Pap tests). Also, the vaccines do not prevent other sexually transmitted infections (STIs). So it will still be important for sexually active persons to lower their risk for other STIs.

Will girls and women be protected against HPV and related diseases, even if they don't get all three doses?

It is not yet known how much protection girls and women get from receiving only one or two doses of an HPV vaccine. So it is very important that girls and women get all three doses.

Safety of the HPV Vaccine

Both vaccines have been licensed by the Food and Drug Administration (FDA) for females aged 9 through 26 years and approved by CDC as safe and effective. Both vaccines were studied in thousands of people around the world and vaccine safety continues to be monitored by CDC and the FDA. These studies showed no serious safety concerns. Common, mild adverse events reported during these studies include pain where the shot was given, fever, dizziness, and nausea.

Fainting can occur after any medical procedure, including vaccination. Recent data suggest that fainting after any vaccination is more common in adolescents. Falls and injuries can occur after fainting.

Adolescents and adults should be seated or lying down during vaccination. Sitting or lying down for about 15 minutes after a vaccination can help prevent fainting and injuries.

More than 35 million doses of HPV vaccine have been distributed in the United States as of June 2011. Almost all doses distributed have been Gardasil.

Why is HPV vaccination only recommended for women through age 26?

HPV vaccines are licensed and recommended for females through age 26 years. Vaccination would have the greatest benefit when administered to girls. As in trials in younger women, a clinical trial of quadrivalent vaccine in women under 26 years found the vaccine to be safe. This study also showed that the vaccine was effective in women without evidence of existing or past infection with HPV vaccine types. However, the study demonstrated no protection against disease in the overall study population. Neither vaccine is licensed in the United States for use in women over the age of 26 years. Although women over age 26 years are not recommended to receive HPV vaccination, they should have cervical cancer screening as currently recommended.

What about vaccinating boys and men?

The quadrivalent vaccine is also safe and effective for males ages 9 through 26 years. It is licensed by the FDA for prevention of anal cancer and genital warts. Since October 2009, the CDC's Advisory Committee on Immunization Practice's guidance has been that the 3-dose series of quadrivalent HPV vaccine may be given to males aged 9 through 26 years to reduce their likelihood of acquiring genital warts. The vaccine is not routinely recommended for administration to males.

Cost and Paying for the HPV Vaccine

As of July 18, 2011, the retail price of the vaccine is about $130 per dose ($390 for full series).

Is HPV vaccine covered by insurance plans?

Most health insurance plans cover the cost of vaccines, but you may want to check with your insurance provider before going to the doctor. If you don't have insurance, or if it does not cover vaccines, the Vaccines for Children (VFC) program may be able to help.

How can I get help paying for HPV vaccine?

The Vaccines for Children (VFC) program helps families of eligible children who might not otherwise have access to vaccines. The program provides vaccines at no cost to doctors who serve eligible children. Children younger than 19 years of age are eligible for VFC vaccines if they are Medicaid-eligible, American Indian, or Alaska Native or have no health insurance. "Underinsured" children who have health insurance that does not cover vaccination can receive VFC vaccines through Federally Qualified Health Centers or Rural Health Centers. Parents of uninsured or underinsured children who receive vaccines at no cost through the VFC Program should check with their healthcare providers about possible administration fees that might apply. These fees help providers cover the costs that result from important services like storing the vaccines and paying staff members to give vaccines to patients. However, VFC vaccines cannot be denied to an eligible child if a family can't afford the fee.

Will girls/women who have been vaccinated still need cervical cancer screening?

Yes, vaccinated women will still need regular cervical cancer screening (Pap tests) because the vaccines protect against most but not all HPV types that cause cervical cancer. Also, women who got the vaccine after becoming sexually active may not get the full benefit of the vaccine if they had already acquired HPV.

Regular cervical cancer screening and follow-up can prevent most cases of cervical cancer. The Pap test can detect cell changes in the cervix before they turn into cancer. Pap tests can also detect most, but not all, cervical cancers at an early, treatable stage. Most women diagnosed with cervical cancer in the United States have either never had a Pap test, or have not had a Pap test in the last five years. There are HPV tests that can tell if a woman has HPV on her cervix, but the HPV tests on the market should only be used to help screen women at certain ages and to help health care providers assess women with certain Pap test findings for cervical cancer. These tests can be used with the Pap test to help your doctor determine next steps in cervical cancer screening.

Are there other ways to prevent HPV?

For those who are sexually active, condoms may lower the chances of getting HPV, if used with every sex act, from start to finish. Condoms may also lower the risk of developing HPV-related diseases (genital warts and cervical cancer). But HPV can infect areas that are not covered by a condom—so condoms may not fully protect against HPV.

People can also lower their chances of getting HPV by being in a faithful relationship with one partner; limiting their number of sex partners; and choosing a partner who has had no or few prior sex partners. But even people with only one lifetime sex partner can get HPV. And it may not be possible to determine if a partner who has been sexually active in the past is currently infected. That's why the only sure way to prevent HPV is to avoid all sexual activity.

Section 49.7

HPV Vaccine Information for Preteens and Teens

This section contains text from "HPV Vaccine for Preteens and Teens," by the Centers for Disease Control and Prevention (CDC, www.cdc.gov), June 2012, and "Are Your Kids Protected from HPV-Related Cancers?" by the CDC, January 2012.

HPV Vaccine for Preteens and Teens

HPV vaccines protect against human papillomavirus (HPV) infection and HPV-related disease.

HPV vaccination is recommended for preteen girls and boys at age 11 or 12 years. If a teenager or young adult (age 13 through 26 years old) has not gotten any or all of the HPV shots when he or she was younger, he or she should ask a doctor about getting them now.

Preteens and teens should get all three doses of an HPV vaccine long before their first sexual contact, so they have time to develop protection from the vaccine. This is also the age they will have the best immune response from the vaccine.

There are two different HPV vaccines (Cervarix or Gardasil) that can be given to girls and young women. Only one HPV vaccine—Gardasil—can be given to boys and young men. Both Cervarix and Gardasil protects against HPV types that cause most cervical cancer and have been shown to prevent cervical cancer. Gardasil has been studied and shown to protect against cervical, anal, vaginal, and vulvar cancers. Gardasil also protects against HPV types that cause most genital warts and has been shown to prevent genital warts.

How Many Shots and When?

HPV vaccine is given in three shots over six months. The second shot is given one or two months after the first, and the third shot is given six months after the first shot. It is very important to complete all of the shots long before sexual activity begins, in order to be fully protected.

The Disease: Human Papillomavirus

Human papillomavirus, also known as HPV, is a very common virus that is spread by skin-to-skin contact during any type of sexual activity with another person. HPV infection is common in people in their teens and early 20s.

There are many different types of HPV. Some types can cause cervical, vaginal, and vulvar cancer in women and penile cancer in men. These HPV types can also cause anal cancer and some head and neck cancers in both women and men. Other types of HPV can cause genital warts in both women and men.

Genital human papillomavirus (HPV) is the most common sexually transmitted infection in the United States. About 20 million people, most in their late teens and early 20s, are infected with HPV. Each year United States, about 18,000 HPV-associated cancers occur in women and cervical cancer is the most common. CDC reports that every year, about 12,000 women are diagnosed with cervical cancer, and about 4,000 women die from it in the United States. About 7,000 HPV-associated cancers occur each year in men in the United States and oropharyngeal cancers are the most common.

Are Your Kids Protected from HPV-Related Cancers?

Protect your sons and daughters from human papillomavirus (HPV)-related cancer and other diseases associated with HPV by getting them the HPV vaccine. It takes three shots to complete the series, so make sure they get all three to be protected.

It's easy to get very busy with school, activities, work, and all of the juggling that parents of preteens and teens do every day. For the sake of your children's health, take the time to get them the life-saving HPV vaccine to protect against HPV-related cancers. Each year United States, about 18,000 HPV-associated cancers occur in women and cervical cancer is the most common. About 7,000 HPV-associated cancers occur each year in men in the United States and oropharyngeal cancers are the most common. Anal cancer caused by HPV affects both men and women, with more women than men diagnosed each year. If we protect our boys and girls now, we could reduce disease and cancer due to HPV.

This is a safe and effective vaccine given in a series of three shots over about a six-month period. The second shot is given one or two months after the first, and the third shot is given six months after the first shot. It is very important to complete all of the shots to be fully protected. More than 40 million doses of HPV vaccine have been safely given across the country.

If your son or daughter is age 11 or 12 years, the American Academy of Pediatrics (AAP), the American Academy of Family Physicians (AAFP), and the Society for Adolescent Health and Medicine (SAHM) recommend you vaccinate now to protect him or her against HPV-related cancer.

If your son or daughter is older than 11 or 12 and has not started these shots, it's not too late to schedule an appointment to begin the series.

About 20 million people, most in their late teens and early 20s, are infected with HPV, the type of virus that causes cervical cancer. That's why it's important to protect preteen and teen boys and girls early through vaccination.

Take advantage of any visit to the doctor—such as an annual health checkup or physicals for sports, camp, or college—to ask the doctor about what shots your preteens and teens need.

Families who need help paying for vaccines should ask their health care provider about Vaccines for Children (VFC). The VFC program provides vaccines at no cost to uninsured and underinsured children younger than 19 years. For help in finding a local health care provider who participates in the program, parents can call 800-CDC-INFO or go to www.cdc.gov/vaccines.

Section 49.8

HPV Vaccine Soon to Be Recommended for Preteen Boys as Well as Girls

Excerpted from an interview with Anne Schuchat, MD, director of the National Center for Immunization and Respiratory Diseases at the Centers for Disease Control and Prevention (CDC, www.cdc.gov), published as "ACIP recommends all 11-12-year-old males get vaccinated against HPV," by the CDC, October 25, 2011.

About 20 million Americans are currently infected with human papillomavirus or HPV. HPV has been associated with several types of cancer. Cancer of the cervix, vulva, vagina, penis, anus as well as head and neck cancer. Each year in the United States about 18,000 HPV-associated cancers affect women. Cervical cancer is the most common type of cancer that HPV can cause in women. About 7,000 HPV-associated cancers each year affect men in the United States. Cancers of the head and neck are the most common type of cancers in men. HPV can also cause most cases of genital warts in both men and women and about one in 100 sexually active adults in the United States have genital warts at any one time. So these are common conditions. Men who have sex with men and people who are infected with HIV [human immunodeficiency virus] are at the highest risk for HPV-related disease. The HPV vaccine is a strong weapon in cancer prevention. The quadrivalent HPV vaccine prevents the types of HPV that cause cervical cancer in women as well as anal cancer and genital warts in both women and men.

In June 2006, the ACIP [Advisory Committee on Immunization Practices] recommended HPV vaccine for 11- to 12-year-old girls and also for teen girls and young women through age 26 who hadn't already received the vaccine. In October 2009, quadrivalent HPV vaccine was also approved for use in boys and young men. The quadrivalent HPV vaccine is covered for both girls and boys through the Vaccines for Children Program. ACIP's 2011 recommendations result from a several-year process where the committee has been reviewing quite a bit of information. The committee recommended that routine vaccination of males aged 11 or 12 years with three doses of quadrivalent HPV vaccine be given to prevent HPV infection and HPV–related disease. They recommended that the vaccination could begin as young as age 9 and that boys and young men 13 to 21 years of age who hadn't already received the vaccine should also be vaccinated. These recommendations to CDC resulted from a careful review of data that's been going on for the past few years. Much of the data became available after the initial permissive recommendation in back in 2009. The new data included clinical trials that have shown quadrivalent HPV vaccine to be very effective for males. The greatest impact can be had when the vaccine is given at ages 11 or 12 where there is a better immune response compared with older ages. The vaccine is most effective when it is given before there is exposure to the virus which occurs through sexual contact. So that's the rationale for recommending this routinely for 11- or 12-year-olds.

Part of the deliberation the committee made was to review trends in cancers associated with HPV types that could be prevented by the quadrivalent vaccine. This vaccine can prevent several different types of cancer. More than 80% of anal cancers are caused by the HPV types included in the vaccine. There have been increases in head and neck cancers and in cancers of the anus over the past few decades. Cervical cancer trends have been decreasing over the past few decades, but the increasing trends in these other cancers was something that was important to the committee. The committee also reviewed the trend in HPV vaccine use among girls. HPV vaccine is not being highly taken up by teenage girls. There's been a disappointing uptake among teen girls we reported earlier this summer. HPV vaccination of males offers an opportunity to decrease the burden of HPV-related disease in both males and females. So in addition to providing direct benefit to boys by preventing future genital warts or anal cancer there is also the potential that vaccinating boys will reduce the spread of HPV from males to females and reduce some of the HPV-related burden that women suffer from.

The committee reviewed a variety of models that looked at the cost effectiveness of different vaccination strategies. This is an important component of what the committee reviews for every vaccine recommendation, but there is no threshold that they use. Male vaccination is most cost effective when coverage of females is low and unfortunately here in the U.S. coverage of females is currently low. The committee also undertook extensive review of data on vaccine safety. Through middle of September nearly 40 million doses of HPV vaccine have been distributed in the United States. The clinical trials that have been carried out in smaller numbers have shown the quadrivalent HPV vaccine to be safe for males as well as for females. The most common adverse events or side effects that can occur following HPV vaccination include injection site reaction, headache, and fever, and those reactions have tended to be mild or moderate in intensity.

The committee reviewed the effectiveness, the disease trends, the cost effectiveness, safety, and also considered practical implementation issues for the providers, parents, and the programs.

Where do we go from here? The ACIP recommendations are delivered to the CDC and there will be a development of written recommendations that will be subject to approval by our agency. Once approved the ACIP recommendations will end up being published in the *MMWR [Morbidity and Mortality Weekly Report]*.

Part Six

Additional Help and Information

Chapter 50

Glossary of Terms Related to Sexually Transmitted Diseases

acquired immunodeficiency syndrome (AIDS): A disease of the immune system due to infection with HIV (human immunodeficiency virus). HIV destroys the CD4 T lymphocytes (CD4 cells) of the immune system, leaving the body vulnerable to life-threatening infections and cancers. Acquired immunodeficiency syndrome (AIDS) is the most advanced stage of HIV infection.[1]

adherence: Taking medications exactly as prescribed. Poor adherence to an HIV treatment regimen increases the risk for developing drug-resistant HIV and virologic failure.[1]

antiretroviral therapy (ART): The recommended treatment for HIV infection. Antiretroviral therapy (ART) involves using a combination of three or more antiretroviral (ARV) drugs from at least two different HIV drug classes to prevent HIV from replicating.[1]

bacterial vaginosis (BV): A vaginal infection that develops when there is an increase in harmful bacteria and a decrease in good bacteria in the vagina.[2]

Definitions in this chapter were compiled from documents published by the following government agencies: Terms marked 1 are from AIDSinfo (aidsinfo.nih.gov), part of the U.S. Department of Health and Human Services; terms marked 2 are from the Office on Women's Health (www.womenshealth.gov), part of the U.S. Department of Health and Human Services; and terms marked 3 are from the Centers for Disease Control and Prevention (CDC, www.cdc.gov).

biopsy: Removal of tissue, cells, or fluid from the body for examination under a microscope. Biopsies are used to diagnose disease.[1]

cervical cancer: A type of cancer that develops in the cervix. Cervical cancer is almost always caused by the human papillomavirus (HPV), which is spread through sexual contact.[1]

chancroid: A sexually transmitted disease caused by the bacterium *Haemophilus ducreyi*. Chancroid causes genital ulcers (sores).[1]

chlamydia: A common sexually transmitted disease caused by the bacterium *Chlamydia trachomatis*. Chlamydia often has mild or no symptoms, but if left untreated, it can lead to serious complications, including infertility. [1]

coinfection: When a person has two or more infections at the same time. For example, a person infected with HIV may be coinfected with hepatitis or tuberculosis (TB) or both.[1]

condom: A device used during sexual intercourse to block semen from coming in contact with the inside of the vagina. Condoms are used to reduce the likelihood of pregnancy and to prevent the transmission of sexually transmitted disease, including HIV. The male condom is a thin rubber cover that fits over a man's erect penis. The female condom is a polyurethane pouch that fits inside the vagina.[1]

drug resistance: When a bacteria, virus, or other microorganism mutates (changes form) and becomes insensitive to (resistant to) a drug that was previously effective.[1]

dysplasia: The development of precancerous changes in cells. Dysplasia can affect various parts of the body, including the cervix or prostate. The extent of dysplasia within body tissue can be mild (grade 1), moderate (grade 2), or severe (grade 3).[1]

genital warts: A sexually transmitted disease caused by the human papillomavirus (HPV). Genital warts appear as raised pink or flesh-colored bumps on the surface of the vagina, cervix, tip of the penis, or anus.[1]

gonorrhea: A sexually transmitted disease caused by the bacterium *Neisseria gonorrhoeae*. Gonorrhea can also be transmitted from an infected mother to her child during delivery. Gonorrhea often has mild or no symptoms. However, if left untreated, gonorrhea can lead to infertility, and it can spread into the bloodstream and affect the joints, heart valves, and brain.[1]

hepatitis B virus (HBV) infection: Infection with the hepatitis B virus (HBV). HBV can be transmitted through blood, semen, or other body fluids during sex or injection-drug use. Because HIV and HBV share the same modes of transmission, people infected with HIV are often also coinfected with HBV.[1]

hepatitis C virus (HCV) infection: Infection with the hepatitis C virus (HCV). HCV is usually transmitted through blood and rarely through other body fluids, such as semen. HCV infection progresses more rapidly in people coinfected with HIV than in people infected with HCV alone.[1]

herpes simplex virus 2 (HSV-2) infection: An infection caused by herpes simplex virus 2 (HSV-2) and usually associated with lesions in the genital or anal area. HSV-2 is very contagious and is transmitted by sexual contact with someone who is infected (even if lesions are not visible). Treatment cannot eradicate HSV-2 from the body, but antiviral therapy can shorten and prevent outbreaks and reduce the risk of transmission.[1]

human immunodeficiency virus (HIV): The virus that causes AIDS, which is the most advanced stage of HIV infection. HIV is a retrovirus that occurs as two types: HIV-1 and HIV-2. Both types are transmitted through direct contact with HIV-infected body fluids, such as blood, semen, and genital secretions, or from an HIV-infected mother to her child during pregnancy, birth, or breastfeeding (through breast milk).[1]

human papillomavirus (HPV): The virus that causes human papillomavirus (HPV) infection, the most common sexually transmitted infection. There are two groups of HPV—types that can cause genital warts and types that can cause cancer. HPV is the most frequent cause of cervical cancer.[1]

injection drug use: A method of illicit drug use. The drugs are injected directly into the body—into a vein, into a muscle, or under the skin—with a needle and syringe. Blood-borne viruses, including HIV and hepatitis, can be transmitted via shared needles or other drug injection equipment.[1]

microbicide: A drug, chemical, or other substance used to kill microorganisms. Increasingly, the term is used specifically for substances that prevent or reduce the transmission of sexually transmitted diseases, such as HIV.[1]

molluscum contagiosum: A common, usually mild skin disease caused by the virus Molluscum contagiosum and characterized by small white, pink, or flesh-colored bumps with a dimple in the center. Molluscum contagiosum is spread by touching the affected skin of an infected person or by touching a surface with the virus on it. The bumps can easily spread to other parts of the body if someone touches or scratches a bump and then touches another part of the body.[1]

mother-to-child transmission (MTCT): When an HIV-infected mother passes HIV to her infant during pregnancy, labor and delivery, or breastfeeding (through breast milk). Antiretroviral (ARV) drugs are given to HIV-infected women during pregnancy and to their infants after birth to reduce the risk of mother-to-child transmission (MTCT) of HIV.[1]

occupational exposure: Contact with a potentially harmful physical, chemical, or biological agent as a result of one's work. For example, a health care professional may be exposed to HIV or another infectious agent through a needlestick injury.[1]

opportunistic infection (OI): An infection that occurs more frequently or is more severe in people with weakened immune systems, such as people with HIV or people receiving chemotherapy, than in people with healthy immune systems.[1]

Pap test: A procedure in which cells and secretions are collected from inside and around the cervix for examination under a microscope. Pap test also refers to the laboratory test used to detect any infected, potentially precancerous, or cancerous cells in the cervical cells obtained from a Pap test.[1]

pelvic inflammatory disease (PID): Infection and inflammation of the female upper genital tract, including the uterus and fallopian tubes. Pelvic inflammatory disease is usually due to bacterial infection, including some sexually transmitted diseases, such as chlamydia and gonorrhea. Symptoms, if any, include pain in the lower abdomen, fever, smelly vaginal discharge, irregular bleeding, or pain during intercourse. PID can lead to serious complications, including infertility, ectopic pregnancy (a pregnancy in the fallopian tube or elsewhere outside of the womb), and chronic pelvic pain.[1]

post-exposure prophylaxis (PEP): Short-term treatment started as soon as possible after high-risk exposure to an infectious agent, such as HIV, hepatitis B virus (HBV), or hepatitis C virus (HCV). The purpose of post-exposure prophylaxis (PEP) is to reduce the risk of infection. An example of a high-risk exposure is exposure to an infectious agent as the result of unprotected sex.[1]

pubic lice: Also called crab lice or crabs, pubic lice are parasitic insects found primarily in the pubic or genital area of humans.[3]

scabies: An infestation of the skin by the human itch mite (*Sarcoptes scabiei* var. *hominis*). The microscopic scabies mite burrows into the upper layer of the skin where it lives and lays its eggs. The most common symptoms of scabies are intense itching and a pimple-like skin rash. The scabies mite usually is spread by direct, prolonged, skin-to-skin contact with a person who has scabies.[3]

semen: A thick, whitish fluid that is discharged from the male penis during ejaculation. Semen contains sperms and various secretions. HIV can be transmitted through the semen of a man with HIV.[1]

sexually transmitted disease (STD): An infectious disease that spreads from person to person during sexual contact. Sexually transmitted diseases, such as syphilis, HIV infection, and gonorrhea, are caused by bacteria, parasites, and viruses.[1]

spermicide: A topical preparation or substance used during sexual intercourse to kill sperm. Although spermicides may prevent pregnancy, they do not protect against HIV infection or other sexually transmitted diseases. Irritation of the vagina and rectum that sometimes occurs with use of spermicides may increase the risk of sexual transmission of HIV.[1]

syphilis: An infectious disease caused by the bacterium *Treponema pallidum*, which is typically transmitted through direct contact with a syphilis sore, usually during vaginal or oral sex. Syphilis can also be transmitted from an infected mother to her child during pregnancy. Syphilis sores occur mainly on the genitals, anus, and rectum, but also on the lips and mouth.[1]

trichomoniasis: A sexually transmitted disease caused by a parasite. It is sometimes called trich.[2]

vaccination: Giving a vaccine to stimulate a person's immune response. Vaccination can be intended either to prevent a disease (a preventive vaccine) or to treat a disease (a therapeutic vaccine).[1]

virus: A microscopic infectious agent that requires a living host cell in order to replicate. Viruses often cause disease in humans, including measles, mumps, rubella, polio, influenza, and the common cold. HIV is the virus that causes AIDS.[1]

yeast infection: A fungal infection caused by overgrowth of the yeast Candida (usually *Candida albicans*) in moist areas of the body. Candidiasis can affect the mucous membranes of the mouth, vagina, and anus.[1]

Chapter 51

Directory of Organizations That Provide Information about Sexually Transmitted Diseases

Government Agencies That Provide Information about STDs

Agency for Healthcare Research and Quality
Office of Communications and Knowledge Transfer
540 Gaither Road
Suite 2000
Rockville, MD 20850
Phone: 301-427-1104
Website: www.ahrq.gov

Centers for Disease Control and Prevention
1600 Clifton Road
Atlanta, GA 30333
Toll-Free: 800-CDC-INFO
(800-232-4636)
Toll-Free TTY: 888-232-6348
Phone: 404-639-3311
Websites:
www.cdc.gov; www.cdcnpin.org
www.cdc.gov/nchhstp
www.hivtest.org/stdtesting.aspx
E-mail: cdcinfo@cdc.gov

Federal Trade Commission
600 Pennsylvania Avenue NW
Washington, DC 20580
Phone: 202-326-2222
Website: www.ftc.gov
E-mail: webmaster@ftc.gov

Resources in this chapter were compiled from several sources deemed reliable; all contact information was verified and updated in June 2012.

Healthfinder®

National Health Information
Center
PO Box 1133
Washington, DC 20013-1133
Toll-Free: 800-336-4797
Phone: 301-565-4167
Fax: 301-984-4256
Website:
www.healthfinder.gov
E-mail:
healthfinder@nhic.org

National Cancer Institute

NCI Office of Communications
and Education
Public Inquiries Office
6116 Executive Boulevard
Suite 300
Bethesda, MD 20892-8322
Toll-Free: 800-4-CANCER
(800-422-6237)
Toll-Free TTY: 800-332-8615
Website:
www.cancer.gov
E-mail:
cancergovstaff@mail.nih.gov

National Center for Complementary and Alternative Medicine

National Institutes of Health
NCCAM Clearinghouse
PO Box 7923
Gaithersburg, MD 20898-7923
Toll-Free: 888-644-6226
Toll-Free TTY: 866-464-3615
Toll-Free Fax: 866-464-3616
Website: www.nccam.nih.gov
E-mail: info@nccam.nih.gov

National Center for Health Statistics

3311 Toledo Road
Hyattsville, MD 20782
Toll-Free: 800-CDC-INFO
(800-232-4636)
Website: www.cdc.gov/nchs
E-mail: cdcinfo@cdc.gov

National Institute of Allergy and Infectious Diseases

6610 Rockledge Drive
MSC 6612
Bethesda, MD 20892-6612
Toll-Free: 866-284-4107
Toll-Free TDD: 800-877-8339
Phone: 301-496-5717
Fax: 301-402-3573
Website: www.niaid.nih.gov
E-mail:
ocpostoffice@niaid.nih.gov

National Institute of Mental Health

6001 Executive Boulevard
Room 8184, MSC 9663
Bethesda, MD 20892-9663
Toll-Free: 866-615-6464
TTY Toll-Free: 866-415-8051
Phone: 301-443-4513
TTY: 301-443-8431
Fax: 301-443-4279
Website: www.nimh.nih.gov
E-mail: nimhinfo@nih.gov

National Institute of Neurological Disorders and Stroke
PO Box 5801
Bethesda, MD 20824
Toll-Free: 800-352-9424
Phone: 301-496-5751
TTY: 301-468-5981
Website: www.ninds.nih.gov

National Institute on Aging
Building 31, Room 5C27
31 Center Drive, MSC 2292
Bethesda, MD 20892
Toll-Free: 800-222-2225
Toll-Free TTY: 800-222-4225
Phone: 301-496-1752
Fax: 301-496-1072
Website: www.nia.nih.gov
E-mail: niaic@nia.nih.gov

National Institutes of Health
9000 Rockville Pike
Bethesda, MD 20892
Phone: 301-496-4000
TTY: 301-402-9612
Website: www.nih.gov
E-mail: NIHinfo@od.nih.gov

National Prevention Information Network
CDC NPIN
PO Box 6003
Rockdale, MD 20849-6003
Toll-Free: 800-458-5231
TTY: 888-232-6348
Website: www.cdcnpin.org/
scripts/contact.asp
E-mail: info@cdcnpin.org

National Women's Health Information Center
Office on Women's Health
200 Independence Avenue SW
Room 712E
Washington, DC 20201
Toll-Free: 800-994-9662
Toll-Free TDD: 888-220-5446
Phone: 202-690-7650
Fax: 202-205-2631
Website: www.womenshealth.gov

Office of Minority Health Resource Center
PO Box 37337
Washington, DC 20013-7337
Toll-Free: 800-444-6472
Phone: 240-453-2882
TDD: 301-251-1432
Fax: 240-453-2883
Website: minorityhealth.hhs.gov
E-mail: info@minorityhealth
.hhs.gov

Substance Abuse and Mental Health Services Administration
PO Box 2345
Rockville, MD 20847-2345
Toll-Free: 877-SAMHSA-7
(877-726-4727)
Toll-Free TTY: 800-487-4889
Fax: 240-221-4292
Website: www.samhsa.gov
E-mail:
SAMHSAInfo@samhsa.hhs.gov

U.S. Department of Health and Human Services

Room 443 H
200 Independence Avenue SW
Washington, DC 20201
Toll-Free: 877-696-6775
Websites: www.hhs.gov
www.AIDS.gov

U.S. Food and Drug Administration

10903 New Hampshire Avenue
Silver Spring, MD 20993
Toll-Free: 888-INFO-FDA
(888-463-6332)
Website: www.fda.gov

U.S. National Library of Medicine

8600 Rockville Pike
Bethesda, MD 20894
Toll-Free: 888-FIND-NLM
(888-346-3656)
Toll-Free TDD: 800-735-2258
Phone: 301-594-5983
Fax: 301-402-1384
Website: www.nlm.nih.gov
E-mail: custserv@nlm.nih.gov

Private Agencies That Provide Information about STDs

Advocates for Youth

2000 M Street NW, Suite 750
Washington, DC 20036
Phone: 202-419-3420
Fax: 202-419-1448
Websites:
www.advocatesforyouth.org;
www.amplifyyourvoice.org/
youthresource

AIDS.org

PO Box 69491
Los Angeles, CA 90069
Website: www.aids.org

AIDS Education Global Information System

32302 Alipaz Street, #267
PO Box 184
San Juan Capistrano, CA
92693-0184
Phone: 949-495-1952
Fax: 949-443-1755
Website: www.aegis.org

AIDS Healthcare Foundation

6255 West Sunset Boulevard
21st Floor
Los Angeles, CA 90028
Phone: 323-860-5200
Website: www.aidshealth.org

American Cancer Society

250 Williams Street NW
Atlanta, GA 30303
Toll-Free: 800-227-2345
Toll-Free TTY: 800-735-2991
Website: www.cancer.org

American Foundation for AIDS Research

120 Wall Street, 13th Floor
New York, NY 10005-3908
Phone: 212-806-1600
Fax: 212-806-1601
Website: www.amfar.org
E-mail:
information@amfar.org

American Medical Association
515 North State Street
Chicago, IL 60654
Toll-Free: 800-621-8335
Website: www.ama-assn.org

American Social Health Association
PO Box 13827
Research Triangle Park, NC 27709
Phone: 919-361-8400
Fax: 919-361-8425
Website: www.ashastd.org
E-mail: info@ashastd.org

American Society for Colposcopy and Cervical Pathology
152 West Washington Street
Hagerstown, MD 21740
Toll-Free: 800-787-7227
Phone: 301-733-3640
Fax: 301-733-5775
Website: www.asccp.org

American Society of Reproductive Medicine
1209 Montgomery Highway
Birmingham, AL 35216-2809
Phone: 205-978-5000
Fax: 205-978-5005
Website: www.asrm.org
E-mail: asrm@asrm.org

Association of Reproductive Health Professionals
1901 L Street NW, Suite 300
Washington, DC 20036
Phone: 202-466-3825
Website: www.arhp.org
E-mail: ARHP@arhp.org

AVERT
4 Brighton Road
Horsham
West Sussex RH13 5BA
United Kingdom
Phone: 011-44-14-321-0202
Website: www.avert.org
E-mail: info@avert.org

The Body
Remedy Health Media, LLC
250 West 57th Street
New York, NY 10107
Website: www.thebody.com

Cleveland Clinic
9500 Euclid Avenue
Cleveland, OH 44195
Toll-Free: 800-223-CARE
(800-223-2273)
Toll-Free: 866-588-2264
(Info Line)
Phone: 216-636-5860 (Info Line)
TTY: 216-444-0261
Website: my.clevelandclinic.org

Engender Health
440 Ninth Avenue
New York, NY 10001
Phone: 212-561-8000
Website:
www.engenderhealth.org
E-mail: info@engenderhealth.org

557

Foundation for Women's Cancer
230 West Monroe, Suite 2528
Chicago, IL 60606
Toll-Free: 800-444-4441
Phone: 312-578-1439
Fax: 312-578-9769
Website: www.foundationfor
womenscancer.org
E-mail: info@foundationfor
womenscancer.org

Gay and Lesbian Medical Association
1326 18th Street NW, Suite 22
Washington, DC 20036
Phone: 202-600-8037
Fax: 202-478-1500
Website: www.glma.org
E-mail: info@glma.org

Gay Men's Health Crisis
446 West 33rd Street
New York, NY 10001-2601
Phone: 212-367-1000
Website: www.gmhc.org

Elizabeth Glaser Pediatric AIDS Foundation
1140 Connecticut Avenue NW
Suite 200
Washington, DC 20036
Toll-Free: 888-499-HOPE
(888-499-4673)
Phone: 202-296-9165
Fax: 202-296-9185
Website: www.pedaids.org
E-mail: info@pedaids.org

Go Ask Alice!
Alfred Lerner Hall, 8th Floor
2920 Broadway, Mail Code 2606
New York, NY 10027
Phone: 212-854-5453
Fax: 212-854-8949
Website:
goaskalice.columbia.edu
E-mail: alice@columbia.edu

Guttmacher Institute
125 Maiden Lane, 7th Floor
New York, NY 10038
Toll-Free: 800-355-0244
Phone: 212-248-1111
Fax: 212-248-1951
Website: www.guttmacher.org

Hepatitis B Foundation
3805 Old Easton Road
Doylestown, PA 18902
Phone: 215-489-4900
Fax: 215-489-4920
Website: www.hepb.org
E-mail: contact@hepb.org

Hepatitis Foundation International
504 Blick Drive
Silver Spring, MD 20904
Toll-Free: 800-891-0707
Phone: 301-622-4200
Fax: 301-622-4702
Website: www.hepfi.org
E-mail:
info@hepatitisfoundation.org

HIV InSite
UCSF Center for HIV
Information
4150 Clement Street
Box 111V
San Francisco, CA 94121
Fax: 415-379-5547
Website: hivinsite.ucsf.edu
E-mail: hivinsite@ucsf.edu

Immunization Action Coalition
1573 Selby Avenue, Suite 234
St. Paul, MN 55104
Phone: 651-647-9009
Fax: 651-647-9131
Website: www.immunize.org
E-mail: admin@immunize.org

iwantthekit.org
Toll-Free: 866-575-5504
Phone: 410-502-0764
Website: www.iwantthekit.org
E-mail: iwantthekit@jhmi.edu

Kaiser Family Foundation
2400 Sand Hill Road
Menlo Park, CA 94025
Phone: 650-854-9400
Fax: 650-854-4800
Website: www.kff.org

National Coalition for LGBT Health
1325 Massachusetts Avenue NW
Suite 705
Washington, DC 20005
Phone: 202-558-6828
Website: www.lgbthealth.net
E-mail:
coalition@lgbthealth.net

National Cervical Cancer Coalition
PO Box 13827
Research Triangle Park, NC 27709
Toll-Free: 800-685-5531
Fax: 919-361-8425
Website: www.nccc-online.org
E-mail: nccc@ashastd.org

National Network for Immunization Information
301 University Boulevard
Galveston, TX 77555-0350
Phone: 703-299-0789
Fax: 409-772-5208
Website:
www.immunizationinfo.org
E-mail: dipineda@utmb.edu

Nemours Foundation Center for Children's Health Media
1600 Rockland Road
Wilmington, DE 19803
Phone: 302-651-4000
Website: www.kidshealth.org
E-mail: info@kidshealth.org

Planned Parenthood
434 West 33rd Street
New York, NY 10001
Toll-Free: 800-230-PLAN
(800-230-7526)
Phone: 212-541-7800
Fax: 212-245-1845
Website:
www.plannedparenthood.org

POZ Magazine
Smart + Strong
462 Seventh Avenue
19th Floor
New York, NY 10018-7424
Phone: 212-242-2163
Fax: 212-675-8505
Website: www.poz.com

Project Inform
273 Ninth Street
San Francisco, CA 94103
Toll-Free: 800-822-7422
(HIV Health InfoLine)
Toll-Free: 877-HELP-4-HEP
(877-435-7443)
(Hepatitis C InfoLine)
Phone: 415-558-8669
Fax: 415-558-0684
Website:
www.projectinform.org
E-mail: info@help4hep.org

Sexuality Information and Education Council of the United States
90 John Street, Suite 402
New York, NY 10038
Phone: 212-819-9770
Fax: 212-819-9776
Website: www.siecus.org

Women Alive
1566 South Burnside Avenue
Los Angeles, CA 90019
Phone: 323-292-1564
Fax: 323-292-9886
Website: www.women-alive.org
E-mail: info@women-alive.org

World Health Organization
Avenue Appia 20
1211 Geneva 27
Switzerland
Phone: 011-41-22-791-2111
Fax: 011-41-22-791-3111
Website: www.who.int
E-mail: info@who.int

Index

Index

Page numbers followed by 'n' indicate a footnote. Page numbers in *italics* indicate a table or illustration.

A

"Abstinence and Sex Education"
(AVERT) 450n
abstinence only sex education,
overview 450–60
access to services, adolescents 76–77
"ACIP recommends all 11-12-
year-old males get vaccinated
against HPV" (CDC) 541n
acquired immune deficiency
syndrome (AIDS)
defined 547
described 20
statistics 33–34, 62–63
symptoms overview 212–13
see also human
immunodeficiency virus (HIV)
acute hepatitis B infection,
described 162–63
acyclovir, genital herpes 155
A.D.A.M., Inc., publications
cervicitis 327n
diagnostic laparoscopy 390n
donovanosis 133n

A.D.A.M., Inc., publications, *continued*
epididymitis 331n
oral herpes 151n
adefovir dipivoxil, hepatitis B 180
adherence
defined 547
described 227–30
adolescents
communication issues 435–38
confidentiality issues 77, 380–81
embarrassing discussions 372–76
HPV vaccine 538–43
sexually transmitted diseases
(STDs) 28–29, 73–78
STD tests 380–81
Advocates for Youth, contact
information 556
Affordable Care Act (2010) 245–46
"The Affordable Care Act and People
Living with HIV or AIDS" (DHHS)
245n
African Americans, sexually
transmitted diseases *31*, 85–92

563

"African Americans and Sexually Transmitted Diseases" (CDC) 89n

Agency for Healthcare Research and Quality (AHRQ)
contact information 553
health discussions publication 366n

AHRQ *see* Agency for Healthcare Research and Quality

AIDS *see* acquired immune deficiency syndrome

AIDS-defining conditions, described 220

AIDS Education Global Information System, contact information 556

AIDS Healthcare Foundation, contact information 556

AIDSinfo, publications
glossary 547n
HIV testing 214n
HIV treatment 219n
HIV vaccines 528n, 531n
post-exposure prophylaxis 492n
pregnancy, HIV transmission 495n

AIDS.org, contact information 556

AIDSVAX vaccine, described 529–30

ALVAC vaccine, described 529–30

ambiguous genitalia, described 16

amenorrhea, described 10

American Cancer Society, contact information 556

American Foundation for AIDS Research, contact information 556

American Medical Association, contact information 557

American Social Health Association, contact information 557

American Society for Colposcopy and Cervical Pathology, contact information 557

American Society of Reproductive Medicine, contact information 557

amiodarone, epididymitis 333

amniotic fluid, described 8

anal sexual activity
HIV transmission 202
human papillomavirus (HPV) 254–56

anergy, HIV infection 196

animal tests, tenofovir 521

antibiotic medications
bacterial vaginosis 299
cervicitis 329
chancroid 116
donovanosis 134
epididymitis 333
neurosyphilis 340
nongonococcal urethritis 125
pelvic inflammatory disease 345–46
resistance overview 393–95
syphilis 289
trichomoniasis 293

antibiotic-resistant gonorrhea, described 144–45

"Antibiotic-Resistant Gonorrhea (ARG) Basic Information" (CDC) 144n

antibodies, described 168–69

antibody test, HIV infection 217–18

antifungal medications, yeast infections 307

antigens, described 168

antimicrobial-resistant gonorrhea 142

antiretroviral medications
HIV infection 192–93, 531–32
versus therapeutic HIV vaccines 531–32

antiretroviral therapy (ART)
defined 547
HIV infection 220, 225

antiviral medications
cervicitis 329
hepatitis C virus infection 176

apoptosis, HIV infection 195

"Approved Drugs for Adults" (Hepatitis B Foundation) 178n

"Are Your Kids Protected from HPV-Related Cancers?" (CDC) 538n

assembly, HIV infection 189

Association of Reproductive Health Professionals, contact information 557

asymptomatic neurosyphilis 339

Atripla, HIV infection 226

autoinoculation, described 311

AVERT
  contact information 557
  publications
    needle exchange programs
      507n
    sex education 440n
    sex education, abstinence 450n
    STDs, symptoms 107n
azidothymidine (AZT)
  HIV infection, pregnancy 497–98
  mother-to-child HIV
    transmission 190
  newborns 502, 503
azithromycin
  chlamydia 129
  gonorrhea 141
  nongonococcal urethritis 125
AZT *see* azidothymidine

B

bacterial vaginosis (BV)
  common symptoms 108–9
  defined 547
  described 18, 354
  lesbians 50
  overview 298–301
  pregnancy *350*
"Bacterial Vaginosis Fact Sheet"
  (Office on Women's Health) 298n
Bactrim, infants 504
Baraclude (entecavir), hepatitis B 180
"Basic Research" (NIAID) 101n
"Basic Statistics" (CDC) 27n
Belshe, Robert 522
biopsy
  abnormal Pap tests 252
  defined 548
Birnkrant, Debbie 397–98
blastocyst, described 7–8
boceprevir, hepatitis C
  virus infection 176
The Body, contact information 557
body art
  HIV infection 419–21
  HIV transmission 208
"Body Art" (NIOSH) 419n
bone marrow, immune system 199

Boston Children's Hospital,
  spermicides publication 479n
breastfeeding
  genital herpes 156
  sexually transmitted diseases 26
bubo, chancroid 117
budding, HIV infection 189
BV *see* bacterial vaginosis

C

cancers
  human papillomavirus
    248–50, 276–80
  men 57–58
Candida albicans,
  described 9, 305, 551
candidiasis,
  common symptoms 113–14
CCR5 receptor HIV infection 187
CD4+ T cells, described
  184, 187–88, 190–91
CD8+ T cells, HIV infection 194
CDC *see* Centers for Disease
  Control and Prevention
cefixime, gonorrhea 142, 144–45
cefotaxime, gonorrhea 142
cefoxitin, gonorrhea 142
cefpodoxime, gonorrhea 145
ceftriaxone
  gonorrhea 142, 144–45
  neurosyphilis 340
Centers for Disease Control
  and Prevention (CDC)
  contact information 341, 553
  publications
    African Americans, STDs 89n
    cervical cancer tests 262n
    chlamydia 120n, 127n
    condoms 470n
    confidentiality 380n
    correctional facilities,
      STDs 97n
    expedited partner
      therapy 484n
    gastrointestinal
      syndromes 314n
    genital herpes 148n
    genital warts 271n

Centers for Disease Control and
  Prevention (CDC), *continued*
publications, *continued*
    glossary 547n
    gonorrhea 138n, 141n
    gonorrhea, antibiotic
      resistance 144n
    hepatitis 162n
    hepatitis C, HIV 174n
    HIV/AIDS 232n
    HIV infection 212n, 214n
    HIV infection transmission
      200n
    HPV infection 248n
    HPV infection, cancer 276n
    HPV infection, men 254n
    HPV tests 264n
    HPV vaccine 533n, 538n, 541n
    human papillomavirus 273n
    injection drug use 421n
    Latinos, HIV/AIDS 93n
    lymphogranuloma
      venereum 281n
    men, HIV/AIDS 62n
    men, HPV infection 56n
    men, STDs 64n
    oral sex, HIV infection 408n
    pregnancy 349n
    pubic lice 316n
    racial disparities, STDs 84n
    risky sexual behaviors 404n,
      405n
    scabies 320n
    STD prevention, youths 448n
    STD statistics 27n
    syphilis 286n
    tests 359n
    trichomoniasis 291n
    women, STDs 44n, 46n
central nervous system (CNS),
  HIV infection 196–97
cephalosporins, gonorrhea 142, 144
Cervarix, described 278, 538
cervical cancer
  defined 548
  human papillomavirus 249–50
  preventive measures 253
  screening tests 262–70
  see also human papillomavirus

"Cervical Cancer Screening"
  (CDC) 262n
"Cervicitis" (A.D.A.M., Inc.) 327n
cervicitis, overview 327–30
cervix
  described 5
  labor and delivery 8
chancre, syphilis 287
chancroid
  defined 548
  overview 115–18
"Chancroid" (Illinois Department
  of Public Health) 115n
"Child Abuse Survivors Have
  Higher Risk for STDs in
  Adulthood Than Non-abused
  Adults" (NIMH) 71n
children, recurrent respiratory
  papillomatosis 260–61
child sexual abuse, sexually
  transmitted diseases 68–72
chlamydia
  adolescents 76
  common symptoms 109
  correctional facilities 98
  defined 548
  described 18–19
  ethnic factors 85
  gay men 65
  lesbians 50
  nongonococcal urethritis 123–26
  overview 120–23
  pregnancy *350*
  racial factor 90–91
  tests *389*
  treatment overview 127–31
  women 47
"Chlamydia - CDC Fact Sheet"
  (CDC) 120n
"Chlamydial Infections" (CDC) 127n
Chlamydia trachomatis
  described 109, 120, 548
  home test kits 382
  lymphogranuloma venereum 281
  treatment overview 127–31
chronic hepatitis B infection
  described 163–64
  treatment overview 178–81
ciprofloxacin, gonorrhea 144

circumcision
  chancroid 117
  described 13
clap *see* gonorrhea
Cleveland Clinic, contact
  information 557
clindamycin, bacterial vaginosis 299
clinical trials
  hepatitis B 179
  Herpevac Trial for Women 522–25
  HIV infection 244
  neurosyphilis 341
  tenofovir 520–21
  therapeutic HIV vaccines 531–32
CMV *see* cytomegalovirus
coinfection, defined 548
colposcopy, abnormal Pap tests 252
"Combating Antibiotic
  Resistance" (FDA) 393n
communication issues
  adolescents 435–38
  condoms 426–28
  expedited partner therapy 484–87
  health care professionals 366–69
  HIV infection status 432–34
  sexually transmitted diseases
    370–71, 429–32
condoms
  bacterial vaginosis 301
  communication issues 426–28
  defined 548
  genital herpes 158, 159
  genital warts 259, 272
  gonorrhea 141
  HIV transmission 204
  human papillomavirus 252, 278
  safer sex 467, 469
  STD prevention 470–74, 475–78
  trichomoniasis 293
"Condoms and STDs: Fact Sheet
  for Public Health Personnel"
  (CDC) 470n
"Confidential and Anonymous
  Testing" (DHHS) 378n
contraception, adolescent
  sexual activity 75
contraceptive foam, described 480
Cooke, David A. 174n, 232n, 359n,
  366n, 411n, 421n, 484n, 528n, 531n

correctional facilities, sexually
  transmitted diseases 97–99
counseling, HIV tests 215–17
crabs *see* pubic lice
crusted scabies, described 320
cytokines, HIV infection 188
"Cytomegalovirus (CMV)"
  (Planned Parenthood Federation
  of America, Inc.) 302n
cytomegalovirus (CMV),
  overview 302–4

D

dental dams
  described 467
  STD prevention 478
Department of Health and Human
  Services *see* US Department of
  Health and Human Services
Department of Justice
  see US Department of Justice
DHHS *see* US Department of
  Health and Human Services
"Diagnostic Laparoscopy"
  (A.D.A.M., Inc.) 390n
"Diagnostics" (NIAID) 101n
direct cell killing, HIV infection 195
disability benefits, HIV infection 242
DNA (deoxyribonucleic acid),
  vaccines 530
donovanosis, overview 133–35
"Donovanosis (Granuloma Inguinale)"
  (A.D.A.M., Inc.) 133n
douching
  bacterial vaginosis 298–300
  candidiasis 113
  cervical cancer 253
  cervicitis 329
  Pap tests 263
  pelvic inflammatory
    disease 344, 346
  STD risk 416–19
  syphilis 290
  thrush 113
  vaginitis 355
  yeast infections 308
"Douching" (Office on Women's
  Health) 416n

doxycycline
  chlamydia 129
  gonorrhea 141
  lymphogranuloma venereum 282–83
  nongonococcal urethritis 125
"Do You Have To Tell?" (DHHS) 432n
"Drug-Associated HIV Transmission
  Continues in the United States"
  (CDC) 421n
drug resistance, defined 548
dysmenorrhea, described 10
dysplasia, defined 548

E

ectopic pregnancy
  chlamydia 121
  described 9
  hospitalizations 49
  pelvic inflammatory disease 344
"Effective HIV and STD Prevention
  Programs for Youth" (CDC) 448n
ejaculatory ducts, described 13
Elizabeth Glazer Pediatric AIDS
  Foundation, contact information 558
embryo, described 8
emergency contraception
  adolescents 75
  sexual assault 491
endometrial biopsy, pelvic
  inflammatory disease 345
endometriosis, described 9
endometrium, described 7–8
Engender Health,
  contact information 557
entecavir, hepatitis B 180
enteritis, overview 314–16
enzyme immunoassay (EIA),
  described 361
epididymis, described 12
epididymitis
  described 15
  overview 331–34
"Epididymitis" (A.D.A.M., Inc.) 331n
Epivir-HBV (lamivudine), hepatitis B
  180
erythromycin
  chlamydia 129
  nongonococcal urethritis 125
estrogen, described 6, 7

ethnic factors
  HIV infection 93–95
  sexually transmitted diseases 29, *31*
expedited partner therapy,
  overview 484–87
"Expedited Partner Therapy in
  the Management of Sexually
  Transmitted Diseases" (CDC) 484n

F

"Fact Sheet: Sexual Health of
  Adolescents and Young Adults
  in the United States" (Kaiser
  Family Foundation) 73n
fallopian tubes, described 6
famciclovir, genital herpes 155
FDA *see* US Food and
  Drug Administration
"FDA Warns: Beware of Bogus
  STD Products" (FDA) 397n
Federal Trade Commission (FTC),
  contact information 553
female condoms
  described 548
  STD prevention 477–78
"Female Reproductive System"
  (Nemours Foundation) 4n
fertilization, described 7–8
fetus, described 8
financial considerations
  hepatitis B medications 181
  HIV infection 241–45
  HPV vaccine 536–37
  sexually transmitted diseases 27
follicular dendritic cells (FDC), HIV
  infection 193
Food and Drug Administration *see*
  US Food and Drug Administration
foreskin, described 13
"For People Who Have Been Sexually
  Assaulted... What You Need to
  Know about STDs and Emergency
  Contraception" (New Jersey
  Department of Health and Senior
  Services) 488n
Foundation for Women's Cancer,
  contact information 558
fraud, STD treatment
  products 397–400

"Free Web-Based Ordering of Home
Test Kits for Sexually Transmitted
Infections Proves Popular and
Effective with Teens and Young
Adults"
(Johns Hopkins Medicine) 381n
"Frequently Asked Questions"
(CDC) 359n
fungal infections *see* yeast infections

G

Gardasil
described 278, 538, 539
men 257
gastrointestinal syndromes,
described 314–16
Gay and Lesbian Medical Association,
contact information 558
Gaydos, Charlotte 382–84
gay men
human papillomavirus 57
sexually transmitted diseases 64–66
Gay Men's Health Crisis,
contact information 558
general paresis 339–40
genital herpes
described 19
lesbians 50–51
overview 148–50
tests *389*
treatment overview 155–59
see also herpes simplex virus
"Genital Herpes - CDC Fact Sheet"
(CDC) 148n
"Genital Herpes Fact Sheet"
(Office on Women's Health) 155n
genital HPV infection,
described 248–49
"Genital HPV Infection -
Fact Sheet" (CDC) 248n
genital warts
common symptoms 109–10
condoms 473
defined 548
men 61, 254–59
overview 271–73
treatment options 274–75
women 249–53
Giardia lamblia, described 314–15

glans, described 13
Global HIV/AIDS Response:
Epidemic update and health sector
progress toward Universal Access -
Progress Report 2011 (WHO) 41n
Go Ask Alice!, contact information 558
gonads, described 6
"Gonococcal Infections" (CDC) 141n
gonorrhea
adolescents 76
common symptoms 110
correctional facilities 98–99
defined 548
described 19
ethnic factors 85–87
gay men 65
lesbians 52–53
overview 138–41
pregnancy *350*
racial factor 91–92
tests *389*
treatment overview 141–43
women 47–48
"Gonorrhea - CDC Fact Sheet"
(CDC) 138n
gp120 molecules, HIV infection 187
granuloma inguinale,
overview 133–35
Guttmacher Institute,
contact information 558

H

HAART (highly active
antiretroviral therapy)
described 192, 225
older adults 82
Haemophilus ducreyi,
described 115, 548
handwashing, molluscum
contagiosum 312
health care professionals
adolescents 372–76
communication issues 366–69
HIV infection 222–23
HIV transmission 205–6
sexually transmitted
diseases 370–71
Healthfinder,
contact information 554

Health Insurance Portability and
    Accountability Act (HIPAA; 1996)
    242, 378
hepatitis
    common symptoms 110
    overview 162–73
"Hepatitis B FAQs for the Public"
    (CDC) 162n
Hepatitis B Foundation
    contact information 558
    hepatitis publication 178n
"Hepatitis B Treatment Information"
    (Hepatitis B Foundation) 178n
hepatitis B virus (HBV) infection
    defined 549
    described 19–20
    lesbians 53
    overview 162–73
    pregnancy *350*
    tests *389*
    treatment overview 178–81
"Hepatitis C Virus and HIV
    Coinfection" (CDC) 174n
hepatitis C virus (HCV) infection
    defined 549
    HIV coinfection 174–77
Hepatitis Foundation International,
    contact information 558
Hepsera (adefovir dipivoxil),
    hepatitis B 180
Heptodin (lamivudine),
    hepatitis B 180
"Herpes - Oral"
    (A.D.A.M., Inc.) 151n
herpes simplex virus (HSV)
    common symptoms 110–11
    Herpevac Trial for Women 522–25
    pregnancy *350*
    RNA interference 426–527
    tenofovir 520–21
    see also genital herpes
herpes simplex virus 2 (HSV-2)
    infection
    defined 549
    oral herpes 151–55
    overview 148–50
Herpevac Trial for Women 522–25
HHS *see* US Department of
    Health and Human Services

HIV *see* human
    immunodeficiency virus
"HIV, AIDS, and Older People"
    (NIA) 79n
"HIV/AIDS 101: Signs
    and Symptoms" (CDC) 212n
"HIV and AIDS Among
    Latinos" (CDC) 93n
"HIV and Its Treatment"
    (AIDSinfo) 219n
"HIV and Pregnancy"
    (AIDSinfo) 495n
HIV infection
    body art 419–21
    communication issues 432–34
    gay men 65
    injection drug users 421–23
    needle exchange
        programs 507–18
    post-exposure prophylaxis 492–93
    pregnancy 495–505
    sexually transmitted diseases 38
    statistics 29–33, 62
    vaccines 528–32
HIV InSite,
    contact information 559
*HIV Surveillance
    Report* (CDC) 62n
"HIV Transmission" (CDC) 200n
Home Access HIV-1
    Test System 361–62
home testing kits
    HIV infection 361–62
    sexually transmitted
        diseases 381–84
hormone therapy, cervicitis 329
Housing Opportunities for
    Persons with AIDS (HOPWA) 245
"HPV and Men Fact Sheet"
    (CDC) 254n
"HPV and Men - Fact Sheet"
    (CDC) 56n
"HPV-Associated Cancers
    Statistics" (CDC) 276n
"HPV Vaccine for Preteens
    and Teens" (CDC) 533n
"HPV Vaccine
    Information for Young Women -
    Fact Sheet" (CDC) 533n

human immunodeficiency
  virus (HIV)
  adolescents 76
  anonymous tests 378–79
  bacterial vaginosis 300
  cause of AIDS 184–97
  condoms 470–72
  defined 549
  described 20
  HCV coinfection 174–77
  lesbians 53–54
  living with HIV 232–40
  older adults 79–82
  pregnancy *350*
  sexual assault 490
  symptoms overview 212–13
  syphilis 288–89, 290
  tests *389*
  transmission 189–90
  transmission overview 200–211
  treatment overview 219–32
  see also acquired immune deficiency
    syndrome; HIV infection
human papillomavirus (HPV)
  adolescents 76
  cancer overview 276–80
  cervical cancer 548
  condoms 471–74
  defined 549
  described 20–21
  lesbians 51–52
  men 56–57, 254–59
  recurrent respiratory
    papillomatosis 259–60
  tests *389*
  treatment options 273–75, 279–80
  vaccine 59–60, 250–51, 278, 533–43
  women 45, 47, 248–53
"Human Papillomavirus (HPV)"
  (CDC) 273n
"Human Papillomavirus
  (HPV) and Genital Warts Fact
  Sheet" (Office on Women's
  Health) 248n, 273n
"Human Papillomaviruses and
  Cancer" (NCI) 276n
hydrocele, described 15
hymen, described 5
hypospadias, described 16

I

Illinois Department of
  Public Health, publications
  chancroid 115n
  nongonococcal urethritis 123n
  vaginitis 353n
immune system, HIV
  infection 197, 198–200
"Immune System 101" (DHHS) 198n
Immunization Action Coalition,
  contact information 559
infertility
  pelvic inflammatory disease 343–44
  STD infections 335–37
"Infertility Fact Sheet"
  (Office on Women's Health) 335n
inguinal hernia, described 16
injection drug users
  defined 549
  HIV infection *31*, 421–23
  HIV transmission 204–5
  needle exchange programs 507–18
integration, HIV infection 188
interferon, hepatitis C
  virus infection 176
interferon alpha, hepatitis B 180
interleukin 6 (IL-6),
  HIV infection 188, 193
intestinal parasites
  overview 309–11
  tests *389*
"Intestinal Parasites"
  (Planned Parenthood Federation
  of America, Inc.) 309n
Intron A (interferon alpha),
  hepatitis B 180
Isentress + Truvada,
  HIV infection 226
ivermectin, pubic lice 318
iwantthekit.org
  contact information 559
  described 384

J

Johns Hopkins Medicine, mail
  order test kits publication 381n
juvenile-onset recurrent respiratory
  papillomatosis (JORRP), described 248

K

Kaiser Family Foundation
  contact information 559
  publications
      adolescents, STDs 73n
      young adults, STDs 73n
killer T cells, HIV infection 190, 195
Knipe, David 527

L

labia, described 5
labor and delivery, described 8
lactic acidosis, nucleoside reverse
  transcriptase inhibitors 502
lamivudine, hepatitis B 180
laparoscopy
  overview 390–92
  pelvic inflammatory disease 345
laryngeal papillomatosis,
  described 259
latex condoms *see* condoms
lentiviruses, described 185
"Lesbian and Bisexual
  Health Fact Sheet" (Office
  on Women's Health) 49n
lesbians
  HIV transmission 207–8
  sexually transmitted
      diseases 49–54
lesions, lymphogranuloma
  venereum 281–82
levofloxacin, chlamydia 129
Lieberman, Judy 526–27
lindane, pubic lice 318
"Living with HIV/AIDS"
  (CDC) 232n
lubricants, safer sex 467–68
lymph nodes
  HIV infection 193–94
  immune system 198–200
lymphocytes,
  immune system 199
lymphogranuloma
  venereum (LGV),
  overview 281–83
"Lymphogranuloma
  Venereum (LGV) - CDC
  Fact Sheet" (CDC) 281n

M

macrophages, HIV infection 187
"Making Sense of Your Pap and
  HPV Test Results" (CDC) 264n
malathion, pubic lice 318
"Male Reproductive System"
  (Nemours Foundation) 11n
Margolis, Leonid 520–21
Medicaid 243
Medicare 242, 244
medications
  chancroid 116
  chlamydia 129–30
  hepatitis B 178–81, 180
  HIV infection, pregnancy 497–502
  oral herpes 153
  recurrent respiratory
      papillomatosis 261
  scabies 322–23
menarche, described 7
men/boys
  HPV vaccine 59–60, 257,
      536, 541–43
  human papillomavirus
      (HPV) 254–59
  reproductive system
      overview 11–16
  sexually transmitted
      diseases 56–66
meningeal neurosyphilis 339
meningovascular
  neurosyphilis 339–40
menstrual cycle, described 7
messenger RNA,
  HIV infection 188–89
metronidazole
  bacterial vaginosis 299
  trichomoniasis 114, 293
microbicide, defined 549
micropenis, described 16
molluscum contagiosum
  common symptoms 111
  defined 549–50
  overview 311–13
  tests *389*
"Molluscum Contagiosum"
  (NCEZID) 311n
monocytes, HIV infection 187
mons pubis, described 5

"More on How HIV
  Causes AIDS" (NIAID) 184n
mother-to-child HIV transmission
  defined 550
  overview 495–505
Multicenter AIDS Cohort
  Study (MACS) 192
Mycobacterium tuberculosis,
  epididymitis 331

N

National Cancer Institute (NCI)
  contact information 554
  HPV infection,
    cancer publication 276n
National Center for
  Complementary and
  Alternative Medicine
  (NCCAM),
    contact information 554
National Center for Emerging
  and Zoonotic Infectious
  Diseases (NCEZID),
  molluscum contagiosum
  publication 311n
National Center for Health
  Statistics, contact information 554
National Cervical Cancer Coalition,
  contact information 559
National Coalition for LGBT Health,
  contact information 559
National Institute for Occupational
  Safety and Health (NIOSH),
  body art publication 419n
National Institute of Allergy
  and Infectious Diseases (NIAID)
  contact information 341, 554
  publications
    behavioral intervention 460n
    genital herpes virus 526n
    Herpevac trial 522n
    HIV/AIDS 184n
    STD research 101n
    syphilis 289n
National Institute of
  Mental Health (NIMH)
  child abuse survivors, STDs
    publication 71n
  contact information 554

National Institute of Neurological
  Disorders and Stroke (NINDS)
  contact information 341, 555
  neurosyphilis publication 339n
National Institute on Aging (NIA)
  contact information 555
  older adults, HIV/AIDS
    publication 79n
National Institute on Deafness and
  Other Communication Disorders
  (NIDCD), recurrent respiratory
  papillomatosis publication 259n
National Institutes of Health (NIH)
  contact information 555
  herpes virus medication
    publication 520
National Library of Medicine *see* US
  National Library of Medicine
National Network for
  Immunization Information,
  contact information 559
National Prevention Information
  Network, contact information 555
National Survey on Drug Use and
  Health (NSDUH) 411–12
National Women's Health
  Information Center (NWHIC),
  contact information 555
NCEZID *see* National Center
  for Emerging and Zoonotic
  Infectious Diseases
NCI *see* National Cancer Institute
"Needle Exchange and Harm
  Reduction" (AVERT) 507n
needle exchange programs,
  overview 507–18
needle sticks, HIV transmission 206–7
Neisseria gonorrhoeae
  gay men 66
  home test kits 382
  treatment overview 141–45
Nemours Foundation
  contact information 559
  publications
    condom discussion 426n
    doctor discussions 372n
    female reproductive system 4n
    male reproductive system 11n
    STD discussion 429n, 435n

neurosyphilis
  overview 339–41
  penicillin 289
"Neurosyphilis" (NINDS) 339n
New Jersey Department of
  Health and Senior Services,
  STD prevention, assaults
  publication 488n
NIA *see* National Institute on Aging
NIAID *see* National Institute of
  Allergy and Infectious Diseases
NIDCD *see* National Institute
  on Deafness and Other
  Communication Disorders
"NIH Researchers Show How
  Anti-HIV Drug Acts to Block
  Herpes Virus" (NIH) 520
NIMH *see* National Institute
  of Mental Health
NINDS *see* National Institute
  of Neurological Disorders
  and Stroke
NIOSH *see* National Institute for
  Occupational Safety and Health
nits, described 316
NLM *see* US National
  Library of Medicine
"Non-Gonococcal Urethritis
  (NGU)" (Illinois Department
  of Public Health) 123n
nongonococcal urethritis
  (NGU), chlamydia 123–26
non-nucleoside reverse
  transcriptase inhibitors
  (NNRTI), pregnancy 501
Norwegian scabies, described 320
nucleoside reverse transcriptase
  inhibitors (NRTI), pregnancy 502
nymphs, described 316

O

occupational exposure, defined 550
Office of Minority Health Resource
  Center, contact information 555
Office on Women's Health,
  publications
  bacterial vaginosis 298n
  douching 416n
  genital herpes 155n

Office on Women's Health,
  publications, *continued*
  genital warts 273n
  glossary 547n
  HIV care 241n
  HPV infection 248n, 273n
  infertility 335n
  lesbians, STDs 49n
  pelvic inflammatory disease 343n
  sexually transmitted diseases 17n
  yeast infections 305n
ofloxacin
  chlamydia 129
  nongonococcal urethritis 125
older adults, sexually transmitted
  diseases 79–82
oligomenorrhea, described 10
opportunistic infections (OI),
  defined 550
oral fluid tests, STDs 361
oral herpes, overview 151–55
oral sex
  condoms 476–77
  HIV infection risk 408–10
  HIV transmission 203–4
  safer sex 466–67
"Oral Sex and HIV Risk"
  (CDC) 408n
OraQuick Advance
  HIV home test 362
ovarian cysts, described 9
ovarian torsion, described 10
ovaries, described 6
Ovide (malathion), pubic lice 318
ovulation, described 7
oxytocin, described 8

P

Pap tests
  cervical cancer screening 262–64
  defined 550
  described 266–68
  HPV vaccine 251–52, 537
  human papillomavirus 251
  vaginitis 354
paraphimosis, described 16
"Paying for HIV Care" (Office on
  Women's Health) 241n
PCOS *see* polycystic ovarian syndrome

Pegasys (pegylated interferon),
  hepatitis B 180
pegylated interferon
  hepatitis B 180
  hepatitis C virus infection 176
pelvic examination
  cervicitis 328–29
  yeast infections 306
pelvic inflammatory disease (PID)
  bacterial vaginosis 300
  defined 550
  infertility 48
  overview 343–47
  tests *389*
"Pelvic Inflammatory Disease
  Fact Sheet" (Office on Women's
  Health) 343n
penicillin
  neurosyphilis 340
  syphilis 289
penile inflammation,
  described 16
penis, described 13
permethrin, pubic lice 318
pets, scabies 323
phimosis
  chancroid 117
  described 16
PID *see* pelvic
  inflammatory disease
piercings
  HIV infection 419–21
  HIV transmission 208
piperonyl butoxide, pubic lice 318
placenta, described 8
Planned Parenthood
  Federation of America, Inc.
  contact information 559
  publications
    cytomegalovirus 302n
    intestinal parasites 309n
    safer sex 464n
    STD testing 386n
plasma HIV RNA test,
  HIV infection 218
Pneumocystis carinii
  pneumonia (PCP) 233
Pneumocystis jiroveci
  pneumonia 220

polycystic ovarian syndrome (PCOS)
  described 10
  infertility 336
"Post-Exposure
  Prophylaxis" (AIDSinfo) 492n
post-exposure prophylaxis (PEP)
  defined 550
  overview 492–93
POZ Magazine,
  contact information 560
precursor cells, HIV infection 196
pregnancy
  adolescent sexual activity 75–76
  bacterial vaginosis 299–300
  chlamydia 122
  cytomegalovirus 304
  doxycycline 283
  emergency contraception 491
  genital herpes 156
  gonorrhea 140
  hepatitis B 172–73
  HIV infection tests 363–64
  HIV medications 226, 238–39
  HIV tests 216–17
  HPV vaccine 534
  human papillomavirus 253, 271
  mother-to-child
    HIV transmission 495–505
  pelvic inflammatory disease 346
  sexually transmitted
    diseases 24–25, 38
  spermicides 479–81
  STD complications 349–52
  syphilis 288, 290
  trichomoniasis 292
premenstrual syndrome (PMS),
  described 7
"Pre-Post-Test Counseling"
  (DHHS) 214n
preteens, HPV vaccine 538–43
"Prevention" (NIAID) 101n
preventive HIV vaccine
  overview 528–530
  versus therapeutic HIV
    vaccine 531
"Preventive HIV Vaccines"
  (AIDSinfo) 528n
Prezista + Norvir + Truvada,
  HIV infection 226

privacy, HIV infection tests 378–79
probenecid, neurosyphilis 340
proctitis, overview 314–16
"Proctitis, Proctocolitis, and
    Enteritis: Sexually Transmitted
    Gastrointestinal
    Syndromes" (CDC) 314n
proctocolitis, overview 314–16
progesterone, described 6, 8
Project Inform,
    contact information 560
prostaglandins, described 7
prostate gland, described 13
protozoan vaginitis 354
pubic lice
    common symptoms 109
    defined 551
    described 21
    lesbians 52
    overview 316–19
    tests *389*
"Pubic Lice Frequently Asked
    Questions" (CDC) 316n
"Pubic Lice Treatment" (CDC) 316n
pyrethrins, pubic lice 318

Q

"Questions and Answers
    Fraudulent STD Products
    Initiative" (FDA) 397n
"Questions and Answers: The
    Herpevac Trial for Women"
    (NIAID) 522n
"Questions Are the Answer"
    (AHRQ) 366n
"Questions to Ask Your Health
    Care Professional" (NLM) 370n

R

racial factor, sexually transmitted
    diseases 29, *31*, 84–92
rapid tests, HIV infection 361
recurrent respiratory
    papillomatosis (RRP)
    described 248
    overview 259–61
"Recurrent Respiratory Papillomatosis
    or Laryngeal Papillomatosis"
    (NIDCD) 259n

recurrent vulvovaginal candidiasis
    (RVVC), described 308
reproductive process,
    described 4, 11
retroviruses, described 185
reverse transcriptase,
    described 185
reverse transcription,
    HIV infection 188
Reyataz + Norvir + Truvada,
    HIV infection 226
ribavirin, hepatitis C
    virus infection 176
risky sexual behaviors,
    overview 404–7
RNA (ribonucleic acid)
    herpes simplex virus 426–527
    HIV infection 185–87
    tests 362
"The Role of STD Detection
    and Treatment in HIV
    Prevention" (CDC) 214n
Ryan White HIV/AIDS
    Program 243–44

S

"Safer Sex" (Planned Parenthood
    Federation of America, Inc.) 464n
safer sex, overview 464–69
"SAFE Studies Show Behavioral
    Intervention Reduces STI in San
    Antonio, Texas (NIAID) 460n
safety considerations
    fraudulent products 397–400
    HPV vaccine 535–36
SAMHSA *see* Substance
    Abuse and Mental Health
    Services Administration
Sarcoptes scabiei var. *hominis*,
    described 111, 320, 551
scabies
    common symptoms 111–12
    defined 551
    overview 320–26
    tests *389*
"Scabies Frequently
    Asked Questions" (CDC) 320n
Schiller test, abnormal Pap tests 252
Schuchat, Anne 541n

scrotum, described 12
Sebivo (telbivudine),
   hepatitis B 180
semen, defined 551
seminal vesicles, described 13
sex education
   abstinence only overview 450–60
   HIV/STD prevention
      programs 448–49
   overview 440–48
   Sexual Awareness for Everyone
      (SAFE) study 460–62
"Sex Education That Works"
   (AVERT) 440n
sexual assault,
   STD prevention 488–91
Sexual Awareness for Everyone
   (SAFE) study 460–62
Sexuality Information and
   Education Council of the United
   States, contact information 560
sexually transmitted diseases (STD)
   child sexual abuse 68–72
   common symptoms 107–14
   communication issues 429–32
   confidentiality issues 77, 380–84
   correctional facilities 97–99
   defined 551
   douching overview 416–19
   female reproductive system 10
   men 56–66
   older adults 79–82
   oral sex 408–10
   overview 17–26
   prevention 23–24
   recent research 101–3
   risk factors 465–66
   sexual assault 488–91
   substance abuse 411–13
   women 44–54
"Sexually Transmitted Diseases
   (STDs)" (NIAID) 101n
"Sexually Transmitted Diseases and
   STD Symptoms" (AVERT) 107n
"Sexually Transmitted Diseases and
   Substance Use" (SAMHSA) 411n
*Sexually Transmitted Diseases
   Treatment Guidelines, 2010*
   (CDC) 127n, 380n

"Sexually Transmitted
   Infections" (WHO) 36n
"Sexually Transmitted
   Infections Fact Sheet" (Office
   on Women's Health) 17n
"Sexual Partners" (DHHS) 432n
"Sexual Risk Behavior: HIV, STD,
   and Teen Pregnancy Prevention"
   (CDC) 404n
Shain, Rochelle 460–61
Sheer Glyde 467
"Shutting Down the Genital
   Herpes Virus" (NIAID) 526n
Sidibé, Michel 518
small interfering RNA
   (siRNA), described 426–527
Social Security Disability
   Insurance Program 242
socioeconomic factors,
   HIV infection 95
Souder, Mark 517
"Special Populations"
   (CDC) 380n
sperm, described 14
spermicides
   defined 551
   overview 479–81
"Spermicides" (Boston
   Children's Hospital) 479n
spleen, immune system 198
sports activities,
   HIV transmission 210–11
stages, syphilis 287–88
statistics
   adolescent
      sexual activity 73–75
   AIDS (acquired immune
      deficiency syndrome) 62–63
   chlamydia 28, 120
   cytomegalovirus 302
   global STDs 36–40
   gonorrhea 28, 138
   hepatitis B infection 163–64
   HIV infection 41–42, 62, 185
   HPV-associated cancers 539–40
   human papillomavirus 249, 541
   infertility 335
   pelvic inflammatory
      disease 343–44

statistics, *continued*
  recurrent respiratory
      papillomatosis 260
  risky sexual behaviors 404
  sexually transmitted
      diseases 27–34
  substance abuse, STDs 411–13
  syphilis 28, 286
  trichomoniasis 291
STD *see* sexually
  transmitted diseases
"STD and Pregnancy"
  (CDC) 349n
"STDs"
  (Nemours Foundation) 435n
"STDs and Child Sexual Abuse"
  (US Department of Justice) 68n
"STDs in Men Who Have
  Sex with Men" (CDC) 64n
"STDs in Persons Entering
  Correctional Facilities"
  (CDC) 97n
"STDs in Racial and Ethnic
  Minorities" (CDC) 84n
"STDs in Women and Infants"
  (CDC) 46n
"STD Testing" (Planned
  Parenthood Federation
  of America, Inc.) 386n
"STD Trends in the United
  States: 2010 National Data for
  Gonorrhea, Chlamydia, and
  Syphilis" (CDC) 27n
stigma, HIV infection 95
substance abuse
  safer sex 468
  sexually transmitted
      diseases 411–13
Substance Abuse
  and Mental Health Services
  Administration (SAMHSA)
  contact information 555
  substance abuse,
      STDs publication 411n
Supplemental Security
  Income (SSI) 242
surgical procedures,
  recurrent respiratory
  papillomatosis 261

Sustiva
  HIV infection 226
  pregnancy 501
syphilis
  common symptoms 112–13
  correctional facilities 99
  defined 551
  described 21
  ethnic factors 87–88
  gay men 65–66
  lesbians 54
  overview 286–89
  pregnancy *350*
  racial factor 92
  tests *389*
  treatment options 289–90
  women 48
"Syphilis - CDC Fact Sheet"
  (CDC) 286n
"Syphilis: Treatment"
  (NIAID) 289n

T

tabes dorsalis 339–40
"Talking to Your Doctor"
  (Nemours Foundation) 372n
"Talking to Your Partner
  about Condoms" (Nemours
  Foundation) 426n
tattoos
  HIV infection 419–21
  HIV transmission 208
telaprevir, hepatitis C
  virus infection 176
telbivudine, hepatitis B 180
"Telling Your Partner
  You Have an STD"
  (Nemours Foundation) 429n
"10 Ways STDs Impact Women
  Differently from Men"
  (CDC) 44n
tenofovir
  hepatitis B 180
  herpes simplex virus 520–21
testicles (testes), described 12
testicular cancer, described 15
testicular trauma, described 15
"Testing for HIV" (AIDSinfo) 214n
testosterone, described 13

tests
  bacterial vaginosis 299, *389*
  cervicitis 329
  chlamydia 128
  confidentiality issues 77, 378–81
  cytomegalovirus 303
  donovanosis 134
  epididymitis 332–33
  genital herpes 150
  hepatitis B 168
  HIV (human immunodeficiency
    virus) 360–64
  HIV infection 214–18
  HIV infection, infants 504
  human papillomavirus 58, 256,
    264–70, 279
  intestinal parasites 310
  oral herpes 153
  pelvic inflammatory
    disease 344–45
  sexually transmitted
    diseases 22, 68,
    359–64, 386–89
  syphilis 288
  trichomoniasis 293
therapeutic HIV vaccine
  overview 531–32
  versus preventive vaccine 528–29
"Therapeutic HIV Vaccines"
  (AIDSinfo) 531n
thrush, common symptoms 113–14
thymus, immune system 198
tinidazole, trichomoniasis 293
"Tips for Using Condoms
  and Dental Dams"
  (US Department of
  Veterans Affairs) 475n
Toerner, Joseph 394
toxic shock syndrome, described 10
toxoplasmosis, AIDS 220
transcription, HIV infection 188
translation, HIV infection 188–89
"Treatment" (NIAID) 101n
"Trends in HIV- and STD-Related
  Risk Behaviors Among High School
  Students - United States, 1991-
  2007" (CDC) 405n
Treponema pallidum, described 112,
  286, 551

Trichomonas vaginalis
  described 114, 291
  home test kits 382
trichomoniasis
  common symptoms 114
  defined 551
  described 21
  lesbians 52
  overview 291–93
  pregnancy *350*
  tests *389*
"Trichomoniasis -
  CDC Fact Sheet" (CDC) 291n
tuberculosis, AIDS 220, 233
tumor necrosis factor (TNF)-alpha,
  HIV infection 188
Tyzeka (telbivudine), hepatitis B 180

U

ultrasound, pelvic inflammatory
  disease 345
umbilical cord, described 8
urethra, described 5, 13
urine tests, STDs 361
US Department of Health and
  Human Services (DHHS; HHS)
  contact information 556
  publications
    anonymous tests 378n
    glossary 547n
    HIV, counseling 214n
    HIV, immune system 198n
    HIV/AIDS, legislation 245n
    HIV status discussion 432n
US Department of Justice, child
  sexual abuse, STDs publication 68n
US Department of Veterans Affairs,
  condoms publication 475n
US Food and Drug
  Administration (FDA)
  contact information 556
  publications
    antibiotic resistance 393n
    bogus STD products 397n
US National Library of Medicine
  (NLM)
  contact information 556
  questions publication 370n
uterus, described 5–6

V

vaccinations, defined 551
vaccines
  hepatitis B 168–72
  HIV infection 528–32
  human papillomavirus
    250–51, 278, 533–43
vagina, described 5
vaginal contraceptive film,
  described 480
vaginal sex, HIV transmission 202–3
vaginal suppositories, described 480
vaginal yeast infections,
  overview 305–8
"Vaginal Yeast Infections Fact Sheet"
  (Office on Women's Health) 305n
"Vaginitis" (Illinois Department of
  Public Health) 353n
vaginitis, overview 353–56
  see also bacterial vaginosis;
    candidiasis; trichomoniasis;
    yeast infections
valacyclovir, genital herpes 155
Valtrex (valacyclovir),
  genital herpes 155
varicocele, described 15
vas deferens, described 12
Videx, pregnancy 502
viral burden, HIV infection 192
viral core, HIV infection 186–87
viral envelope, HIV infection 186
viral load test, HIV infection 218
Viramune, pregnancy 501
Viread (tenofovir), hepatitis B 180
virus, defined 551
vulva, described 5
vulvovaginitis, described 9

W

water warts
  see molluscum contagiosum
"What Patients Should Know
  When They Are Diagnosed with
  Genital Warts" (CDC) 271n
WHO *see* World Health
  Organization
Widom, Cathy S. 71
Wilson, Helen W. 71
womb, described 5–6
women/girls
  HIV infection 238
  HPV vaccine 533–40
  reproductive system
    overview 4–10
  sexually transmitted
    diseases 44–54
World Health Organization (WHO)
  contact information 560
  publications
    HIV/AIDS statistics 41n
    STD statistics 36n

Y

yeast infections
  defined 551
  overview 305–8
Youth Risk Behavior
  Surveys (YRBS) 405–7

Z

Zeffix (lamivudine), hepatitis B 180
Zerit, pregnancy 502
zidovudine, mother-to-child HIV
  transmission 190

Health Reference Series

Adolescent Health Sourcebook, 3rd Edition

Adult Health Concerns Sourcebook

AIDS Sourcebook, 5th Edition

Alcoholism Sourcebook, 3rd Edition

Allergies Sourcebook, 4th Edition

Alzheimer Disease Sourcebook, 5th Edition

Arthritis Sourcebook, 3rd Edition

Asthma Sourcebook, 3rd Edition

Attention Deficit Disorder Sourcebook

Autism & Pervasive Developmental Disorders Sourcebook, 2nd Edition

Back & Neck Sourcebook, 2nd Edition

Blood & Circulatory Disorders Sourcebook, 3rd Edition

Brain Disorders Sourcebook, 3rd Edition

Breast Cancer Sourcebook, 4th Edition

Breastfeeding Sourcebook

Burns Sourcebook

Cancer Sourcebook for Women, 4th Edition

Cancer Sourcebook, 6th Edition

Cancer Survivorship Sourcebook

Cardiovascular Disorders Sourcebook, 4th Edition

Caregiving Sourcebook

Child Abuse Sourcebook, 2nd Edition

Childhood Diseases & Disorders Sourcebook, 3rd Edition

Colds, Flu & Other Common Ailments Sourcebook

Communication Disorders Sourcebook

Complementary & Alternative Medicine Sourcebook, 4th Edition

Congenital Disorders Sourcebook, 2nd Edition

Contagious Diseases Sourcebook, 2nd Edition

Cosmetic & Reconstructive Surgery Sourcebook, 2nd Edition

Death & Dying Sourcebook, 2nd Edition

Dental Care & Oral Health Sourcebook, 4th Edition

Depression Sourcebook, 3rd Edition

Dermatological Disorders Sourcebook, 2nd Edition

Diabetes Sourcebook, 5th Edition

Diet & Nutrition Sourcebook, 4th Edition

Digestive Diseases & Disorder Sourcebook

Disabilities Sourcebook, 2nd Edition

Disease Management Sourcebook

Domestic Violence Sourcebook, 4th Edition

Drug Abuse Sourcebook, 3rd Edition

Ear, Nose & Throat Disorders Sourcebook, 2nd Edition

Eating Disorders Sourcebook, 3rd Edition

Emergency Medical Services Sourcebook

Endocrine & Metabolic Disorders Sourcebook, 2nd Edition

Environmental Health Sourcebook, 3rd Edition

Ethnic Diseases Sourcebook

Eye Care Sourcebook, 4th Edition

Family Planning Sourcebook

Fitness & Exercise Sourcebook, 4th Edition

Food Safety Sourcebook

Forensic Medicine Sourcebook

Gastrointestinal Diseases & Disorders Sourcebook, 2nd Edition

Genetic Disorders Sourcebook, 4th Edition

Head Trauma Sourcebook

Headache Sourcebook

Health Insurance Sourcebook

Healthy Aging Sourcebook

Healthy Children Sourcebook

Healthy Heart Sourcebook for Women

Hepatitis Sourcebook

Household Safety Sourcebook

Hypertension Sourcebook

Immune System Disorders Sourcebook, 2nd Edition

Infant & Toddler Health Sourcebook

Infectious Diseases Sourcebook